Teaching Epidemiology

Teaching Epidemiology

SECOND EDITION

Edited by

Jørn Olsen

Rodolfo Saracci

Dimitrios Trichopoulos

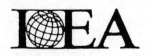

Association
Internationale d'Epidemiologie

EEPE: The European Educational Programme in Epidemiology

OXFORD
UNIVERSITY PRESS

OXFORD

UNIVERSITY PRESS

Great Clarendon Street, Oxford OX2 6DP

Oxford University Press is a department of the University of Oxford.
It furthers the University's objective of excellence in research, scholarship,
and education by publishing worldwide in

Oxford New York

Auckland Bangkok Buenos Aires Cape Town Chennai
Dar es Salaam Delhi Hong Kong Istanbul Karachi Kolkata
Kuala Lumpur Madrid Melbourne Mexico City Mumbai Nairobi
São Paulo Shanghai Taipei Tokyo Toronto

Oxford is a registered trade mark of Oxford University Press
in the UK and in certain other countries

Published in the United States
by Oxford University Press Inc., New York

© Oxford University Press, 2001

First edition published (edited by Jørn Olsen and Dimitrios Trichopoulos) 1992
Reprinted 1993
Second edition published 2001
Reprinted 2003

A catalogue record for this title is available from the British Library

Library of Congress Cataloging in Publication Data
(Data available)

ISBN 0-19-850969-3 (hbk)
ISBN 0-19-263066-0 (pbk)

10 9 8 7 6 5 4 3 2 1

Typeset in Minion
by EXPO Holdings, Malaysia
Printed in Great Britain
on acid-free paper by
Biddles Ltd
www.biddles.co.uk

Preface

Teaching epidemiology is a task that requires skill and knowledge. The overriding requirement is knowledge, which, however, should be combined with a clear teaching strategy and good pedagogic skills. The general advice is simple: if you are not an expert on a topic, try to enrich your background knowledge before you start teaching it. In this book we help you to locate the most important sources of knowledge you need to study before you start.

In addition, we provide expert teachers' advice on how best to structure teaching – what has worked in their hands. You should not, however, expect that these guidelines will automatically work for you. You have to find your own personal style and use examples of relevance for your audience. It is, nevertheless, always useful to make sure your teaching follows a predefined logical sequence. The book will help you to set up this structure.

Most experienced epidemiologists are able to write a satisfactory paper by complying with the established rules for scientific writing. Teaching is different because you also have to establish personal contact. Without personal contact, teaching may well be replaced by reading or computer-assisted learning. Personal contact requires that the teacher wants to teach and that the students are at least willing to give it a try. Evaluation of your success as a teacher includes assessment of your knowledge as well as how the teaching was received. Any serious evaluation takes both aspects into consideration and this book will help you improve your knowledge as well as your teaching skills.

Epidemiology is an old discipline, but its concepts and principles are still evolving. We provide guidelines from different perspectives. Teachers have different ideas as to what the level of sophistication in methods should be and where to focus the attention of the students. We have not sought consensus when inviting the authors to contribute. Science is not driven by consensus but rather by diversity.

We advise you to read and make your own judgements. Identify your coordinates and develop your preferred trajectory. But first, see what older and more experienced colleagues have to offer. Then – but only then – you can throw it away.

This book is a second edition of *Teaching Epidemiology*, first published in 1992. The structure, as well as the content, has changed substantially since the first version. The first edition was published by Oxford University Press and the Commission of the European Communities. This version is published by Oxford University Press in collaboration with the International Epidemiological Association (IEA) and the European Educational Programme in Epidemiology (EEPE).

We would like to thank all authors who, without hesitation, agreed to share their experience and knowledge with their less experienced colleagues. Without their contributions there would not have been any book. We also thank Inge Børven for her important administrative support.

Jørn Olsen
Rodolfo Saracci
Dimitrios Trichopoulos

Advisory board

All chapters have been reviewed by members of the advisory group which comprised the following members: Haroutune K. Armenian (Department of Epidemiology, Johns Hopkins University, Baltimore, USA), Robert Beaglehole (University of Auckland, New Zealand), Charles Florey (Department of Epidemiology and Public Health, Ninewells Hospital and Medical School, Dundee, UK), Jørn Olsen (Danish Epidemiology Science Centre, Statens Serum Institut, Copenhagen and University of Aarhus, Aarhus, Denmark), Rodolfo Saracci (National Research Council, Pisa, Italy and International Agency for Research on Cancer, Lyon, France), Chitr Sitthi-Amorn (College of Public Health, Chulalonkorn University, Thailand), Dimitrios Trichopoulos (Department of Epidemiology, Harvard School of Public Health, Boston, and Department of Hygiene and Epidemiology, University of Athens, Athens).

Contents

Outcome oriented epidemiology

Pedagogies

Contributors

Joseph H. Abramson
Department of Social Medicine, Hebrew University — Hadassah School of Public Health and Community Medicine, PO Box 12272, Jerusalem, Israel

Anders Ahlbom
Karolinska Institutet, Institute of Environmental Medicin, Division of Epidemiology, Box 210, Stockholm S171 77, Sweden

Per Kragh Andersen
Department of Biostatistics, University of Copenhagen, Panum Instituttet, Blegdamsvej 3, DK-2200 Copenhagen N, Denmark

Haroutune Armenian
Department of Epidemiology, Johns Hopkins School of Hygiene and Public Health, 615 N Wolfe Street, Baltimore, MD 21205, USA

John A. Baron
Section of Biostatistics and Epidemiology, Dartmouth-Hitchcock Medical Center, 7927 Rubin Building, Lebanon, NH 03756, USA

Olga Basso
Danish Epidemiology Science Centre, Institute of Epidemiology and Social Medicine, Aarhus University, Vennelyst Boulevard 6, DK-8000 Aarhus C, Denmark

Jako Bue Bjørner
National Institute of Occupational Health, Lersø Park Allé 105, DK-2100 Copenhagen Ø, Denmark

Paolo Boffetta
Unit of Environmental Cancer Epidemiology, International Agency for Research on Cancer, 150 cours Albert-Thomas, 69008 Lyon, France

Annie R. Britton
Department of Public Health Policy, London School of Hygiene and Tropical Medicine, Keppel Street, London WC1E 7HT, UK

Harry Campbell
Public Health Sciences, Department of Community Health Sciences, The University of Edinburgh Medical School, Teviot Place, Edinburgh EH8 9AG, Scotland

Paul Elliott
Imperial College School of Medicine, Department of Epidemiology and Public Health, St Mary's Campus, Norfolk Place, London W2 1PG, UK

Charles Florey
Department of Epidemiology and Public Health, Ninewells Hospital and Medical School, University of Dundee, Dundee DD1 9SY, UK

Linda M. Frazier
Department of Preventive Medicine, University of Kansas School of Medicine — Wichita,
1010 N Kansas, Wichita, Kansas 67214-3199, USA

Rebecca Fuhrer
University College London (UCL) Medical School, Department of Epidemiology and Public Health, 1–19 Torrington Place, London WC1E 6BT, UK

Amanda L. Golbeck
Kansas Board of Regents,
700 SW Harrison Suite 1410 Topeka,
KS 66603-3760, USA

Susan Jick
Boston Collaborative Drug Surveillance
Program, Boston University, School of
Medicine, 11 Muzzey Street, Lexington,
MA 02421, USA

Japhet Killewo
Reproductive Health Programme,
ICDDR,B, GPO Box 128 Dhaka –– 1000,
Bangladesh

Pagona Lagiou
University of Athens School of
Medicine, Department of Hygiene and
Epidemiology, 115 27 Athens, Greece

John M. Last
Department of Epidemiology and
Community Medicine, University of
Ottawa, 451 Smyth Road, Ottawa ON
K1H 8M5, Canada

Anthony J. McMichael
Department of Epidemiology and
Population Health, London School of
Hygiene and Tropical Medicine, Keppel
Street, London WC1E 7HT, UK

Olli S. Miettinen
McGill University, Department of
Epidemiology and Biostatistics, 1020
Pine Avenue West, Montreal PQ, Canada
H3A 1A2

Craig A. Molgaard
Department of Preventive Medicine,
University of Kansas School of Medicine
–– Wichita, 1010 N Kansas, Wichita,
Kansas 67214-3199, USA

Norman D. Noah
Department of Infectious Diseases,
London School of Hygiene and Tropical
Medicine, Keppel Street, London WC11
7HT, UK and Communicable Disease
Surveillance Centre, 61 Colindale
Avenue, London NW9 5EQ, UK

Jørn Olsen
Danish Epidemiology Science Centre,
Aarchoas University and
Statens Serum Institut, Artillerivej 5,
DK-2300 Copenhagen S, Denmark

Neil Pearce
Centre for Public Health Research,
Massey University Wellington Campus,
Private Box 756, Wellington, New Zealand

Eleni Petridou
University of Athens School of
Medicine, Department of Hygiene and
Epidemiology, 115 27 Athens, Greece

Charles Poole
Department of Epidemiology
(CB#7400), University of North
Carolina School of Public Health,
McGavran-Greenberg Hall, Pittsboro
Road, Chapel Hill, NC 27599-7400, USA

Kenneth J. Rothman
Department of Epidemiology,
Boston University School of Public
Health, 715 Albany Street, Boston, MA
02118, USA

Nathaniel Rothman
Occupational Epidemiology Branch,
Division of Cancer Epidemiology and
Genetics, National Cancer Institute,
Executive Plaza South 8116, Bethesda
MD 20892, USA

Jonathan Samet
Department of Epidemiology, School of
Hygiene and Public Health, Johns
Hopkins University, Baltimore MD, USA

Anita Sandström
Framnäsbacken 9, 6tr., 17166 Solna,
Sweden

Rodolfo Saracci
National Research Council, Pisa, Italy
and International Agency for Research
on Cancer (IARC), 150 Cours Thomas,
69008 Lyon, France

Flemming Scheutz
The Royal Dental College, Vennelyst
Boulevard 9, DK-8000 Aarhus C,
Denmark

Lowell Sever
The University of Texas School of Public
Health, 1200 Herman Pressler Suite
E1023, Houston TX 77030, USA

Aubrey Sheiham
Department of Epidemiology and Public
Health, University College London,
London, UK

Alkistis Skalkidou
University of Athens School of
Medicine, Department of Hygiene and
Epidemiology, 115 27 Athens, Greece

Henrik Toft Sørensen
Department of Clinical Epidemiology,
Aarhus University Hospital, Vennelyst
Boulevard 6, Building 260, DK-8000
Aarhus C, Denmark

Michael Thompson
MPH Program, School of Hygiene and
Public Health, Johns Hopkins University
and Public Health Program, American
University of Armenia.

Dimitrios Trichopoulos
Harvard School of Public Health, 677
Huntington, Avenue, Boston MA 02115,
USA

Walter C. Willett
Harvard School of Public Health,
Department of Nutrition, 665
Huntington Avenue, Boston MA 02215,
USA

Context

Chapter 1

Introducing the history of epidemiology

Rodolfo Saracci

Nature cannot know its own history, humans can

Introduction

Why teach the history of epidemiology?

'Know yourself': this Socratic maxim expresses the rationale for learning the history of epidemiology. Self-knowledge and a critical but positive attitude towards the discipline is fostered by the study of the historical development of epidemiology, which enables the epidemiologist/teacher to highlight several salient features. (A professional historian of science may adopt a more personalized view arising from his/her research.) These salient features include:

♦ The common elements unifying all branches of epidemiology as a population health science beyond today's subdivision into specialized areas.

♦ The relationship of epidemiology to other scientific disciplines and its methodological specificities, strengths and weaknesses in respect to them.

♦ The emergence of key concepts, either methodological as 'risk', or substantive as the modes of diffusion of pathogens in the community. This cumulative but irregular accrual of knowledge is characterized by controversies, blind alleys, and sheer errors as well as by material hurdles and personal and institutional conflicts. It may appear long when time is measured in years but is much less when a generation of scientists is, more appropriately, taken as the time unit.

♦ The influence of the demographic, health, social, cultural, and economic context on the development of epidemiology and of epidemiological methods.

♦ The role of epidemiology in society through its impact in the health field, largely mediated through the essential functions of epidemiology within public health.

♦ The roots and dynamics of present trends in epidemiology and the options for reinforcing, contrasting, or inflecting them.

None of these features are going to be entirely missed by anyone working in epidemiology without much concern for remote or proximate historical antecedents. However, as in epidemiology follow-up studies – which explicitly embody the time dimension – are much more informative than cross-sectional studies, so the historical dimension can provide a wider and clearer perspective on the nature of the discipline and on the role of its practitioners in society. At a time when all scientific activities have increased (and increasingly recognized and debated) the implications of an economic, social, and ethical nature of the historical perspective may become more of a necessity than a curiosity.

As history can be learnt so it can be taught. In this respect a basic consideration is that historical knowledge changes in time not only because of cumulative advances, as for all theoretical or empirical sciences, but also because the point of observation of the historical past moves continuously forward with time and the landscape that becomes visible to the eye of the observer changes in consequence. As a reconstruction of the past, history is to a non-negligible extent a function of the present and of what the present allows or does not allow us to discern. This unavoidable bias may be grossly amplified when the past is reconstructed primarily to justify particular aspects and views of the present: for instance, rudimentary and lopsided reconstructions of mankind's evolutionary history have been abundantly and tragically employed to support racist theories and practices.

Whom to teach?

The teaching as outlined here is primarily addressed to students following Master and PhD courses who intend to become full-time epidemiologists or make a large use of epidemiology in their professional work; for example, public health practitioners, clinicians, and occupational physicians.

This teaching can only be regarded as preliminary for students who may wish to proceed in one of two directions: first, historical epidemiology as a description and analysis of health and diseases in given areas and past periods of time; second, the history of epidemiology as the reconstruction of the development of theories, concepts, methods, and practices, including the study of the role of individuals and institutions.

At a number of medical schools students follow a course in epidemiology or epidemiological methods lasting 20–40 hours: in this context a short (1-hour) historical overview should be offered.

How and when to teach?

This chapter is a guide for the preparation of a short introductory module of 8–10 hours within a Master or PhD programme; it does not provide a script for lectures. In many epidemiology programmes historical notes are confined to occasional (if any) comments within the body of other modules. This module aims instead at presenting structured material as an individualized teaching block to students provided they have already followed at least one or more modules in general epidemiology and epidemiological methods. Important points to which the teacher should pay attention are features in the development of epidemiology particular to their country. An effort should be made to take these into account, lest elements essential to the understanding of the present situation are missed.

Teaching objectives

The objective of the module is to focus and raise the motivation of students for the historical perspective in epidemiology, promoting the exercise of asking and answering – when confronted with a methodological or substantive issue – questions such as: How has the issue developed overall? Was it recognizable and in what form, for example, at the beginning of the twentieth century? What were its antecedent and related issues? How was it tackled within the framework of existing knowledge? Did it induce critical advancements in knowledge? Was it instrumental for the development of approaches and methods more widely applicable? Were there any social, economic, political, and ethical factors which had non-trivial influences on it? Were any social, economic, political, and ethical consequences derived from its treatment within epidemiology? What can a historical exploration tell us about the present status and future evolution of the issue?

Of course, similar questions arise in daily work, typically when reviewing the literature on a specific research topic. Looking at these historically means expanding questions and answers in two ways: first, in time, going back not only a few years or a couple of decades (which may, however, be perfectly adequate for the strict needs of the research topic at hand); and second, in extent, tracing connections of the issue internally within epidemiology and other sciences, and externally to the societal context.

Structure of course

The module includes five parts:

1. An overview of the history of epidemiology (one lecture with brief discussion in plenary).
2. The modern history of tobacco and health: scientific aspects (one lecture with extended discussion in plenary).
3. The modern history of tobacco and health: societal aspects (one lecture with extended discussion in plenary).
4. A paper from the past (paper reading followed by extended discussion in plenary).
5. Present trends linking past and future (reading of papers followed by extended discussion in plenary).

The total time required for the module is between 8 and 10 hours, to be split over 2 or more days. Papers for reading can be distributed in advance. A class of more than ten to fifteen students should be split into smaller subgroups. Reading can be completed and some discussion developed within subgroups in preparation for a plenary session in which each subgroup presents for general discussion the issues they have identified as important. A written outline of each part with essential references should be prepared for distribution.

Teaching contents

Material for the five components of the module can be found and selected for assemblage and teaching in:

1. The historical sketch.
2. The key references listed at the end of the chapter.
3. The other references reported at the chapter end.

Following the historical sketch (pp. 4–15), content indications (with specific references) for each of the five parts are provided (pp. 15–17). *The key references should be readily available to the teacher as they are a primary source of material for all parts of the module.*

A historical sketch

As the name implies this 'sketch' is not a synthesis of an analytical and scholarly work: more simply, and much less ambitiously, it aims to offer the teacher a broad framework and some illustrative material for the module.

To review the yesterday, today, and tomorrow of epidemiology (here seen with a bias towards Europe) it may be convenient, though somewhat arbitrary, to consider three periods: (1) early epidemiology, extending from the fifth century BC to around 1830; (2) classical epidemiology, from around 1830 to the 1940s; (3) new epidemiology, from the 1940s to the present.

Yesterday: a bird's eye view

Early epidemiology This long stretch of time ran for more than two millennia, from Hippocrates (c.470–c.400 BC) to the first third of the nineteenth century. Numerous and keen epidemiological observations were made and have been handed down in surviving documents, based at best on simple or crude methods of investigation (when unfairly judged by our contemporary methodological standards). Epidemiological theories were also elaborated to explain the spreading of diseases, notably those recurrently striking and decimating populations ('epidemics').

Hippocrates developed the medical approach by providing concise, accurate, and complete descriptions of actual clinical cases, including diseases such as tetanus, typhus, and phthisis. This remained 'without parallel until the late seventeenth century' (Singer and Underwood, 1962). However, in his book on *Air, Waters and Places*, he clearly identified – as a seminal environmental scientist – the general dependence of health not on magical influences but on an identifiable array of natural external factors (Table 1.1).

The reawakening of *clinical* observation in the seventeenth century, epitomized by the 'English Hippocrates' Thomas Sydenham (1624–1689), brought attention back to the circumstances surrounding the occurrence of clinical cases, thus not only reviving the Hippocratic tradition but adding to it. In the year 1700, Bernardino Ramazzini (1633–1714) wrote in his *De Morbis Artificum Diatriba* (Ramazzini, 1982):

> The physician has to ask many questions of the patients. Hippocrates states in *De Affectionibus* 'When you face a sick person you should ask him from what he is suffering, for what reason, for how many days, what he eats and what are his bowel movements'. To all these questions one should be added 'What work does he do?'

Table 1.1

Whoever wishes to investigate medicine properly should proceed thus: in the first place to consider the seasons of the year, and what effects each of them produces. Then the winds, the hot and the cold, especially such as are common to all countries, and then such as are peculiar to each locality. In the same manner, when one comes into a city to which he is a stranger, he should consider it situation, how it lies as to the winds and the rising of the sun; for its influence is not the same whether it lies to the north or the south, to the rising or to the setting sun. One should consider most attentively the waters which the inhabitants use, whether they be marshy and soft, or hard and running from elevated and rocky situations, and then if saltish and unfit for cooking; and the ground, whether it be naked and deficient in water, or wooded and well watered, and whether it lies in a hollow, confined situation, or it elevated and cold; and the mode in which the inhabitants live, and what are their pursuits, whether they are fond of drinking and eating to excess, and given to indolence, or are fond of exercise and labor.

Hippocrates
On Airs, Waters and Places

Besides being an acute clinician Ramazzini moved from the observation of individual cases to the consideration of similar cases sharing work circumstances.

Ramazzini is today regarded as the founder of occupational medicine, a key section of the larger field of environmental medicine and epidemiology. A contemporary of Ramazzini was Giovanni Maria Lancisi (1654–1720), anatomist and clinician, whose *De Subitaneis Mortibus* (1707), in which he reports a detailed pathological investigation of a series of sudden deaths in Rome, is probably the first epidemiological study of a non-communicable condition (Lebowitz, 1970). The study was commissioned by the Pope, to whom Lancisi was the personal physician (there were no grant applications!).

On a rather different, essentially *demographic* approach, are the developments that were already taking place in the late Middle Ages and Renaissance Italy in the latter part of the fourteenth and in the fifteenth centuries. For instance, in Florence and Venice the counting of deaths and some early form of death certification specifying the cause in broad terms (e.g. 'plague' or 'not plague' during such epidemics) were current and established practices (Carmichael, 1986). The major step forward from recording, counting, and accounting to a quantitative analysis of the data was the later accomplishment of John Graunt (1620–1674) in London, who can be regarded as the founder of demography. His *Natural and Political Observations Upon the Bills of Mortality* (1662) was based on a series of weekly bills covering individual deaths and their causes in the London area back to 1603. His treatment of the data included three key innovations (Dupaquier and Dupaquier, 1985): (1) a critical examination of the sources, attempting to address issues of biased recording; (2) the use of frequencies, e.g. of deaths and ratios rather than absolute numbers in his analysis, which allowed several correct comparisons to be made; (3) the application of methods to tackle concrete problems which prompted him, for instance, to conclude that homicides were indeed rather rare, that mortality rates in the first year of life were higher in males than in females, thus compensating the slightly higher number of males at birth; and that, apart from plague, chronic conditions were killing more people than were acute conditions. After Graunt, demographic studies progressed with the invention of the first empirical life tables (E. Halley, 1656–1742), while, particularly in France, mathematical tools were being developed for dealing with chance events and probabilities (initially arising out of games), which were soon seen as equally applicable to the study of such collective phenomena as births, deaths, etc.

The third approach, *theorization*, concerning in particular the fact that the most frequent and murderous diseases appeared obviously 'communicable', either from person to person or from fomites, has a forerunner in the Latin poet Lucretius (first–second century BC). In his poem *De Rerum Natura* he hints that 'seeds' of disease can pass from a sick to a healthy individual. It was, however, only much later that Gerolamo Fracastoro (1478–1553), in his *De Contagione et Contagiosis Morbis* (1546), presented the first clear and coherent germ theory of disease, 'a mountain peak in the history of aetiology, perhaps unequalled by any other writer between Hippocrates and Pasteur' (Winslow, 1980). Fracastoro theorized that a variety of diseases are caused by transmissible, self-propagating entities (germs) which, however, were conceived more as substances akin to present day viruses than to bacteria. Correctly, he thought that these agents were specific to each disease and could spread from person to person or through infected articles (fomites) or at a distance. He went as far as arguing that treatment should consist of the destruction of the germs by either heat or cold (which is obviously correct), or of their evacuation from the body, or by checking the putrefaction processes caused by these germs, or by neutralizing them by antagonistic substances (which again was correct, but unfortunately these were not available). He is also on record as having not only described, but also given the name to a new disease making ravages in his time – syphilis (1530).

The three streams in early epidemiology, medical, demographic and theoretical, coalesced in an effective way only towards the end of the eighteenth and beginning of the nineteenth centuries, giving rise to epidemiology as we recognize it today, an investigation of diseases and their aetiology at the population level. What had been missing during the very long early phase was not so much the individual components of the epidemiological approach as the integrated and systematic process of empirical observations, quantitative description, hypothesis formulation, deductive reasoning and empirical testing on new observational or experimental data. This started in science with Galileo Galilei (1564–1642) at the beginning of the seventeenth century and gradually spread from physics to other branches of study. In biology an early high point in this combination of observation, experiment and quantitative reasoning was the discovery of the circulation of blood by Willliam Harvey (1578–1657), a contemporary of Galilei.

Classical epidemiology With the advent of the industrial transformation of western Europe, starting in Great Britain and propagating from the mid-eighteenth century to the continent in the next decades, 'crowd diseases' emerged which struck the populations amassed in the slums of the fast-growing centers of industrial development: London, Glasgow, Manchester, Paris, Lyon, Berlin, etc. This provided the decisive stimulus and at the same time the observational field for epidemiology, which developed as the investigation facet of a vast public health movement. Only a few landmarks and figures can be briefly cited.

In Great Britain medical registration of deaths had been introduced in 1801 and in 1838 William Farr (1807–1883) introduced a national system of recording causes of death. Once the mechanism started to work it provided a wealth of data which Farr himself first analyzed with great skill, making full use of life table techniques (close in most details to those in present day use) and of procedures for standardizing rates. He was also instrumental in building up a classification of diseases for statistical purposes, both national and international. His analyses, published from the Registrar General's Office at regular intervals, gave a picture of the evolving health condition of the population of Great Britain and drew the attention of all social investigators during the Victorian period, including Marx and Engels. The work of John Snow (1813–1858), a contemporary of William Farr, is generally quoted as an example of a brilliant analytical investigation which can lead to the identification of a pathogenic agent and its elimination from the environment. Cholera (Asiatic cholera) had started to rage in India and then moved westwards, the first epidemic hitting Great Britain in 1831–32, causing at least 60 000 deaths. Snow directly investigated the subsequent major epidemic episodes in London in 1849 and 1854, focusing attention on the role that polluted water might have played in the spread of the disease. Among a number of other observations he noted (Table 1.2) that, while in 1849 and 1854 roughly the same number of deaths had occurred in the London districts supplied by the water company of Southwark and Vauxhall, a marked reduction in deaths had occurred in those districts supplied by the Lambeth company. No major change in population had occurred between 1849 and 1854 but, unlike Southwark and Vauxhall, the Lambeth company had changed its sources of water supply, moving higher up the Thames, probably above, as Snow conjectured, the greatest source of contamination by city sewage. Indeed, when he computed death rates from cholera (Table 1.3), they were more than 20 times lower for the districts supplied by the Lambeth company in respect to those supplied by Southwark and Vauxhall. Strong corroboration of these findings came from a more refined investigation: in some areas the water supplies for the two companies happened to be closely intermixed, some houses receiving their water from the Lambeth company and others from Southwark and Vauxhall. The number of houses and the size of the pertinent populations belonging to each company were known, but a door to door inquiry was needed, and was indeed carried out by Snow, on all cholera cases to ascertain to which company the water supply of their

Table 1.2 Mortality from cholera in the areas of London supplied by the Southwark and Vauxhall, and Lambeth Water Companies in 1849 and 1854*

Districts with water supplied by	Number of deaths attributed to cholera	
	1849	1854
Southwark and Vauxhall Company	2261	2458
Lambeth Company	162	37
Both companies	3905	2547

* From Snow, 1853

Table 1.3 Mortality from cholera in the districts of London supplied by the Southwark and Vauxhall, and the Lambeth Companies, July 8 to August 26, 1854*

Districts with water supplied by	Population 1851	Deaths from cholera	Cholera death rate per 1000 population
Southwark and Vauxhall Company	167,654	844	5.0
Lambeth Company	19,133	18	0.9
Both companies	300,149	652	2.2

* From Snow, 1853

homes belonged. This allowed the correct calculation of valid rates of cholera occurrence. The results are shown in Table 1.4, which clearly demonstrates that even within the same physical area the origin of the water supply separates in a clearcut way those populations with high and low rates of disease occurrence. All of these observations can be seen, in fact (Winkelstein, 1995), as the test of a lucid theory of the etiology of communicable diseases that Snow had elaborated and presented in 1853 in a paper entitled 'On continuous molecular changes', along the lines of previous work by the German pathologist Jacob Henle (1809–1885).

In France the influence of great mathematicians such as D'Alembert, Condorcet, the Swiss Euler and Bernoulli family, Lagrange and Laplace who worked to various extents on probability and statistics during the eighteenth and early nineteenth century was strongly felt in the medical field. A central figure in this development was the physician Pierre Louis (1787–1872), who introduced the 'numerical method' in medicine and produced statistical evidence that the then widespread practice of bloodletting was virtually ineffective or even dangerous. That the scientific climate in the first half of the

Table 1.4 Mortality from cholera in London, July 8 to August 26, 1854, related to source of individual water supply in three groups of districts*

Group of districts with water supplied by	Water supply of individual houses	Population 1851	Deaths from cholera	Cholera death-rate per 1000 population
Southwark and Vauxhall Company	Southwark and Vauxhall Company	167,654**	738	4.4
Lambeth Company	Lambeth Company	19,133**	4	0.2
Both companies	Southwark and Vauxhall Company	98,862	419	4.2
	Lambeth Company	154,615	80	0.5
Rest of London		1,921,972	1,422	0.7

* From Snow, 1855

** Overestimated by a small amount, since this figure includes population with no water supply

nineteenth century had become favorable to a quantitative study of medical phenomena is shown by the substantial number of articles published in most of the European countries dealing with problems in quantitative biology or in the clinical or public health domains (Buck *et al.*, 1988). Even in a country like Italy, which by that time had become, after an illustrious past, rather peripheral in scientific development, one finds evident traces of this atmosphere. For instance, at the first Congress of Italian Scientists, in Pisa in 1838 (Atti della prima riumione degli scienziati italiani 1939), it was proposed that to compare different treatments the best method would be to administer them in different wards of large hospitals to which access of patients would be on a strict rotation basis without any possibility of choice on the part of the physicians. The outcome of each treatment would then be carefully recorded and counted and the whole process, as well as the interpretation of the results identifying the superior treatment (if any), would be strictly monitored and reported by a steering committee.

The highest degree of synthesis between experimental science, medicine, simple but penetrating demographic investigation, and public health concern was probably achieved in the unique personality of the German scientist Rudolf Virchow (1821–1902). His work in pathology is regarded as a cornerstone of modern medicine. Not only is he the acknowledged founder of (microscopic) cellular pathology, but he also wrote and was very active in the field of public health, based on his belief that 'medicine is a social science'. It is interesting to see how the flow of communication took place at that time and how, for instance, an agreed system of classification of diseases, basic to any epidemiological work, was shaping up. At the International Congress of Statistics in 1855, Rudolf Virchow stated (Virchow, 1985):

> The form of the bulletin indicated by Mr. Farr can be recommended from the practical and medical point of view, because it contains one column for the disease, and another for the consequences of the diseases that have been the immediate cause of death; for it is one of the most important aims of statistics to know not only the direct causes of death but also the indirect ones, i.e. the pathological state which produces the truly lethal alterations. The mechanism itself of death is of interest for practical statistics only in the case of crime, or of a lesion due to violence, or of accident. In contrast, practical hygiene is most interested in appraising the aetiology of mortality.

One can clearly recognize here the basic concept and structure of current death certification, separating underlying causes from proximate causes, as well as the separate classification of accidents and traumatic events even now present in the International Classification of Diseases (ICD). It fell to another German scientist, Robert Koch (1843–1910), in the wake of the fundamental discovery of microorganisms by Louis Pasteur (1822–1895), not only to contribute to the discovery of the agents of several diseases (including the actual identification of the major disease tuberculosis), but also to formulate a set of criteria for establishing causality in epidemiological studies. With the new ability to isolate from healthy and diseased people a wide variety of microorganisms, an entirely new problem arose at that time of sorting out the few capable of causing a disease from the majority of innocent passengers. Koch's criteria, among others, addressed this issue in a sharp way, stating that, to be regarded as a causative agent of a disease, a microorganism:

(a)   should be found in all subjects with the disease;

(b)   should be grown *in vitro* (in a suitable medium);

(c)   should be capable of reproducing the disease in some animal species.

While the first criterion is formulated in a strictly deterministic way and therefore looks at a glance radically different from our contemporary probabilistic concepts, one may doubt whether it has ever been applied as such without in practice making allowance for a margin of error in what one would regard as 'all subjects' (99%? 95%?). Perhaps it is the third criterion which more sharply differs from those nowadays quoted in the literature, following the guidelines put forward by A. B. Hill, which include as one element supporting causality 'the biological plausibility'. This is much weaker and less strict than the ability to reproduce the disease in some animal species, which reflects an attitude of giving full weight to the result of experiments in animals, a feature which became somewhat blurred with the advent of the 'new epidemiology' in the 1940s. Indeed, while the further evolution of epidemiology after Pasteur and Koch throughout the last part of the nineteenth and first part of the twentieth centuries largely occurred hand in hand with parallel experimental and laboratory developments in the field of microbiology, the new epidemiology addressing the unknown causes of non-infectious diseases went back to rely, as for instance Snow had done before the microbiological era, pre-eminently on direct observations in human groups.

The new epidemiology Individual studies on cancer, non-rheumatic cardiovascular diseases, and psychiatric diseases, can be traced well back in time, but one can take as a convenient turning point for the rise of the new epidemiology the period around the Second World War. A major stream in the development of the new epidemiology is what could be labeled as the 'tobacco and health story'. Initial observations were either of a statistical nature or of a clinical one. Among the first one can mention is a short and remarkable paper by Pearl (Pearl, 1938) using insurance data showing that the expectation of life for smokers was substantially reduced in respect to non-smokers. Among the second, one might single out the observation by Ochsner and De Bakey (Ochsner and De Bakey, 1939) of high frequency of smokers among the lung cancer patients coming to their hospital in those early days of thoracic surgery. These were followed by still other statistical findings of a general nature pointing to a dramatic increase of lung cancer rates in men throughout the 1940s, in particular in the US and the UK. In 1950, three hospital-based case control studies were almost simultaneously published (Levin *et al.*, 1950; Wynder and Graham, 1950; Doll and Hill, 1950) which clearly showed an association 'most probably' (at that time) causal, between tobacco smoking and lung cancer.The paper by Levin *et al.* used information available in clinical records at one cancer center starting from 1938. The other two investigations collected *ad hoc* information on hospitalized cases and controls. Interestingly, when Doll and Hill set forth to investigate the etiology of lung cancer, which had become a common disease in the UK, they were thinking of air pollution, at that time very severe in London (the 'London Fog'), as an even more plausible candidate than tobacco smoke. As it turned out, the results of their study neatly caused the role of tobacco smoke to emerge, with that of air pollution much less evident. These three studies were the first in a long sequence of case control and cohort studies carried out in different countries relating tobacco smoking to various diseases. Doll and Hill themselves added another well known investigation, following a cohort of British doctors prospectively and reporting the results first in 1964 (Doll and Hill, 1964). This cohort, which has now been observed for 40 years (Doll *et al.* 1994), provided strong support to the etiological role of tobacco, not only on lung cancer but on a spectrum of neoplastic and non-neoplastic diseases. It is interesting to note (Saracci, 1995) that the survival curves from age 35 to 100 years for the 6813 subjects insured in the US observed by Pearl in the late thirties and for the cohort of 34 439 British doctors followed from 1951 to 1971 by Doll and coworkers show a closely similar loss in median survival (4.9 and 5 years, respectively). When lifetime smokers are compared to lifetime non-smokers, however, with the prolongation of the follow-up until 1991 the loss increased to 7.5 years in the British cohort.

One can safely state that by 1964, the date of publication of the results of the cohort study by Doll and Hill and of the first US Surgeon General's report on Smoking and Health (the 'Terry Report' from the name of the Surgeon General) (Smoking and Health, 1964), the role of smoking in the causation of a number of lethal diseases can be regarded as soundly established. The Terry Report is an extremely valuable document, which can still be read with profit by anyone interested in assessing large amounts of disparate data bearing on an etiological problem. It is interesting from the methodological viewpoint to know that the inability in the initial periods of study to reproduce neoplasms in animals by exposing them to tobacco smoke was regarded – in line with Koch's third criterion – as an important element for questioning the validity of the conclusions drawn from the epidemiological studies. It is certainly not coincidental that at about this time epidemiologists felt compelled to rethink the criteria used to infer causality in general (rather than in infectious diseases) and that A. B. Hill produced a set which can still be used as a reference (Hill, 1965). As already noted, this changes the requirement of an agent to be able to reproduce the disease in animals to the more general and optional requirement of biological plausibility. This perspective on causality had the unintended consequence of downplaying almost completely in some circumstances and epidemiological circles the value of animal experiments (incidentally, it can be noted that, using better experimental set-ups, tobacco smoke has produced cancers in experimental animals): this result was an unfortunate one and in flat contradiction to all thinking and practice in biology.

This phase of the development of epidemiology received new input from the two-way exchange between epidemiology and clinical medicine, which has been a constant feature in the history of the subject. As previously exemplified Ramazzini, a clinician, and Snow, a physician (pioneering anesthesia), had enlarged clinical observations by looking for causes of disease at the population level; conversely, Louis had brought the methods of population studies into the clinical domain to evaluate the effects of medical acts in patient populations. The 'new epidemiology' clearly highlights this dual exchange. In Great Britain, John Ryle (1899–1950), Professor of Medicine at Cambridge, moved from the clinic to become the first director of the Institute of

Social Medicine at Oxford, established at the time of the Second World War to investigate the influence of social, genetic, environmental, and domestic facors on the incidence of human diseases and morbidity. He was a key motivator of the work of the post-war generation of British epidemiologists, who made crucial contributions to the identification of causal factors of chronic diseases. In a parallel and opposite move, epidemiological methods were showing their value for clinical research and were increasingly incorporated into a growing stream of 'clinical epidemiology', namely studies of diagnostic, prognostic, therapeutic, and rehabilitative procedures in populations of sick subjects. A yardstick in this development was the publication in 1972 by Archie Cochrane (1909–1988); (Cochrane, 1972) of a brilliant essay advocating a systematic use of the randomized trial method to evaluate procedures in the areas of clinical and health services.

Today: epidemiology in the making

Today, as yesterday, epidemiology as a population approach to health and disease embraces two bodies of knowledge: first, epidemiological methods of investigation (which are part of scientific methodology), and, second, epidemiological substantive notions developed by application of such methods (these notions become part of medicine in its biological and social facets).

Both bodies of knowledge have undergone substantial expansion since World War II with the development of the 'new epidemiology'. A simple comparison of early with recent editions of any one of the classical textbooks of medicine (*Cecil Textbook of Medicine*, 9th edition, 1955, 19th edition, 1992, Philadelphia, Saunders) shows how epidemiology has contributed to change and increased, sometimes dramatically, our understanding of the time and space evolution, etiology, and opportunities for control (preventive or therapeutic), of major classes of diseases such as ischemic heart disease, chronic obstructive lung disease, asthma, cancers at several sites, not to mention newer entities like toxic shock syndrome, AIDS, Legionnaires' disease, or *Helicobacter* infections. This progress has been matched by the emergence, *de facto* or formally recognized, of a wide spectrum of subspecialties (cancer epidemiology, pediatric epidemiology, genetic epidemiology, clinical epidemiology, etc.) within epidemiology itself. On the methodological side it is sufficient to remember that no text specifically devoted to epidemiological methods was available before 1960, when the book by MacMahon and coworkers was published (MacMahon *et al.*, 1960), whereas today methodology provides enough matter for 10 or 20 major books with different degrees of completeness and complexity. Study design methods and statistical methods of analysis have been developed in and from the context of problems in epidemiology, rather than by borrowing them from other areas of applied methodology and statistics. Also, in recent years, a unified approach to the analysis of occurrence data (incidence and mortality rates), which has implications for study design, has been developed based on the unifying principle of likelihood inference. These developments have taken place concurrently within an accelerated evolution in the whole field of biology and health, and one can single out four traits, particularly salient in Europe and other economically developed areas of the world.

1. The unprecedented advances of research in some domains, fundamental to all other fields of biology and medicine, like immunology, the neurosciences, and, most prominently, molecular genetics and cell and developmental biology. Clearly, switching the study of higher organisms, including humans, from the anatomy and physiology of the phenotype (as has been the case until recently) to the direct study of the anatomy and physiology of the genotype opens an entirely new perspective, the implications of which (preventive, therapeutic, and ethical) are not yet fully perceptible.

2. The advances in clinical medicine at the diagnostic and therapeutic levels. Until 60 or 70 years ago effective treatments could be counted on the figures of one hand, so that the only way open for disease control – in many cases effective – was prevention. Nowadays, treatments capable of effectively influencing length and quality of survival are available for a number of serious conditions, both infectious and non-infectious. As a consequence, the balance and the competition between the preventive and curative approach needs to be seen in a fresh light and critically reassessed. A relevant example is mortality rates from ischaemic heart disease, the marked decrease of which in several western countries appears to be in part due to decreased incidence and in part to decreased lethality because of better treatment options.

3. The escalating costs of all health care delivery systems, whether private, public or mixed, have brought to the forefront issues of effective and efficient use of available resources which were of negligible importance, or almost unknown, three or four decades ago.

4. The renewed awareness among professionals and the general public of the dependence of health (of humans as well as of other living organisms) on the environment, material and social, personal, local or general. In parallel with this goes the realization that tangible deterioration of the environment does take place because of shortsighted human activities.

These developments and their interrelationship change the pattern of the factors capable of promoting, damaging or restoring health, and impose a virtually continuous reappraisal and adaptation of the health care system and, more generally, of all plans of action aimed at influencing health.

Tomorrow's horizon

Three major challenges stand on the horizon of epidemiology and epidemiologists in the coming decades entailing, as with any challenge, both opportunities and risks.

The challenge of evolving biology Few would disagree with a comment by Sir Richard Doll (Doll, 1993):

> Classical methods of epidemiological research are proving less and less productive as the simple problems are being successfully solved. They will doubtless continue to be used to make new discoveries from time to time ... but without some brilliant new inspirations, the rate of discovery of new facts of any importance by the use of these classical methods must be expected to slow down.

A major way to maintain momentum is certainly to incorporate concepts and techniques evolving at an impressive pace from such basic disciplines as immunology and molecular biology and genetics. For instance, epidemiology can improve its resolving power by using biological markers of exposures (e.g. DNA or protein adducts with toxic xenobiotics) rather than continue to rely in the future mostly on questionnaire assessment of exposure. The study of individual susceptibility, genetic or acquired, can help to identify the most vulnerable subgroups. More generally, the mechanistic study (pathogenetic study) of how different factors cooperate in producing a disease can be of help in identification of specific etiological agents (etiological study). For instance, if an investigation combining epidemiology with immunology and biochemistry isolates a specific air pollutant as responsible for the induction of asthma attacks, control measures can be addressed specifically to the sources of that pollutant (a more generic approach to all pollutants in the air may simply not be possible). There is, however, the danger that studies of pathogenesis may become attractive *per se* (indeed, they are) rather than as one more way of elucidating controllable etiological factors. It will be for epidemiologists to bring back to the level of etiology and prevention the wealth of investigations that the convergence of epidemiology and modern biology is now making possible.

The challenge of evolving society Society in most developed countries, and particularly in Europe, is characterized by an ageing population, reproduction rates that are below the population replacement rates, current flow of immigration from less developed countries (which is likely to continue in the coming decades), and persistent inequalities in health conditions between different sections of society, in particular gender, occupation, and socioeconomic categories. Monitoring trends and identifying causal factors in this area, which could be labeled 'social epidemiology', has been a longstanding concern of epidemiologists, characterizing in a major way their involvement in public health, both from the scientific and, when required, from the campaigning for health viewpoint. Whether this will retain substantial and sustained attention in epidemiological research or be left mostly to other professionals (e.g. sociologists) while epidemiologists become almost exclusively concentrated in the biomedical area, is an open issue.

The challenge of diversification *versus* integration As in all other scientific and technical branches of activity, epidemiology has been recently, and continues to, specialize along different axes. A first axis is methodology *versus* substantive studies; areas of current and future development in methodology are, for example, the treatment of exposure measurements and errors of measurement to reduce misclassification and improve study power, methods in genetic epidemiology, modeling of the exposure–response relationship with multiple longitudinal measurements. A second axis is diversification of different fields of substantive interest; for instance, cancer epidemiology, epidemiology of ageing, etc. A whole area of specialization is 'clinical epidemiology', the application of epidemiological methods within the clinical domain, both for studies evaluating diagnostic, prognostic, therapeutic, and rehabilitative procedures and for evolving formal methods of optimal clinical decision-making.

Stemming from this is the rapidly growing branch of 'evidence-based medicine' (EBM), which employs formal methods to assemble and evaluate the existing evidence on the effects of medical interventions. A final axis of diversification tends to separate those who specialize in investigative aspects for routine or research purposes from those who plan and implement interventions. In clinical medicine this has produced a variety of specialists in purely diagnostic activities (clinical chemists, clinical pathologists, diagnostic radiologists, imaging specialists), different from the therapist who decides and acts on the basis of the diagnosis; similarly, in the public health area the epidemiologist may become more and more a pure specialist in etiological and evaluative investigations, leaving others to decide what to do.

This unavoidable trend raises three major issues : (1) to what extent a global view can be preserved jointly with specialized or 'subspecialized' technical skills; (2) to what extent, side by side with epidemiologists specializing in different areas, the figure of the generalist can be maintained (again, the analogy with clinical medicine is pertinent, with one of the most difficult present day problems being the survival and role of the general physician or of the internist); (3) how epidemiologists can best cooperate in teams of specialists (epidemiologists with special skills and other professionals), including those in charge of taking public health decisions.

In its historical evolution epidemiology's successes have largely derived from its working as the investigative component of public health, studying the distribution and determinants of health and diseases in populations. This essence should continue to be preserved in the foreseeable future by incorporating into epidemiological research the new opportunities currently arising in particular from the fields of genetics, environmental sciences, clinical medicine, and health care.

Content indications for the five parts of the module

Overview of the history of epidemiology

The historical sketch can be used as a basis for this overview. The interest of the students is heightened if examples are produced from the national and local context. The bulk of significant scientific advances in epidemiology has been concentrated in a relatively small number of countries. However, isolated but important discoveries – often related to special traits of local health and diseases – have come from many more countries and there is virtually no country in which the echo of scientific advance has not been received in some form. It is these aspects which can be exploited for illustrative purposes.

The modern history of tobacco and health: scientific aspects

The identification of the causal role of tobacco smoking in a variety of diseases is a prime success of the new post-World War II epidemiology. The historical sketch (see The new epidemiology, above) contains an outline to be fleshed out using material from the quoted sources. The focus can be on the controversy on the etiological role of tobacco smoking, in particular on lung cancer, and on the emergence, under the stimulus of the controversy, of methodology for data analysis and of criteria for inferring causation in epidemiology. These aspects are covered in the 'Smoking and Health

' report (1964), especially in Chapters 8 and 9 and in some of the publications, cited in the report, by eminent critics of the smoking causal hypothesis such as R. A. Fisher, a founder of modern statistical methodology, and J. Berkson, a leading medical statistician.

The modern history of tobacco and health: societal aspects

The direct link between epidemiology and prevention is commonly stated as one of the merits of the epidemiological approach. Once causation has been established, as from the early 1960s for tobacco smoking and various pathological conditions, preventive actions can be implemented even without knowledge of the biological mechanisms leading to the condition. This logical sequence often breaks down in practice as the transition from sufficient knowledge for action to actual action is strongly influenced by a number of social, economic, cultural, and psychological factors. First, simply comparing the local or national tobacco smoking patterns and trends with the available established knowledge on health effects over time, and also comparing these with legislative and health promoting-actions is instructive. Second, as documented and discussed by Proctor (1999), the crucial role played in prevention by factors other than sound science and epidemiology is highlighted by the case of Nazi Germany, where vigorous anti-smoking campaigns were conducted, inspired by strong ideological reasons. Moreover, informative epidemiological evidence gathered during the Nazi period went ignored until recently for reasons mostly foreign to science. Third, the adverse health effects of passive exposure to environmental tobacco smoke (ETS), particularly lung cancer (Hackshaw et al.. 1997; Boffetta et al., 1998), have radically changed the prospects of preventive measures. Unlike (partially) voluntary active smoking, ETS exposure is wholly involuntary and there is general agreement that involuntary exposure should be controlled, mainly through legal restrictions. Hence, simply denying any material health effect of ETS became a major priority for tobacco producers, fought with organized and often unscrupulous means, as documented by Ong and Glantz (Ong and Glantz, 2000). This offers a lesson first on how powerful and well structured economic interests can lead to misinterpretation of scientific evidence to the point of active disinformation and, second, on how inherently liable to distortion by extrascientific forces the judgement of experts (who think of themselves as independent) may in fact be (Maggi, 2000).

A paper from the past

A paper addressing a substantive epidemiological issue with the methodological armamentarium available at the time of writing will provide a measure of the methodological gap separating the past from the present. Papers can be selected from those in the Key references: one example is the article on sickness and stress in operational flying in the Royal Air Force during World War II (Reid, 1948). In reading this article (or any other article selected for the exercise), students should focus in particular on:

(a) key issues of design; whether and how issues of confounding, bias, and chance were dealt with at the design and analysis stages; how inferences about causation were developed;

(b)   how they would design today, within the limits of the database available to the author, a study addressing the same issue and how they would conduct and analyse it.

From a comparison of (a) and (b) the conclusions in the article may be assessed as: credible neither at the time of writing nor today; credible to a degree that one may even wish to specify (e.g. as 'moderately credible, credible, highly credible'), at the time of writing but not today in the light of new methodological criteria judged as non-dispensable; or credible at the time of writing as well as today, notwithstanding the inherent limitations deriving from the past status of the art.

Present trends linking past and future

This topic is discussed in the sections Today: epidemiology in the making and Tomorrow's horizon of the historical sketch. Taking as the occasion the turn of the century, many conferences and papers have been devoted to the role and future of epidemiology. At the international level a supplement of the *International Journal of Epidemiology* (The Future of Epidemiology, 1999) contains a series of papers providing a spectrum of views on the evolution of epidemiology. Two or three of these papers can be distributed to students for reading: each student should extract from each paper two lists of key points on which he or she agrees or disagrees. These points, with supporting arguments, will be discussed in plenary. An alternative way is to ask each student (before distributing any relevant paper) to prepare an outline of how they see, on one hand, the likely and, on the other, the desirable evolution of epidemiology as a scientific endeavour and as a practice within society. The outlines can then be presented to the class for discussion and compared with published essays.

Areas for consideration when looking from past and present into the future come under three main headings: (1) information sources (items such as population disease registries and stores of biological specimens: organization, access, use, protection, ethical and legal implications); (2) methodology (items such as methods to improve exposure and endpoint assessment, new study designs, multilevel analyses, pooled data analyses and meta-analyses, and risk modeling); (3) aims and uses of epidemiology (items such as the role of epidemiology in clinical medicine, environmental and occupational health, public health, prevention and reduction of inequalities in health between and within countries, priorities for research, communication of results and the role of epidemiologists in decision-making in the health area, responsibilities of epidemiologists).

Assessing students' achievements

As stated, the objective of the module is to focus and raise the interest and motivation of students for the historical perspective on epidemiological themes, not to develop the skills necessary to gain this perspective (this would require a more sustained didactic endeavour). Students should be asked using a miniquestionnaire how they rate (on a 'poor, fair, good, excellent' scale) the module in respect to four aspects: increase in knowledge; usefulness for work; stimulation of interest for the historical perspective; motivation for personally engaging in historical exercises.

Key references

Books

Porter, R. (1997). *The greatest benefit to mankind: a medical history of humanity from antiquity to the present*. Fontana Press, London.

A history of health and medicine, seen both in its internal development and in its relationship to society, as a background to the history of epidemiology.

Rosen, G. (1993). *A history of public health* (Expanded edn). The Johns Hopkins University Press, Baltimore.

A standard reference, comprehensive and highly readable.

Collections of articles and essays

American Journal of Epidemiology (1995), Vols 141 and 142. On the occasion of its 75th anniversary the journal has reprinted in the issues of 1995 a number of articles published from the late 1930s to the late 1970s which are regarded to be of historical relevance. Each is accompanied by a short commentary.

Buck, C., Llopis, A., Najera, E. and Terris, M. (1988). *The challenge of epidemiology: issues and selected readings*. Pan American Health Organization, Washington.

An indispensable collection of papers from Hippocrates to present day.

Greenland, S., ed. (1987). *Evolution of epidemiologic ideas: annotated readings on concepts and methods*. Epidemiology Resources Inc., Chestnut Hill.

A collection of methodological papers published between 1945 and 1977 covering issues of causal inference and developments in theory and quantitative methods. Each paper is accompanied by a commentary placing it in historical perspective.

Lilienfeld, A. M., ed. (1980). *Times, places and persons. Aspects of the history of epidemiology*. The Johns Hopkins University Press, Baltimore.

A series of essays, most of them scholarly documented, by historians and epidemiologists: topics range from numerical methods in the 1830s to the history of eradication of small-pox.

Smoking and Health (1964). *Report of the Advisory Committee to the Surgeon General*, PHS, US Department of Health, Education & Welfare, Washington DC.

A landmark report: it establishes the etiological role of tobacco smoking in a number of diseases through a rigorous examination of the evidence, mostly epidemiological. Still instructive from a methodological angle.

Other references

Atti della prima riumione degli scienziati italiani, 1838., 4th edn (1939). Pisa, Nistri-Lischi, (reprinted).

Boffetta, P., Agudo, A., Ahrens, W. *et al.* (1998). Multicenter case-control study of exposure to environmental tobacco smoke and lung cancer in Europe. *J Natl Cancer Inst*, **90**, 1440–50.

Carmichael, A. G. (1986). *Plague and the poor in Renaissance Florence*. Cambridge University Press, Cambridge.

Cochrane, A. L. (1972). *Effectiveness and efficiency. Random reflections on health services*. The Nuffield Provincial Hospitals Trust, London.

Doll, R. and Hill, A. B. (1950). Smoking and carcinoma of the lung: preliminary report. *BMJ*, **ii**, 739–48.

Doll, R. and Hill, A. B. (1964). Mortality in relation to smoking: ten years' observation of British doctors. *BMJ*, **i**, 1399–1410 and 1460–7.

Doll, R. (1993). Lecture at the 6th summer course of the European Educational Programme in Epidemiology, Florence.

Doll, R., Peto, R., Wheatley, K., Gray, R., and Sutherland, I. (1994). Mortality in relation to smoking: 40 years' observation in male British doctors. *BMJ*, **309**, 901–10.

Dupaquier, J., and Dupaquier, M. (1985). *Histoire de la demographie*. Perrin, Paris.

Hackshaw, A. K., Law, M. R. and Wald, N. J. (1997). The accumulated evidence on lung cancer and environmental tobacco smoke. *BMJ*, **315**, 980–8.

Hill, A. B. (1965). The environment and disease: association or causation. *Proc R Soc Med*, **58**, 295–300.

Lebowitz, J. O. (1970). *The history of coronary heart disease*. Wellcome Institute of the History of Medicine, London.

Levin, M. L., Godstein, H. and Gerhardt, P. R. (1950). Cancer and tobacco smoking: a preliminary report. *JAMA*, **143**, 336–8.

MacMahon, B., Pugh, T. F. and Ipsen, J. (1960). *Epidemiologic methods*. Little, Brown and Company, Boston.

Maggi, L. (2000). Bearing witness for tobacco. *J Public Health Policy*, **21**, 296–302.

Ochsner, M., and De Bakey (1939). Primary pulmonary malignancy.Treatment by total pneumonectomy; analyses of 79 collected cases and presentation of 7 personal cases. *Surg, Gynecol Obstet*, **68**, 435–51.

Ong, E. K. and Glantz, S. A. (2000). Tobacco industry efforts subverting International Agency for Research on Cancer's second-hand smoke study. *Lancet*, **355**, 1253–59.

Pearl, R. (1938). Tobacco smoking and longevity. *Science*, **87**, 216–17.

Proctor, R. N. (1999). *The Nazi war on cancer*. Princeton University Press, Princeton.

Ramazzini, B. (1982). *De morbis artificum diatriba* (Italian translation by I. and V. Romano and F. Carnevale). La Nuova Italia Scientifica, Firenze.

Reid, D. D. (1948). Sickness and stress in operational flying. *B J Soc Med*, **2**, 123–31.

Saracci, R. (1995). Smoking and death. *BMJ*, **310**, 600 and 672.

Singer, C. and Underwood, E. A. (1962). *A short history of medicine*. (2nd edn). Clarendon Press, Oxford.

The Future of Epidemiology (1999). *Int J Epidemiol*, **25**, S996–S1024.

Virchow, R. (1985). *Collected essays on public health and epidemiology*. Vol. 1.(L. T. Rather, ed.), Science History Publications, Canton, MA.

Winkelstein, W. Jr. (1995). A new perspective on John Snow's communicable disease theory. *Am J Epidemiol*, **142**, S3–S9.

Winslow, C. E. A. (1980). *The conquest of epidemic disease*. The University of Wisconsin Press, Madison.

Wynder, E. L., and Graham, E. A. (1950). Tobacco smoking as a possible etiologic factor in bronchiogenic carcinoma: a study of 684 proved cases. JAMA, **143**, 329–36.

Chapter 2

Epidemiology and public health

John M. Last

Introduction

The *raison d'être* for all teaching is to help learners to acquire the knowledge and skills that are pertinent to the topic being taught. Good teaching also creates and enhances attitudes towards learning as a lifelong process; it encourages a critical, sceptical attitude to dogma and *ex cathedra* opinion statements, and insistence on seeing the evidence for all conclusions. Good teachers have been doing this since the days of Socrates. Educators, especially those who teach teachers, have produced handbooks on how to do it well, e.g. Postman and Weingartner's *Teaching as a Subversive Activity* (1969). This is an unsettling book, aimed at dislodging dogma, detecting and eliminating nonsense, and discovering truths that are sometimes evaded or buried – in short, a book every teacher should read. Above all, teaching is not for the teachers, it is for the learners – although of course teachers can and often do learn a great deal both from the teaching itself, and in preparing for teaching. The teaching–learning dyad should be enjoyable for learners and teachers alike. It works best when it is fun for everyone. It is a dismal failure if it leaves learners, or their teachers, feeling bewildered, angry or sad.

In many fields of scholarly activity there can be more than one interpretation of the evidence, more than one conclusion based on the interplay of axioms or principles with the facts derived from observation and original investigation. This often occurs with ethical problems. It occurs in environmental epidemiology, when evidence from studies that have used different methods and procedures yield discordant results. For example, some studies of the long-term effects of exposure to polyhalogenated hydrocarbons show evidence of harm to human health and other studies do not. When the evidence is equivocal, political or economic pressures can intrude and influence public health policy decisions, which then tend to be based on subjective criteria rather than on an objective interpretation of the evidence. Debates about contentious issues may be matters for postgraduate study, but medical students too need to become acquainted with the real world where these controversies exist.

Teaching objectives

Learning objectives have three components: knowledge, skills, and attitudes. The body of knowledge that comprises epidemiology is set out in elementary textbooks and advanced monographs, including several that are oriented towards public health applications (Beaglehole *et al.*, 1993; Lilienfeld and Stolley, 1994). The relevant skills

Table 2.1 Sample behavioral objectives for public health component of epidemiology course for medical students. (These are examples; this is not a comprehensive list.)

Knowledge

At the end of the course students will be able to:

Describe and explain how community health is measured

List the strengths and weaknesses of commonly used health indicators (vital and health statistics)

Describe epidemiological methods – observational, analytic and experimental i.e. randomized controlled trials (RCTs)

List the strengths and weaknesses of case control and cohort studies

Explain the distinction between association and causation

Describe how disease surveillance works in practice

Outline the procedures for investigation of an epidemic

Explain the epidemiological principles of screening programs

Describe the uses of epidemiology in public health policy, planning, and evaluation

Skills

At the end of the course, students will be able to:

Calculate specified rates and proportions, e.g. mortality rates, standardized mortality ratios (SMRs), incidence, prevalence

Interpret the data from epidemiological studies and arrive at a logical conclusion

Distinguish valid from flawed study designs

Calculate the sensitivity and specificity of screening tests from samples of relevant data

Attitudes

At the end of the course, students will:

Be sceptical of, and demand evidence for, opinion statements

Examine data sources thoroughly before using them

Demonstrate appreciation of the balance between rights of individuals and collective needs

Act responsibly in conducting sensitive public health functions, e.g. STD contact tracing

Respect privacy and protect confidentiality of personal data

are also well described in monographs, some of which include exercises for readers to test their own skills and reasoning capacity (Ellwood, 1998; Friedman, 1995). The body of knowledge and the relevant skills are best expressed as behavioral objectives. Attitudes or values are the most difficult part to communicate and to acquire, and to summarize. Table 2.1 offers examples of behavioral objectives. The list can easily be expanded, especially in the domain of attitudes.

Knowledge

At the end of the public health component of the teaching of epidemiology, students should be able to describe and explain how epidemiological methods are used to identify public health problems, to discover their causes, to control these problems, and to evaluate the efficacy of control measures. These aims and objectives apply at both undergraduate and graduate levels, although the emphasis differs. Undergraduates require an overview of the body of knowledge that is pertinent to the application of epidemiology in public health practice. They should be able to describe the essential principles and methods of epidemiology. They should be able to demonstrate that they understand and can interpret epidemiological evidence contained in scientific papers and reports, and that they know what they must do when they encounter a problem that has an epidemiological aspect, such as a case of a dangerous communicable disease or a possible cluster of cases of cancer among children living in a polluted environment. They must understand their obligations regarding official statistics, and why accurate certification of vital events (births, stillbirths, and deaths) is important. Students need to appreciate that when they are in practice they will be the ultimate source of such information at community or hospital level. They must be able to use evidence-based medicine (Sackett *et al.*, 2000) in patient care, and must understand that much of the evidence is acquired by the use of epidemiological methods. Although they will be able to function in most branches of medical practice without possessing the skills required to conduct an epidemiological study, students should know what those skills comprise so they can discriminate between well and poorly performed studies when reading accounts of them.

Skills

Students who have completed a course in epidemiology should be able to take part in the investigation of an epidemic or other occurrence of illness. They should understand and be able to interpret basic kinds of epidemiological evidence such as the data of a case control or cohort study, and the results of randomized controlled trials. Postgraduates require more; they must possess and be able to use a range of pertinent epidemiological skills, and know which method to use in particular circumstances. Brownson and Petitti (1998) provide a good introduction to what is best called practical epidemiology, the application of epidemiological methods in public health practice. The ability to conduct a competent case control study, to take part in, ultimately to plan and execute a cohort study, or to manage a community-based survey that yields reliable and valid results, are the hallmarks of a thorough understanding of the epidemiological methods without which public health services cannot function effectively. Demonstration of the ability to make imaginative and effective use of all available sources of data and information about the public health (Morris, 1964; 1975) is another feature of effective postgraduate training. Fully trained postgraduate students must also be able to defend epidemiological evidence when it is used in tort claims in a law court. This requires an advanced and sophisticated grasp of all epidemiological methods, including the strengths and weaknesses of each (Rothman and Greenland, 1998).

Attitudes

As teachers, we want undergraduate students to become aware of the importance of public health – to believe that the first priority of all health professionals is to preserve and protect the health of individuals and populations, and to understand that epidemiology is absolutely essential in the pursuit of this goal. We want postgraduates to acquire a set of attitudes or beliefs (something almost akin to instincts) about what epidemiology is, what it does, what it can do, and what it ought to do. The role of the teacher at postgraduate level therefore requires much more than a cookbook approach.

Epidemiologists who take pride in their work speak of core values of the calling. The education of the epidemiologist is incomplete if it does not include a module on the ethical foundations of epidemiological practice and research (Coughlin and Beauchamp, 1996; Last, 1994; 1996a). How do we protect the personal privacy of individuals and safeguard the confidentiality of information about them that is obtained in the process of tracing contacts and treatment for sexually transmitted diseases? What harms may befall the people who are studied by epidemiologists? Does attaching 'labels' such as overweight, indolent or smoker to high-risk individuals and groups stigmatize them? Can this lead to victim-biaming? The popular student exercise on the investigation of an outbreak of food poisoning after a social function should, in passing, ponder the guilt feelings of the good lady who made the potato salad that was the vehicle for staphylococcal enterotoxin, and the diarrhea and vomiting that kept many who attended the event up all night (this ethical question is for undergraduates). Graduates, particularly those destined for a career in public health, where paternalist attitudes are not uncommon, need to be acquainted with other aspects of the core values of epidemiology. What is the epidemiologist's role and duty with regard to the community, colleagues, the service of which they are part, the nation, the science itself, the students who are embarking on careers in this field? What constitutes professional misconduct? How do we avoid conflicts of interest? Why do we do epidemiology anyway? What is its purpose in the great mosaic of human life?

Role of mentors

Education, especially at graduate level, works best if teachers are mentors, guides, and friends to their students. Mentors, but not pedantic or didactic teachers, can discuss questions like those in the preceding paragraph and communicate core values to those whom they encounter in their professional role (Swenson et al., 1995). This is an essential aspect of the attitudes required of a well rounded epidemiologist in public health practice, more so even than an epidemiologist in academia, where the distance separating epidemiologists from the public is greater. It takes an evangelist to convey in a classroom setting what the 'right attitudes' should be. Even the most charismatic lecturer may be unable to infect the unconverted with values that we hope all practising epidemiologists will possess. It is easier for mentors to demonstrate these attitudes than for anyone to describe them in words. Values need demonstration and discussion.

Epidemiology in the context of public health practice will introduce students to practising public health workers who use epidemiological methods in their work, and they can be excellent mentors. It isn't enough to 'expose' learners only to scholarly PhD epidemiologists who know all the smartest statistical tricks but have never dealt with an epidemic or a public health emergency. Learners need to encounter and experience epidemiology in practice, by dealing with current problems that are confronting public health practitioners. These may be 'acute' problems such as an outbreak of a communicable disease, or 'chronic' (long-term) problems such as evaluation of intervention tactics to reduce disparities in health levels between high- and low-risk population groups in a community. If learners are assigned to public health practitioners who act as mentors as well as teachers, the stage is set for rich learning experiences that can convey attitudes (values) as well as knowledge and skills.

Teaching contents

The content of educational programs in epidemiology is summarized in the Table of Contents of textbooks such as those mentioned above, and displayed as behavioral objectives in Table 2.1. An excellent way to introduce the content is a historical progress through the evolving epidemiological approaches to dealing with public health problems (Greenland, 1987). This leads from descriptive epidemiology that began with logical inferences derived from empirical observations to the development of analytic and experimental methods. Systematic analysis of observational studies can begin with William Farr's use of simple mathematical models, digress if appropriate through mathematical epidemic theory and its modern application in HIV/AIDS control programs (Hamer, 1906; Fine, 1993), and continue with consideration of case control and cohort studies. Other essential components of a comprehensive course in epidemiology include randomized controlled trials and their use in evidence-based medicine, the hierarchical nature and quality of epidemiological evidence, the use of large data files, record linkage, and the emerging interfaces between epidemiology and molecular biology, behavioral sciences, genetics, environmental sciences, etc.

Historical perspectives

The specific aims and objectives of the public health component in the teaching of epidemiology are beautifully demonstrated in the historical development of the science (Evans, 1993; Flinn, 1968; Porter, 1997). Epidemiology was born because 19th century physicians and public health workers, concerned about the oppressive burden of disease that afflicted so many people in the expanding industrial cities and towns, needed information about the distribution of disease and needed to know what caused these diseases so that they could figure out how to control them. Epidemiology thereby became the essential basic science without which public health could not function. Its central role has been demonstrated innumerable times, in investigating and controlling global public health problems such as smallpox (Henderson, 1980) and in control of localized epidemics such as outbreaks of food poisoning.

A brief discourse on the early developments in epidemiology in the 19th century, especially the work of John Snow (Snow, 1855) and William Farr (Humphrys, 1885) is an excellent way to introduce students to epidemiology as a fundamental public health science. John Snow's *On the Mode of Communication of Cholera* is a superb introductory textbook. There is no better demonstration of the elegance and power of epidemiology than a step-by-step progress through Snow's logical analysis of the facts at his disposal, and his subsequent investigations of cholera. Snow's work during the outbreak in Soho in 1854 demonstrated the capacity of simple descriptive epidemiology, aided by the insights of an informed mind, to clarify the cause. His investigation of the 1854 epidemic in London beautifully illustrates how 'shoe leather' epidemiology can point the way towards the solution of public health problems. Many teachers have used these accounts as the basis for exercises in introductory epidemiology.

The 'public health' component of epidemiology is summarized in Table 2.2 (Last, 1997). This detail is beyond the scope of undergraduate teaching unless curriculum time is unusually generous, but everything listed in this table, and more, should

Table 2.2 Epidemiology teaching content and Essential Public Health Functions

Prevention, surveillance, and control of communicable and non-communicable diseases
Disease surveillance (descriptive epidemiology)
Immunization schedules (applied epidemiology)
Disease outbreak control (applied epidemiology)
Monitoring the health situation
Monitoring morbidity and mortality rates (observational epidemiology)
Monitoring determinants of health (observational epidemiology)
Evaluation of health promotion, disease prevention, and health service programs
Assessment of effectiveness of public health programs (analytic studies)
Assessment of population needs (analytic studies)
Health risk assessment (case control and cohort studies)
Environmental protection
Food and water safety
Environmental epidemiology
Epidemiological methods
Descriptive and analytic epidemiology, use of information technology, etc.
Cross-sectional studies (surveys)
Case control and cohort studies
Randomized controlled trials
Public health management
Use of scientific evidence
Public health and health systems research methods
Specific public health services
Maternal and infant care services
School health services, etc.
Public health laboratory services

form part of graduate courses in epidemiology, particularly for graduates destined for careers in public health practice. This is derived partly from the Essential Public Health Functions defined by a delphi network under the auspices of the World Health Organization (Bettcher *et al.*, 1998). Public health functions that require knowledge of, and ability to use, epidemiological methods include epidemiological surveillance, monitoring of morbidity and mortality rates, monitoring of health determinants, program evaluation, needs assessment, evidence-based program planning and management, and health systems research. Undergraduates in both industrial and developing countries require a broad understanding of surveillance epidemiology, including not only the nuts and bolts of how it is done, but also what their roles and responsibilities will be when they are in practice. All practising doctors must be aware of the clinical indicators of all diseases of public health importance. Graduate education in public health aspects of epidemiology includes in addition an introduction to methods of identifying, measuring, and assessing environmental and behavioral determinants of health and the other aspects of essential public health functions identified in the WHO list of Essential Public Health Functions. However, this list does not include some aspects of epidemiology that are ingredients of competency in public health practice. An understanding of epidemiological methods of identifying causes and assessing health risks, i.e. descriptive and analytic epidemiology, may be the single most important component in epidemiology teaching that is intended to acquaint learners with public health concepts, principles, and methods. In industrial nations, public health services include occupational and environmental health, and therefore epidemiological applications in these aspects require emphasis (National Research Council, 1991; Last, 1997). In developing countries there must be greater emphasis on communicable disease epidemiology and control, maternal and infant care, and family planning programs, and on the applications of epidemiology in needs assessment and program evaluation for these services (Vaughan and Morrow, 1989). Regardless of the level of development of the country, epidemiology teaching has to be connected to practical, real world problems, not only as perceived in public health departments but also in laboratory and clinical services of the medical school.

Teaching method and format

Methods of teaching vary greatly and are determined by traditions, convenience, and pragmatism. They are rarely, until recently, based on evidence on what works and what doesn't.

Evidence-based education

The most significant development in clinical medicine in the final quarter of the 20th century was the birth of evidence-based medicine (Sackett *et al.*, 2000). Evidence-based public health is just as important (Brownson *et al.*, 1999). Public health practice, especially the basic science components of epidemiology and vital statistics, must be unequivocally evidence-based, cut loose from the received wisdom and outmoded rules that still drive some of our decisions at the beginning of this new century.

In public health, the evidence includes findings from pertinent studies, precise descriptions of all the steps in the reasoning processes, and clear statements about the rationale for decisions. Why is one course of action chosen rather than another? Why can we trust the results of one study but not those of another? In short, the essential evidence for every statement used to arrive at decisions must be plain for all to see. And – very important – how do we distinguish between conclusions derived from logical analysis of the evidence and statements of opinions unsubstantiated by facts? The evidence comes from demography, sociology, economics, and other pertinent sources as well as from epidemiology, and published studies that have been peer-reviewed are always preferable to those that have not. In a teaching program a critical attitude towards evidence can be demonstrated by analysis of imperfect studies or scientific papers that on careful review can be shown to contain flawed data or faulty reasoning or logic. Unfortunately, there is no shortage of such papers.

Epidemiology sets the scene for evidence-based public health practice when it addresses questions on policy decisions about, for instance, the value of routine restaurant inspections. The available evidence suggests these are no more efficacious, and probably less cost-effective, than routine periodic health examinations. On the other hand, evaluation of home visits to mothers of newborn infants has been shown by epidemiological evidence to be efficacious and cost-effective (Edwards and Sims-Jones, 1997).

Teaching aids

There is a preoccupation with 'teaching aids' among many teachers in universities and technical colleges. The vogue for audiovisual props such as slide-tape shows and video presentations has receded, but electronic props, especially PowerPoint presentations, have replaced those earlier crutches to help teachers over the difficult jumps. They have the advantage that the visual displays can easily be printed and distributed as handouts. Do they help learners to learn? It is important to evaluate their efficacy. It is as difficult to become wise or well educated by studying handouts as it is to become wealthy collecting handouts of small change on a city street. It is essential for all handouts to be peer-reviewed, preferably by someone outside the department whence they emanated. And it is important for learners to discuss and argue with each other and with their teachers about the content of this material, not merely learn it by rote to regurgitate in response to multiple choice examination questions.

Classroom exercises

Practical exercises for medical students, based on the sequence of steps taken in the investigation of an epidemic or the evaluation of a public health program have been designed by several well known teachers, such as Milton Terris, and the Epidemiology Program Office of the US Centers for Disease Control and Prevention (CDC). These exercises can demonstrate eloquently and economically to medical students the utility of basic epidemiological skills, without necessarily having to apply the skills in practice.

Exercises come in all shapes and sizes. Those that focus on real problems and are constructed as problem-solving exercises, for example the excellent exercises that are used in the CDC Epidemic Intelligence Service Officer training program, fulfil the purpose for which they were designed, demonstrating what epidemiology is and how it is done. Many others have developed similar exercises. They are a useful and sometimes stimulating and provocative way to introduce elementary epidemiology to a large class of students.

It is obviously better, however, to teach epidemiology to small groups, and this is especially true of problem-solving exercises. Any university department that is affiliated with a local or regional public health unit should have an inexhaustible supply of practical examples to illustrate the basic principles of surveillance epidemiology, case finding, epidemic control, etc. Material may be available from past or current experience; for instance, on evaluation of public health programs such as health education of school children and home visits to isolated old people.

Problem-based learning

Problem-based learning (PBL) has revolutionized life in medical school for teachers and students alike. PBL obliterates the compartments into which medical education has traditionally been divided by confronting students with problems that transcend conventional disciplinary boundaries. This means that epidemiology is not taught as a discrete entity that differs in various ways from basic and clinical sciences, but is like all other branches of biomedical sciences and arts, an inseparable part of becoming a complete physician.

A problem I helped to design and implement illustrates this. The starting point is a young woman who gave birth 1 week earlier to a baby with a severe lumbosacral neural tube defect (open spina bifida). The baby is in constant pain, will never have bladder or bowel control or sexual capacity. With heroic plastic surgical reconstruction and long-term intensive care, costing an estimated $1M per annum, life expectancy is only a few years. So one challenge is to confront very difficult ethical problems, including euthanasia, tough decisions about resource allocation, and experimental surgical repair of congenital malformations. There are several physiological, embryological, and anatomical aspects of the problem. The epidemiological aspects include the voluminous and confusing studies of the epidemiology of neural tube defects, and the epidemiological evidence for folic acid supplements as a public health measure aimed at preventing neural tube defects. We gave this problem to medical students in the second week of their first year, and observed with approval that these new recruits to the medical profession acquitted themselves with the competence and maturity that might be expected of students on the point of graduating.

Assessing students' achievements and evaluating teaching

Examinations in epidemiology take many forms: essays, short answer and multiple choice questions, and problem-solving exercises. The traditional essay examination question has many variations. The questions can be designed in ways that require structured responses. Multiple choice questions can be arranged in clusters, in which the answer to the first in a series determines the response to the second, the response to the second determines the response to the third, and so on. These questions work well in communicable disease epidemiology and control. The first question could describe the symptoms and signs of the index case in an outbreak and the answer, the correct diagnosis, is required before proceeding to the second question which deals with the relevant investigations, followed by surveillance and control measures, and so on. At the postgraduate level, examination committees of the Royal College of Physicians and Surgeons of Canada have designed many such clusters, reinforced by clinical findings displayed in X-rays, pathology reports, etc. to comprise objective structured clinical examinations (OSCEs). The degree of difficulty of OSCEs varies, and thus they can be used to rank candidates or grade them on an honours/pass/fail scale.

We have to be concerned about evaluation of ourselves as teachers to at least the same extent as we are preoccupied with assessing how much our students have learned. How can we evaluate our own teaching (as opposed to learning)? Objective criteria are preferable to subjective ('satisfaction' surveys). If students vote with their feet by staying away from classes, this is an unmistakable sign that the teacher is not providing what the learners want and need. Structured questions that demand specific answers, such as 'Did you learn this from your teacher, from textbooks, from journals, from the World Wide Web, from fellow students?' are preferable to open-ended questions that ask students to rate their level of satisfaction with a course and those who taught it. Performance in examinations is in itself a form of evaluation of the quality of teaching, but there are obviously many confounding factors.

Conclusion: the philosophy of education in epidemiology

Epidemiology is the essential basic and applied science without which public health services cannot function. The reverse is almost true: epidemiology can function as a science that has little or no contact with public health, but it tends to become a sterile academic exercise, focused more on minutiae than the 'big picture,' preoccupied with tasks such as refining methodology as an end in itself – an activity that has been called a form of intellectual masturbation. For this reason, the teaching of epidemiology should give a central place to its role and function in public health, and in the evaluation of aspects of health services provision and delivery.

All teaching of epidemiology, especially the aspects most pertinent to public health, must emphasize that epidemiology is not an abstract science for science's sake; it is action-oriented. This is made explicit in the final clause of the definition in the *Dictionary of Epidemiology*: '… and the application of this study to the control of health problems' (Last, 1983). Zbigniew Brzeziúski insisted on having this final clause in the definition: we can't separate control from surveillance (Last, 1996b). This reality should be emphasized in teaching. In many teaching exercises it is there anyway, as a subliminal or even explicit message.

Does this mean that we should avoid getting drawn into debates about methodological refinements that rely on use of complex mathematical formulae that many non-mathematicians find incomprehensible? Not quite. The late Reuel ('Stony') Stallones was eloquently scornful of these methodological refinements (Stallones, 1980):

> … concern for methods, and especially the dissection of risk assessment, that would do credit to a Talmudic scholar and that threatens at times to bury all that is good and beautiful in epidemiology under an avalanche of mathematical trivia and neologisms.

Yet we must ensure that our methods are sound; there is a role for methodological refinements and, more important, a role for application of rigorous logic à la John Snow to all the epidemiological evidence. It can be a challenge to steer a course between oversimplification and excessive complexity when we base our teaching of epidemiological problems on data from public health practice, especially when emotions and political realities enter the equation.

References

Beaglehole, R., Bonita, R., Kjellström, T.: *Basic epidemiology*. Geneva: WHO, 1993.

Bettcher, D., Yach, D., Sapirie, S.: Essential public health functions. *Wld Hlth Statist Quart* 1998, **51**, 21–32.

Brownson, R. C., Petitti, D. B.: *Applied epidemiology*. New York: Oxford University Press, 1998.

Brownson, R. C., Gurney, J. G., Land, G.: Evidence-based decision-making in public health. *J Pub Health Manag Pract* 1999, **5**, 86–97.

Coughlin, S. S., Beauchamp, T. L.: *Ethics and epidemiology*. New York: Oxford University Press, 1996.

Edwards, N. C., Sims-Jones, N. A.: A randomized controlled trial of alternative approaches to community follow-up for postpartum women. *Can J Public Health* 1997, **88**(2), 123–8.

Ellwood, M.: *Critical appraisal of epidemiological studies and clinical trials*, 2nd edn. Oxford: Oxford University Press, 1998.

Evans, A. L.: *Causation and disease; a chronological journey*. New York: Plenum, 1993.

Farr, W.: *Vital Statistics*; a posthumous collection, edited by Noel Humphrys. London: Stanford, 1885; reprinted New York Academy of Medicine, 1975; re-edited by M. W. Susser and A. Adelstein.

Fine, P. E. M.: Herd immunity; history, theory, practice. *Epidemiol Rev* 1993, **15**, 265–302.

Flinn, M. W.: *Public health reform in Britain*. London: St Martin's, 1968.

Friedman, G. D.: *Primer of epidemiology*, 4th edn. New York: McGraw Hill, 1995.

Greenland, S. (Ed.): *Evolution of epidemiologic ideas*. Chestnut Hill, M. A.: Epidemiology Resources, Inc, 1987.

Hamer, W.: Epidemic disease in England. *Lancet* 1906, **i**, 733–9.

Henderson, D. A.: The eradication of smallpox, in Last J. M. (Ed.): *Maxcy-Rosenau Public Health and Preventive Medicine*, 11th edn. New York: Appleton Century Crofts, 1980: 95–110.

Last, J. M.: Epidemiology, society and ethics, in Gillon R., Lloyd A. (Eds): *Principles of health care ethics*. Chichester: John Wiley & Sons, 1994: 917–32.

Last, J. M. (Ed.): *A dictionary of epidemiology*. New York: Oxford University Press, 1983; also 4th ed, 2001, p. 62.

Last, J. M.: Professional standards of conduct for epidemiologists, in Coughlin, S. S., Beauchamp, T. L. (eds) *Ethics and epidemiology*. New York: Oxford University Press, 1996a: 53–75.

Last, J. M.: Making the Dictionary of Epidemiology. *Int J Epidemiol* 1996b, **25**, 1098–1101.

Last, J. M.: Public Health and Human Ecology, 2nd edn. Stamford CT: Appleton & Lange, 1997.

Lilienfeld, D. E., Stolley, P. D.: *Foundations of epidemiology*, 3rd edn. New York: Oxford University Press, 1994.

Morris, J. N.: *Uses of epidemiology*, 2nd edn. Edinburgh, London: Churchill Livingstone, 1964; see also 3rd edn, 1975.

National Research Council, Committee on Environmental Epidemiology (Miller, A. B., Chairman): *Environmental Epidemiology; Public Health and Hazardous Wastes.* Washington DC: National Academy Press, 1991.

Porter, R.: *The greatest benefit to mankind; a medical history of humanity from antiquity to the present.* London: Harper Collins, 1997.

Postman, N., Weingartner, C: *Teaching as a subversive activity.* New York: Dell, 1969.

Rothman, K. J., Greenland, S.: Modern epidemiology, 2nd edn. Philadelphia: Lippincott-Raven, 1998.

Sackett, D. L., Richardson, W. S., Rosenberg, W. *et al.*: *Evidence-based medicine – how to practice and teach EBM*, 2nd edn. London: Churchill Livingstone, 2000.

Snow, J.: *On the mode of communication of cholera*, 2nd edn. London: Churchill, 1855; reprinted with introduction by Wade Hampton Frost, New York, Commonwealth Fund, 1936,

Stallones, R. A.: To advance epidemiology. *Annu Rev Pub Health* 1980, **1**, 69–82.

Swenson, J. R., Boyle, A., Last, J. M., Pérez, E. L., Rassall, J. A., Josselin, J. Y.: Mentorship in medical education. *Ann Roy Coll Phys Surg Canada* 1995, **28**, 165–71.

Vaughan, J. P., Morrow, R. H.: *Manual of Epidemiology for District Health Management.* Geneva: WHO, 1989.

Chapter 3

Important concepts in epidemiology

O. S. Miettinen

Introduction

As is evident from the preceding two chapters, epidemiology was originally solely a discipline of the practice of health care, specifically community medicine, but it then also evolved to be a research discipline; throughout, in both meanings, it has had a close relation and, indeed, subservience to public health.

As we in epidemiology continue our commitment to public health, it is important that we adopt a tenable concept of public health. As it is, the concepts of public health, community medicine, and social medicine are commonly taken to be essentially the same (Public Health in England, 1988; Last, 1995). On the other hand, some authorities (quite some time ago) came to recognize that the advent of national health insurance called for dramatic updating of the concept of public health, to encompass the societal aspects of clinical medicine as well (World Health Organization, 1957). I side strongly with the latter view, noting that, in the context of national health insurance, society is by no means simply the payer of health care; it takes an active role in all policy aspects of it, research policy included (Epstein, 1990; Eisenberg, 1998).

Under the traditional concept of public health, epidemiologic research has principally been etiologic, inquiry into the causation of illnesses, with a view to opening avenues for preventive interventions in the practice of community medicine. Selectively, such research has been supplemented by studies directly addressing the effects of the interventions that etiologic research suggests.

Insofar as the more modern and comprehensive concept of public health is adopted, epidemiologic research is naturally taken to be concerned with the advancement of the knowledge-base of whatever aspect of health care, the vast bulk of which is clinical. General knowledge bears on practice in its knowledge–practice interface, of course; and this I term 'gnosis', encompassing diagnosis, etiognosis, and prognosis, with the effects of interventions accounted for under prognosis. The research that provides the knowledge-base of 'gnosis' I view as being quintessentially applied medical research, all of it epidemiologic in nature (Miettinen, 1998).

Not everything that is now termed epidemiologic research is scientific by the criterion of addressing universals, topics devoid of reference to particular places and times. In particular, a major concern in modern public health is quality assurance in health care, seeing to it that care conforms to acceptable standards of quality. This

requires healthcare 'research' in the meaning of quality assessments specific to particular settings of care in particular administrative regions and with reference to the
present time (Relman, 1988). These assessments, too, are epidemiologic in nature; so
are, of course, morbidity surveys etc. conducted as a part of the practice of community medicine in community diagnosis, inherently concerned with the level of
morbidity for a particular illness.

This chapter is concerned with epidemiologic research in its scientific meaning
only, and with the idea that research is aiming to be pragmatic in the sense of advanc-
ing the knowledge-base of the practice of health care, whether in clinical or community medicine. While the general flavor of this volume is that of principal concern for
community medicine, the more general outlook adopted in this chapter is, I hold,
directly applicable to community medicine as well.

The level of the content here is introductory, oriented to fundamentals. At the same
time, though, the content is somewhat exceptional, a bit avant-garde in nature, as epidemiologic research is still evolving even in respect to its fundamental concepts and
principles. The content thus is principally directed to the beginning of students epidemiologic research, whether already committed to a career in it or just considering
the possibility; it should also be of interest to those whose professional interests only
interface with epidemiology. On the other hand, experience shows that the content
outlined below is of great interest to even senior epidemiologists.

Teaching objectives

The course prepares the student to understand what epidemiologic research is about
in general, to follow presentations of epidemiologic studies, written and oral, and to
engage in thinking about epidemiologic research. However, it does not provide for
thinking that is both learned and critical, as that requires study not only of the concepts but also the principles of epidemiologic research.

Teaching contents

Concepts are the elements with which thought operates. They are thus preparatory to
all thought, including that in epidemiologic research.

A concept is the shared essence of particular instances of something, epidemiologic
research for example. It is the basis on which particular instances, 'singulars' of the
concept, can be grouped together as representing the same entity or category –
abstract, placeless and timeless. This essence is demarcated by the concept's definition,
and the concept is referred to, or expressed, by a term – a word ('significant', 'categore-
matic') or a set of words.

The concepts that pertain to epidemiologic research may be classified, most broadly, as those that have to do with the general context of epidemiologic research and
those that are ones of epidemiologic research itself.

Among the contextual concepts, pre-eminent are those that have already been discussed above: medicine, or healthcare (professional), and its broadest subcategories,
clinical medicine and community medicine, together with the societal aspect of all of
this, public health.

Allusion has also been made to the broadest concern in medicine, to ill-health or illness, although not to its principal subordinate concepts of disease (Lat. *morbus*, a process of ill-health), defect (Lat. *vitium*, a state) and injury (Gr. *trauma*). While in clinical medicine the concern is with particular instances of illness, actual or potential, it has been noted that in community medicine the counterpart of this is concern with the frequency of the occurrence of illness, morbidity.

In the practice of medicine, the practitioner's first responsibility is to have knowledge of the client's (individual's, community's) health. For this knowledge, the term adduced above is gnosis (Miettinen, 1998), and allusion was made to the component concepts of diagnosis, etiognosis, and prognosis. As indicated, these concepts are of central import to epidemiologic research, as it is in the context of these that general knowledge, scientific and other, bears on the practice of medicine.

Before discussing concepts specific to epidemiologic research, it is, I hold, essential to grasp the general concept of science and that of knowledge in the scientific meaning (Niiniluoto, 1984), and to understand that, contrary to common belief, even the scientific practice of medicine is a matter of art, not of science (Miettinen, 1999a).

Among the specific concepts, epidemiology and epidemiologic research are pre-eminent, already touched on above. As epidemiologic research is inquiry into the frequency of occurrence of states and events of health (of health 'outcomes' in epidemiologic jargon) in human domains, the first-order focus needs to be on concepts pertaining to rates of occurrence. A distinction is made between rates of prevalence (of states) and rates of incidence (of events), and between empirical rates (documented) and theoretical rates (abstract, of scientific interest). Proportion-type empirical rates are distinguished from mere common fractions (vulgar fractions), a distinction that extends to incidence density also. In the context of all rates the concept of a rate's referent or domain is important: for a proportion-type empirical rate a series of person-moments (instances in this sense); for a density-type empirical rate an aggregate of population-time (consisting of an infinite number of person-moments); and for a theoretical rate a category (abstract). The concept of empirical incidence density adduces that of population, involving the important duality in types of population – the distinction between cohorts and dynamic populations, or closed (for exit) and open (for exit) populations.

Further on rates, one distinguishes between the overall rate for a particular domain and the specific rates referring to subdomains of this, proceeding to the concept of a crude overall rate as a weighted average of the component-specific rates with the sizes of the subdomains providing the weights for the respective specific rates. This naturally leads to the concept of adjusted rate and this, in turn, to that of mutually standardized rates. The concept of 'indirectly standardized' rate is to be either ignored or explained as being malformed.

The concept of theoretical rate varying among subdomains leads to the epidemiologic concept of determinant. In this, the distinction between descriptive and causal determinant, or between the descriptive (acausal) and causal interest in a determinant, needs to be made. The latter in particular leads to the concept of determinant contrast, involving a defined index category and its defined reference category of the determinant. Focus on a contrast, in turn, leads to the concept of comparative measures of occurrence and to the component concepts of rate difference and rate ratio first and foremost, each of these either empirical or theoretical, and to that of odds ratio besides. From these particulars one naturally proceeds to the broader concept of occurrence relation and to the idea that, in general, epidemiologic research is about occurrence relations in human domains, whether descriptively or causally.

When interest focuses on a determinant contrast and, hence, on a comparative measure of occurrence, the issue of potential modification is inescapable: is the theoretical value of the comparative measure to be thought of as single, characterizing the entire domain, or is one to distinguish among subdomains according to one or more modifiers of this magnitude? If the contrast is of interest with a view to causal interpretation of the measure's magnitude, the question is whether all codeterminants of the outcome's occurrence (potential confounders) have suitably balanced distributions across the contrast (within a modifier-based subdomain perhaps). This leads to the concepts of crude and adjusted/standardized comparative measures (of occurrence relation).

Whereas rates characterize the frequency of occurrence of states and events, outcome entities of the all-or-none type on a binary scale, the student needs to come to understand that epidemiologic research is not restricted to the study of rates, extended to ordinal-scale outcomes by focus on a particular category on such a scale. As for quantitative outcomes in particular, the principal interest is in the median of its distribution, readily interpretable in terms of the rates of occurrence of values higher and lower than this. The concept of median extends to the comparative concepts of median difference and median ratio, the latter in the context of a ratio scale only. Moreover, where the research has rates as the immediate objects, mediately the interest may be in the distribution of time to an event, as in the construction of life tables.

The student is now ready to apprehend concepts generally involved in the object of an epidemiologic study, in its formulation or definition in successive stages. At the first stage, concern is with the entities involved in the definition of the occurrence relation and its domain. The second stage adduces the very important concept of scientific time and that of the definitions of those elements on the scale of scientific time. As the third stage, the student is brought to understand that epidemiologic research generally can, and commonly must, be thought of as regression research; this leads to the need to introduce concepts of regression models. At the outset, the important conceptual distinction is made between the scales for scientific entities on one side and the statistical variates that, on the other side, are adopted (*ad hoc*) to represent these and realizations of these (always numerically). In the end, the object of study is understood to be the entire set of regression coefficients (in a descriptive study) or perhaps only a subset of these (in a causal study).

Next to the concepts surrounding the object of a study it is most natural to introduce those having to do with the result of the study. Most broadly, the result is characterized by its form – that of the object of the study – together with empirical content of that form. The latter involves, first, the concept of the empirical or fitted (to the data) value for a parameter of interest, and consideration of whether the empirical value is justifiably a/the 'point estimate' of the parameter (given possible bias and whatever prior knowledge). Closely related to the concept of empirical values is that of their referent, the study base. In addition, the concept of imprecision and its related concepts of replication of the study, replication distribution of an empirical value, and those of standard error and confidence interval are involved. In this context it is valuable to introduce the idea that the value of a parameter (theoretical) is a rather loose concept because of undefined distributions of latent determinants in a descriptive object and of latent modifiers of a comparative measure (typically in a causal study), taking away from the reproducibility of even a totally 'precise' result (hypothetical). The concept of 'chance' and its proper understanding in epidemiologic science (as distinct from sample surveys) is related to this.

The concept of study result is closely related to that of evidence and inference. The former involves the component concepts of study design and protocol, along with study execution, documentation included, jointly leading to the result as its final element. As for inference, the duality between frequentist and Bayesian ideas needs to be introduced, also addressing the question of whether inference is part of a study or only a concern for members of the scientific community facing the evidence from individual studies or from a systematic review, possibly including meta-analysis.

As the concept of study design thus comes up, it requires explanation. Is object design part of of it or merely a prerequisite for study design, with the latter specifically a methods concept? Either way, are some aspects of the 'design' actually givens rather than results of designing? Is the conventional distinction between study design and data analysis intellectually tenable, or is it instead that study design and protocol should be understood to encompass all of the scientifically relevant aspects of the study, including defining the statistical model(s) and the calculation of the parameters' empirical values and their associated measures of imprecision? One must not forget that the topic of regression models naturally comes up in the object design already (c.f. above); surely there is to be a close interdependence, coherence and a hierarchy even, between object(s) of study and the scientifically relevant aspects of the methods, inclusive of the methods of 'data analysis' (the term being a misnomer).

The methods aspect of a study involves a number of important concepts. Most intimately connected to any result of a study is that of the referent of this, the study base. Pursuit of this leads to the procedural concepts of source population (to be distinguished from target population in epidemiologic fact-finding) and its follow-up, first and foremost. In this follow-up, the concepts of process – and hence topics of design – include, most importantly, those of admissibility/eligibility, admission (or inclusion/enrolment), experimentation or experimental procedure (including in descriptive studies), and documentation. It is important to understand that while a source population is always involved, this is not necessarily the case for a study population: the study base may be a series of person-moments, of instances of the study domain. This is different from the members of a study population in that these instances are not in motion over time.

Of primary importance to the design of both the object and the methods of an epidemiologic study is the concept of fundamental types of epidemiologic study, types not in the sense of alternative options but as a-priori givens. The most proximal given is the genre of study objective, according to whether the intended advancement of the knowledge-base of practice has to do with diagnosis (of a particular illness), etiognosis (of a particular illness in respect to possibly causal antecedents), prognosis as it depends on descriptive determinants, or prognosis in causal relation to options for prospective intervention. The respective objectives of diagnostic, etiognostic, descriptive-prognostic and intervention-prognostic studies imply the corresponding generic types of study object; the latter, in turn, imply their corresponding fundamental types of study proper, the diagnostic study etc., each of them singular in structure. The concept of the etiologic/etiognostic study necessitates, in today's culture, addressing the malformed concepts of 'cohort study' and 'case control study' (Miettinen, 1999b). Upon solid understanding of the fundamental types of pragmatic – gnosis-oriented – epidemiologic study, select variants of, and types beyond, these may be addressed.

With the design of the study object and study methods thus generally a matter of designing the particulars in an a-priori framework for each, concepts having to do with the quality of study need to be introduced. As for the objects, principal among these are scientific admissibility (objectivity, rationality) and relevance to, or applicability in, practice. In respect to methods, the quality desiderata of validity and efficiency need to be defined. The former is best accomplished by defining the broadest types of possible bias – admission, documentation, confounding and overparametrization biases. Beyond the principal desiderata for quality, those for quantity of study – study size – need to be introduced, principal among them the desirability of size zero for a study the qualitative aspects of which involve remediable deficiencies. The malformed concept of 'sample size determination', still very prevalent, requires critical consideration, especially in the modern context of future meta-analysis representing the hoped-for destiny of the evidence from a study.

I said in the beginning that concepts are the elements with which thought operates. I close with two thoughts. First, the concepts involved in thought about epidemiology remain less than fully developed, including in my own case; second, that the first-order application of concepts-based thought in epidemiology is the development and critical adoption of principles of epidemiology. Even though epidemiology, like morphology etc., is not a science *per se* but an aspect of a multitude of health sciences, I wish to quote what the great humanist Isaiah Berlin said about the prerequisites for science (Berlin, 1997, p. 61):

> Where the concepts are firm, clear and generally accepted, and the methods of reasoning and arriving at conclusions are agreed between men (at least the majority of those who have anything to do with these matters), there and only there is it possible to construct a science, formal or empirical.

Teaching method and format

Implicit in the section above is the essence of the syllabus for a course given the title Epidemiologic Research I: Concepts, which is preparatory for Epidemiologic Research II: Principles. Both these courses are directed to general orientation before specialized courses, each of the latter focusing on a single genre of gnosis, a single fundamental category of objects and corresponding methods of epidemiologic research.

Explicitly, my most up-to-date plan for the next course on Epidemiologic Research I: Concepts, following the flow in the section above, involves the following syllabus specific for a 5-day full-time study:

Day	Session	Topic
1	1	Self-introductions; course overview
1	2	Science, medicine, medical science
1	3	Public health, epidemiology, epidemiologic research
1	4	Rates, empirical *versus* theoretical; respective referents/domains
1	5	Subdomains 1: focus on overall rate, crude, adjusted, standardized
1	6	Subdomains 2: focus on specific rates; determinant; contrast; comparative measures; occurrence relation/function
2	1	Q & A
2	2	2/1 continued
2	3	Comparative measures: subdomains by modifiers; confounding
2	4	Overall comparative measures, crude, standardized
2	5	2/4 continued
2	6	Occurrence concerns beyond rates
3	1	Q & A
3	2	Object of study 1: scientific entities, scientific time; entities temporally defined
3	3	Object of study 2: scientific entities *versus* statistical variates; object of study as one of regression analysis; regression models
3	4	Result of study: empirical value(s), its (their) referent(s); measures of imprecision, their referent
3	5	Evidence from a study; inference; systematic review; meta-analysis
3	6	Study design: what should the concept encompass?
4	1	Q & A
4	2	The study process, from source population follow-up to documentation of the result(s)
4	3	Types of study: orientation
4	4	The diagnostic study
4	5	The descriptive-prognostic study
4	6	The intervention-prognostic study
5	1	Q & A
5	2	The etiologic/etiognostic study
5	3	5/2 continued

5	4	Desiderata in object design: scientific admissibility, relevance
5	5	Desiderata in methods design: validity, efficiency; 'sample size determination'
5	6	Retrospective overview

For the course, the written materials consist of four elements, starting with a succinct description of the course, followed by the course syllabus. These are followed by something like the Introduction and Teaching Contents sections above. The fourth element is a series of definitions of epidemiologic concepts, presented in the natural sequence of the teaching – and understanding – of these. The teaching itself is expository yet interactive rather than a matter of lecturing. When a course like this is given in a hotel-type setting in which the students stay, a very useful adjunct to the class sessions are student discussion group sessions in the evenings, with designated rapporteurs bringing questions to the Q & A session the next morning.

Assessing students' achievements

For a long time, my method of assessing students' learning has been asking them to comment on the correctness/incorrectness of a set of propositions, the commentary having to do with the rationale presented or implied by me, the teacher. Such a set of propositions also serves to highlight the contents of the course, and to this end it is made more effective by me distributing the teacher's own commentaries immediately upon completion of the examination.

References

Berlin, J. *The Proper Study of Mankind*. London: Chatto and Windus, 1997.

Eisenberg, J. Agency for Health Care Policy and Research. *Annals of Epidemiology* 1998; **8**, 283–5.

Epstein, A. M. The outcomes movement – will it take us where we want us to go? *New England Journal of Medicine* 1990; **323**, 266–9.

Last, J. M. (ed.). *A Dictionary of Epidemiology*, 3rd edn. New York: Oxford University Press, 1995.

Miettinen, O. S. Evidence in medicine: invited commentary. *Canadian Medical Association Journal* 1998; **158**, 215–21.

Miettinen, O. S. Ideas and ideals in medicine: fruits of reason or props of power? *Journal of Evaluation in Clinical Practice* 1999a; **5**, 107–16.

Miettinen, O. S. Etiologic research: needed revisions of concepts and principles. *Scandinavian Journal of Work, Environment & Health* 1999b; 25 (6, special issue): 484–90.

Niiniluoto, I. *Is Science Progressive?* Dortrecht: D. Reidel Publishing Company, 1984.

Public Health in England. *The Report of the Committee of Inquiry into the Future Development of the Public Health Function*. Cmnd 289. London: HMSO, 1988.

Relman, A. S. Assessment and accountability: the third revolution in medical care. *New England Journal of Medicine* 1988; **319**, 1220–2.

World Health Organization. *Report of WHO Conference on Public Health Training of General Practitioners*. TRS 140, 1957.

Chapter 4

Study design

Jørn Olsen and Olga Basso

Introduction

In our experience it is easy and rewarding to teach design principles at every level. The most basic concepts and principles are understood by the majority of the students early in the course and the topic can be made as complex as the skills of teacher and students permit. At all levels there are challenging and important issues to discuss, and there are still many things we do not know. It is important for the students to know about this uncertainty.

A study is a process – documented throughout from design to execution – that aims to provide empirical evidence on a given issue. An epidemiologic study may start with a public health problem, a hypothesis concerning the etiology of a disease, or it may be initiated by the available research opportunities. It is important, however, to give some thought to whether it is worthwhile pursuing the hypothesis. A study could be undertaken because of a health problem that needs a solution, or because a new, or differently formulated, hypothesis may lead to a better understanding of a phenomenon. Also, a study may be worthwhile doing if it is aimed at providing data of better quality for exploring an existing hypothesis. The 'first' study on a new hypothesis is often very important, since subsequent studies may be biased by the results of that study. For example, when it was first reported that vasectomy may increase the risk of prostate cancer, a number of men who had undergone vasectomy were checked for prostate cancer (either at the patient's request or because the physician was alerted to the problem). This phenomenon may produce a higher number of diagnoses of prostate cancer in men who have been vasectomised, while a number of men who had not had a vasectomy would not receive this diagnosis, thus making any successive study relying upon diagnosed cases potentially biased. To overcome this problem and achieve equal accuracy of information the first principle to follow is to define as cases only those that are typical and severe. When designing a study to address a novel hypothesis, ensure that it is done with great care.

In any case, the study design should be dictated by its aim(s). The challenge is to find a study design that most effectively and validly addresses the research hypothesis. If the optimal design is not feasible for ethical or practical reasons, it is important to consider if it is worthwhile pursuing the study at all.

The main aim of the teaching should be to focus on the logical link between the study aim(s) and its design. Key issues in teaching study design are related to how you will formulate the entities (determinants, outcome, confounders, and modifiers) under study and whether the results will provide the evidence for which they are designed.

Teachers should try to remember what was most difficult to understand at the time when they themselves were students of the discipline. This is often a good indicator of what needs particular attention in the teaching. All teaching should be didactic. Let the students interrupt. Insist on questions from the students at regular intervals. Ask questions yourself to test the level of understanding.

At the undergraduate level students should be taught the core concepts of the basic epidemiological study design and be able to describe and characterize these accurately. For postgraduate students teaching should incorporate new and more specialized study design and methods.

Epidemiology usually rests on observations of occurrence of disease as a function of its potential determinants. For ethical reasons these determinants cannot in most cases be manipulated by the researcher. Most of the research, at least within public health epidemiology, is therefore non-experimental. In clinical epidemiology it is, however, possible to manipulate treatment in a way that makes scientific inference less vulnerable to bias, as in the randomized controlled trial. The randomized controlled trial should not, however, be taken as a model for research on disease causation, and disciplines like demography, sociology, and economics may, on occasion, offer the epidemiologist more appropriate study designs than the randomized trial.

Epidemiologic research aims to capture the experience within a population of the occurrence of illness according to life style factors, treatment, environmental exposures, etc., and at making inference from such experience. All study designs, therefore, share this aim and, rather than focusing upon dissimilarities, the teacher should focus on the similarities of the various designs. All designs are aimed at capturing the underlying population experience, for different purposes and with different efficiency (and accuracy). The general aim is to maximize validity at the lowest possible cost.

An epidemiologic study is always a simplification of reality (e.g. one outcome, often binary, and a limited number of determinants). Since no study can specify all modifiers and confounders this is acceptable, and possibly the best way to proceed in many situations, but it is important to be aware of this. We think that the teacher should stress that they are never addressing the natural complexity.

Theoretical epidemiology, that is, research into the concepts and methods of the discipline, has developed rapidly during the last 30 years (Miettinen, 1985a; 1998; 1999), leaving many of the disease- or exposure-oriented epidemiologists behind. This need not cause problems if the researcher sticks to basic and well defined concepts and principles. Many (perhaps most) of the important epidemiologic studies are performed by people with limited skills in theoretical epidemiology and biostatistics, because the idea is by far the most important part of the study. The rise and fall of the new methodology has made it difficult to reach consensus on proper textbooks. Many of the textbooks, even some of the new ones, are hopelessly outdated, especially concerning the understanding of case control studies (Axelson, 1979; Miettinen, 1985b; 1999). These developments are mostly related to achieving more rigorous ways of collecting the available information and a more precise understanding of the ability to estimate the occurrence relation measure of choice in the underlying population.

Teaching objectives

We do not expect undergraduate students to be able to design a complicated study themselves, but they should be aware of the core concepts and of the strengths and weaknesses of the basic designs within epidemiology. Undergraduate students should be able to read epidemiological news critically, whether the source is a drug company, a newspaper or a scientific report. They should also be able to read articles that use standard designs and to comment on the relevance of the design in the light of the aim of the study. Students should be aware of the major potential sources of bias and be able to identify them in individual studies. They should be able to explain how randomization, blinding and placebo administration operate in minimizing bias and confounding in randomized controlled trials.

Students should be able to suggest an appropriate design when the researcher wants to learn about the frequency of an outcome as a function of a given determinant or about the etiology of a disease that may cluster in time or space (Prentice and Sheppard, 1995; Steel and Holt, 1996).

Undergraduate students should also be aware of how epidemiological designs may be used to monitor health care interventions over time, like new screening activities or other interventions. They should know the strengths of these designs in comparison with unsystematic reporting of side effects of drugs, accidents, etc. They should of course be familiar with concepts like prevalence, incidence, relative risk, risk difference, incidence rate ratio, rate difference, etc.

Students should also understand the meaning of the basic concepts of measuring observation time in epidemiology and be aware of the demarcation line between epidemiology and statistics. They should be able to define epidemiological problems and know the difference between medical sociology or medical psychology and epidemiology. It is epidemiologic research to study the health consequences of smoking, but not why smokers smoke or why people engage in unsafe sex.

Postgraduate students in epidemiology should have a more detailed knowledge of different design options and be able to design classical studies themselves. They should be able to understand the concepts of validity, precision, efficiency, and study power. At the end of the course they should be able to peer-review a paper and write a study protocol using one of the standard designs in epidemiology. They should also be familiar with the principles of *Good epidemiology practice* (IEA/The European Epidemiology Group), data documentation, and data protection.

Since epidemiologists often try to identify causes of diseases or ill-health, the teaching should include a session on the concept of causation and counterfactuals, and its consequences for the design and interpretation of the results (Rothman, 1976; Susser, 1991; Olsen J, 1993; Hill, 1965; Lewis, 1973).

Teaching contents

Rather than simply classifying designs as randomized controlled trials, follow-up studies, case control studies, cross-sectional studies, and correlation studies, students at all levels should be taught about the key parameters that characterize a given design. These are discussed in the following sections.

The unit of observation

This could be an individual or a group of individuals (microepidemiology or macro-epidemiology). When the units of observation consist of an aggregate of individuals, the study is often called an ecological or correlation study. Individuals or groups of individuals are the usual units of observation, which may, however, also be events rather than individuals (e.g. pregnancies).

Type of population

Populations studied in epidemiology can be of two main types: closed cohort (membership is defined by a given event, and no exit is possible), and dynamic population (where a given state defines membership, and exit occurs when that state terminates).

Allocation of the exposure under study

The allocation may either be performed by the researcher to learn about health consequences of a given exposure (experimental design) or by nature, self-selection, imposed by others, etc. without the primary intention of making scientific inference as to the consequences of this exposure. In the latter case, the researcher attempts to organize the observations in such a way as to learn about the effect of such exposures without interfering with the allocation (non-experimental design).

A 'natural experiment', like the Chernobyl accident, is not an experiment in the scientific sense of the word. Although this specification may seem obvious, it is important to make the students properly understand what characterizes an experiment and what does not.

The timing of the observations

Since diseases occur over time we normally expect a *longitudinal* recording of exposures and disease, as in the follow-up study and in the case control study. If the exposures, health conditions, and other factors are recorded at the same point in time using prevalence data without attempting to reconstruct the exposure history we usually talk about a *cross-sectional* study.

Definition of the relevant etiologic time window

Based upon the available knowledge of the condition under study and of the hypothesized effect of the exposure, the appropriate etiologic time window must be defined (i.e. cigarette smoking cannot be the only cause of lung cancer in subjects who started smoking 6 months before being diagnosed).

Definition of the study base

The study base is the actual person–time experience that is the referent of the occurrence relation (Miettinen, 1985a). It is a *primary* study base when the source population is defined before the case series is identified, and the challenge is then to obtain complete ascertainment of the cases. It is *secondary* when the case series is identified first, and the challenge is then to identify the study base that originated *that* case series (which is, by definition, complete).

For example: if one wishes to study the effect of a given exposure on sperm production without setting up a follow-up, there are at least two options. The first is to set up population surveys in a well defined area and to identify *all* incident infertile males (through, say, sperm samples obtained from all). In this case the study base is primarily ascertained and well defined, but this option may be unfeasible because of the cost.

A second option is to identify the case series first by enrolling all couples presenting themselves to clinical centres for infertility and identify the males who carry the problem. Once the case series is identified, they define the study base for this case series, namely males that would seek help had they had the problem in question. Since males in the case series had volunteered to go to the infertility centres, and not all infertile men do, this factor has to be taken into consideration when defining the secondary study base. The option which best avoids selection bias may be to enrol couples who went to infertility centres and it then turned out that the female had the problem. The study base is, thus, properly defined secondarily (Rachootin and Olsen, 1983).

Sampling the study base

When the study base is sampled according to the exposure status, e.g. exposed *versus* unexposed, we usually talk about a *follow-up* study. If we first identify cases and then sample from the study base, the study is defined as a case control.

The type of data

If data are collected for the purpose of the current study we talk about primary data or *ad hoc* data. If data are collected primarily for other purposes, e.g. data from medical files, registers, etc., we describe these data as secondary or antecedent data.

The terms prospective and retrospective have been used in many different ways in the past in connection with epidemiologic studies and it may, for this reason, be best to avoid these terms altogether. At least one should avoid using the term with respect to causal inference. Causal inference is always forward in time and in the case control study we reconstruct the occurrence of the putative determinants in the past to learn about its consequences. We do not make inference from the effect to its possible cause. A case control study is therefore not a retrospective study from the perspective of causal reasoning, and the term 'trohoc' study (cohort spelled backwards; Feinstein, 1973) bears witness to the misunderstanding of the proper structure of this design.

It may be useful to illustrate the use of different designs in the evaluation of a hypothesis by means of an example. This particular example illustrates studies that often progress from inexpensive to more expensive and from simple to more complex designs.

We may, for example, observe that birth weight tends to be higher in areas with a high fish intake (Olsen SF, 1993).

This hypothesis could, at first, be inexpensively tested with a correlation study, since birth weight data are often available and dietary surveys or sales of food items may provide exposure data. Such a simple macroepidemiological study, or correlation or ecological study, could show that birth weight tends to increase in populations characterized by a high fish intake, but fish intake need not be causally related to birth weight (as we have no information on whether it was the fish eaters who had the largest babies). The association could also be caused by genetic factors, differences in smoking habits, social status or gestational weight gain, etc. It could, of course, be due to growth promoting factors in fish or factors that delay the onset of labour. This type of study will not in itself provide any effect measures related to individual risks.

The next type of study could be a case control study based on post-term born babies or babies born with a high birth weight. Controls could be samples from all pregnant women and we could then try to reconstruct dietary habits during pregnancy. In this study we would seek information on smoking, social conditions, and other determinants of gestational age and birth weight during pregnancy. We would use the information to adjust the intake of fish from correlates to fish consumption that may confound the results. If such a study showed an association we would be more convinced, but we would probably still doubt the quality of the data on dietary habits and we would have no control of confounding by unknown factors.

The next step would be to set up a follow-up study where we select pregnant women with a high fish intake recorded during the entire pregnancy and compare newborns in this group with newborns of pregnant women who did not eat fish during pregnancy. The non-exposed group provides the expected gestational age and birth weight in the exposed cohort, had the exposed cohort not been exposed (counterfactual reasoning: i.e. a given factor is causal if, in its absence, the effect would not have occurred at that point in time; Lewis, 1973). If needed, we could make this group comparable to the exposed group by taking potential confounders into consideration. In this study we have better dietary habits, but we would still not solve the possible problem with unknown determinants of fetal growth and pregnancy duration that may correlate with fish intake.

The final logical step would be to set up a randomized controlled trial in which pregnant women would be allocated to high and low intakes of fish, or the presumed active components in fish (n-3 fatty acids). If such a trial could be blinded (perhaps possible with the n-3 fatty acids), it would be highly unlikely that those who were randomly allocated to receive the active component would differ from those who received placebo. If the placebo provided a similar energy supply, the effects on birth weight should also be similar if the null hypothesis is true (n-3 fatty acids have no effect except that associated with the energy intake). If this study were to show an effect it would provide a strong case, but no certainty. In general, we only provide evidence that will press personal beliefs towards high or low values, never to probabilities of 0 or 1.

This simple teaching experiment illustrates the sequential progression of studies moving from inexpensive to more expensive designs. At the same time complexity in analysis and inference move from complicated to less complicated. The randomized controlled trial is in theory the most simple to design, analyse, and interpret. For logistic reasons it is, however, often the most difficult to conduct well, especially if it is of long duration.

Teaching should be based on updated concepts and methods, and the teacher needs to know some of the basic literature in theoretical epidemiology, at least from the last decades (MacMahon and Trichopoulos, 1996; Rothman and Greenland, 1998). Teachers must be familiar with concepts like bias, confounding, and effect modification (Miettinen, 1981; Hennekens and Buring, 1987; Miettinen, 1988; Weinberg, 1993).

Students need to know how the three cornerstones in the randomized control trial help to isolate the effect of exposure. Randomization will make the groups comparable at baseline (no confounding) when the study is large and replicated many times. Blinding will make compliance and outcome measurements comparable on average (no differential misclassification), and placebo use will make circumstances comparable by controlling for the placebo effect. Any differences in the outcome in a well conducted trial must be because of an effect of the difference in exposure or between the groups to be compared, or chance. Lack of exposure contrast is a major problem if compliance is low or if the drug is available for those receiving placebo treatment. More details on the randomized controlled trial are available in Feinstein (1989a, b), Greenland (1990), and Senn (1991).

The randomized controlled trial is a follow-up study. Non-experimental follow-up studies have to rely upon counterfactual reasoning to isolate the effect of the exposure. The reference category provides the expected occurrence parameter in the exposed category had the exposure been absent (or without effect).

In qualitative studies we usually want to make the exposure contrast as large as possible to answer the question: does this exposure have an effect or not? In studies in which we wish to estimate the quantitative nature of the association, we usually need to compare several levels of exposure to answer the question: at what level does the exposure have an effect, and what is the dose–response relationship?

We should use the principle of deconfounding when contrasting the groups to be compared by identifying the study base in such a way that members are similar in aspects other than those we are able to measure. People of similar age and educational background have many habits in common. In general, we want as little variation as possible in potential confounders, but as much variation as possible in exposures and modifiers. These two principles are often in conflict in a non-experimental study and a balance has to be reached according to the specific purpose of the study and practical considerations.

Students very often have problems in understanding the distinction between effect modification and confounding, and it is important for teachers to be aware of this. Effect modification is the phenomenon for which the (theoretical) rate of a given illness varies across different categories of the determinant (e.g. the incidence of esophagus cancer is higher in smokers with a high alcohol consumption than in smokers with a low alcohol consumption). Effect modification may be model-dependent, as it can be on the multiplicative or additive scale depending upon the model that is chosen to describe the association (rate ratio or rate difference). The presence of effect modification on one scale does not necessarily imply the presence on the other scale, and vice versa.

Effect modification as defined by a deviation from an additive model, may be a main target for study since the lay people concept is usually additive. That is best studied in a well balanced design that uses the principles of factorial design in the randomized control trial (Armitage and Berry, 1994).

Confounding is a matter of *unbalanced* distribution of determinant(s) of the outcome associated with the exposure, and a potential effect modifier may or may not be a confounder. A given variable may or may not be a confounder in a given study depending upon its association with the determinant under study. On the other hand, an effect modifier is not study-dependent.

Students should be aware of follow-up studies based on fixed cohorts or cohorts with open entry or exit. We usually use fixed cohorts to study the effect of a given exposure localized in time or independent of time, e.g. when we study people who are exposed to contaminated food. We use cohorts with an open entry in, for example, studies of occupationally exposed people who enter the cohort as soon as they become exposed. If exposure duration is unrelated to the occurrence of the disease under study and has a short incubation time, follow-up may end as soon as the exposure ends, but usually members of a cohort are followed-up until the end of the study regardless of the duration of exposure. Measurement of the exposure usually has to be updated if the follow-up is long. Proper effect measures are rates that take follow-up time from exposure into consideration.

Students at the postgraduate level should also be taught more complicated designs where longitudinal recording of exposure is necessary to take a changing exposure status into consideration. They should be familiar with some of the designs used in genetic epidemiology, such as the case only studies, twin studies or other family studies.

When introducing the case control study it is important to stress that this design tries to capture the information in underlying populations by using a different sampling strategy from that of the classical follow-up study. The aim is to estimate the relative effect measures during follow-up without studying the entire population. The aim is not to compare cases and controls as in John Stuart Mill's causal reasoning (Mill, 1862), which apparently called for comparison of similarities among the cases and differences from the controls.

If we are imagining an underlying fixed cohort without loss to follow-up we have the data for all the relative effect measures, as illustrated in the following table.

Exposure	Diseased	Not diseased	Start of follow-up	Observation time
+	a	b	N_+	t_+
−	c	d	N_-	t_-

The relative risk (RR) is: $\dfrac{a/N_+}{c/N_-}$ or $\dfrac{a/c}{N_+/N_-}$

The incidence rate ratio (IRR) is: $\dfrac{a/t_+}{c/N_-}$ or $\dfrac{a/c}{t_+/t_-}$

The odds ratio (OR) is: $\dfrac{a/b}{c/d}$ or $\dfrac{a/c}{b/d}$

If we assume that a registry captures all the cases from this underlying population and we are able to reconstruct valid data on the exposures, we can estimate the numerators from the columns marked 'Start of follow-up' and 'Observation time' for the relative effect measures. 'Controls' should bring us estimates of the denominators which, for the relative risk, are the exposure distributions in the entire study base at the start of follow-up (N_+/N_-). If the follow-up is based on members of a registry or a biological bank and the follow-up time is short, a random sample from this study base will estimate the exposure distribution of interest. We call this design a case cohort study. Its merits are mainly that one control sample may be used for several case groups (Prentice, 1986; Greenland, 1986).

If there is loss to follow-up or if our study base is a dynamic population we need to estimate the distribution of exposed and unexposed time during follow-up. If the underlying population is a closed cohort, like members of a biological bank, we could let members of the cohort be represented by units of their exposed and unexposed follow-up time and sample among these units. In other situations we would sample from the population at risk at the time period when cases were detected and accept that controls may be sampled more than once, and that controls enter the case group if they get the disease under study. We call this design the case base study.

In the case cohort study we would sample controls that would include cases since cases have the same probability of being selected as non-cases. In the second situation we could sample controls that later could become cases. It is important to accept that the same subjects may be represented as both cases and controls. Sometimes this requires refinement of the normal statistical procedures, but these simple sampling procedures bypass the 'rare disease assumption' (that ORs only estimate the proper effect size for rare diseases) often mentioned in textbooks. We obtain unbiased estimates of RR and IRR regardless of the frequency of the disease.

Only for the case–non-case study in which cases are sampled from those who remain disease-free during follow-up does the rare disease assumption apply. This is only if we want the OR to estimate the RR or IRR, since the exposure OR ($\frac{a/c}{b/d}$) always estimates the disease OR ($\frac{a/b}{c/d}$).

For postgraduate students the teaching should also include more detailed sampling strategies and the principles that have to be used if not all cases are detectable from a given population. Sometimes the study base has to be based upon the case series (secondary base). A number of designs are based upon case-only studies. The most important of these is the case crossover study which is especially useful when studying immediate treatment effects or effects which happen shortly after the exposure and when trying to avoid confounding by stable time factors (MacLure, 1991; Mittleman et al., 1995; Greenland, 1996). If patients only use a given drug occasionally the incidence rate of a particular potential side effect while using the drug may be compared with the incidence rate in periods of no treatment. The ratio between these two incidence rates reflects the association between treatment and the potential side effect, and this information may be captured by studying those with side effects only (cases). By comparing drug use prior to the outcome with drug use at a reference time period for the same persons, the underlying IRRs can be ascertained for members of the study.

Almost all designs that address etiologic problems, i.e. the occurrence of an illness as a function of a given determinant, must be based upon a longitudinal recording of determinants and outcomes, perhaps with the exceptions of exposures that do not change over time, like some genetic factors or prenatal exposures.

Cross-sectional surveys are usually employed in the context of descriptive studies that aim at estimating the prevalence of a specific illness at a given time in well defined populations. For this type of study the principles of random sampling from a target population apply. The study aims at making inference for a specific population and it is particularistic in the sense that results are valid for that population only and at a given point in time. When we estimate effect measures in analytic designs we usually do not have a target population in mind and we expect (or hope) the results to be valid for other populations or for other time periods unless unspecified effect modifiers are part of the causal field leading to the disease.

The students should be aware that cross-sectional associations often have no scientific value since we know nothing about the direction of the causation. At a more advanced level the problems related to using cross-sectional data as part of a longitudinal recording in a follow-up or a case control study should be discussed.

Teaching method and format

In our experience design issues are best taught by using a mixture of different teaching methods.

The logical structure of the design, criteria for writing a protocol, and good epidemiological practice may be presented in lectures.

Published articles could be presented to the students and discussed with respect to the used design and the authors' conclusions in light of the stated objective. The students can take part in an open discussion about the appropriateness of the authors' design, the validity of the study, and the conclusions. This is usually a successful exercise as it focuses the students' attention on important aspects of the subject as well as stimulating critical assessment. It is also preparatory for the following step.

Published papers could be read and discussed by the students according to standard criteria for a peer review (Elwood, 1998) and this discussion should be brought forward to a plenary debate.

Students at a more advanced level should be asked to write a protocol on a specific topic and have this protocol discussed in plenary. PhD courses could use participants' own protocols as a point of reference for teaching.

It is important at all levels to illustrate the pitfalls in all designs, especially in designs that deviate from routine principles. Mistakes made at the design stage are frequent and may often have serious consequences.

Assessing students' achievements

Most students find design problems interesting and take active part in the discussions, but there is a difference between being able to discuss the problems and understanding the basic concepts. Since the teaching has to move from basic principles to more advanced topics, it is important to implement an ongoing assessment procedure and make sure the students master a topic before the lectures move forward to the next.

At the end of the course students should be evaluated on the understanding of the concepts rather than on the learning of specific details.

We personally prefer oral examinations or written essays to multiple choice types of exams since the latter emphasizes details rather than the overall picture. Such questions furthermore indicate that the teachers know the 'truth', which is never the case.

For undergraduate students we aim to establish that they have a firm grasp of design options and are able to discuss problems of confounding and bias inherent to these designs competently. At a more advanced level we would seek evidence that students can review study protocols and appraise published papers critically.

References

Armitage, P. and Berry, G. (1994). *Statistical methods in medical research*. Blackwell Science Ltd, Cambridge.

Axelson, O. (1979). The case-referent (case-control) study in occupational health epidemiology. *Scand J Work Environ Health*, **5**, 91–9.

Elwood, J. M. (1998). *Critical appraisals of epidemiological studies and clinical trials*. Oxford University Press, Oxford.

Feinstein, A. R. (1973). Clinical biostatistics. XX. The epidemiologic trohoc, the ablative risk ratio, and 'retrospective' research. *Clin Pharmacol Ther*, **14** (2), 291–307.

Feinstein, A. R. (1989a). Epidemiologic analysis of causation: the unlearned scientific lessons of randomized trials. *J Clin Epidemiol*, **42** (6), 481–9.

Feinstein, A. R. (1989b). Unlearned lessons from clinical trials: a duality of outlooks. *J Clin Epidemiol*, **42** (6), 497–8.

Greenland, S. (1986). Adjustment of risk ratios in case-base studies. *Stat Med*, **5**, 579–84.

Greenland, S. (1990). Randomization, statistics, and causal inference. *Epidemiology*, **1** (6), 421–9.

Greenland, S. (1996). Confounding and exposure trends in case-crossover and case-time-control designs. *Epidemiology*, **7**, 231–9.

Hennekens, C. H. and Buring, J. E. (1987). *Epidemiology in medicine*. Little, Brown and Company, Boston.

Hill, A. B. (1965). The environment and disease: association or causation? *Proc R Soc Med*, **58**, 295–300.

IEA/The European Epidemiology Group. *Good epidemiological practice: proper conduct in epidemiologic research*. http://www.dundee.ac.uk/iea/euro_Contents.htm.

Lewis, D. (1973). Causation. *Journal of Philosophy*, **70**, 556–67.

MacLure, M. (1991). The case-crossover design: a method for studying transient effects on the risk of acute events. *Am J Epidemiol*, **133**, 144–53.

MacMahon, B. and Trichopoulos, D. (1996). *Epidemiology. Principles and methods*. Little, Brown and Company, Boston.

Miettinen, O. S. (1981). Confounding: essence and detection. *Am J Epidemiol*, **114**, 593–603.

Miettinen, O. S. (1985a). *Theoretical epidemiology*. John Wiley and Sons, New York.

Miettinen, O. S. (1985b). Design options in epidemiologic research. An update. *Scand J Work Environ Health*, **8** (1), 7–14.

Miettinen, O. S. (1988). Striving to deconfound the fundamentals of epidemiologic study design. *J Clin Epidemiol*, **41**, 709–13.

Miettinen, O. S. (1998). Evidence in medicine: invited commentary. *Can Med Assoc J* **158**, 215–21.

Miettinen, O. S. (1999). Etiologic research: needed revisions of concepts and principles. *Scandinavian Journal of Work, Environment and Healt*, **25** (6, special issue), 484–90.

Mill, J. S. (1862). *A system of logic, ratiocinative and inductive*. Parker, Son and Bowin, London.

Mittleman, M. A., MacLure, M. and Robins, J. M. (1995). Control sampling strategies for case-crossover studies: an assessment of relative efficiency. *Am J Epidemiol*, **142**, 91–8.

Olsen, J. (1993). Some consequences of adopting a conditional deterministic causal model in epidemiology. *Eur J Public Health*, **3**, 204–9.

Olsen, S. F. (1993). Marine n-3 fatty acids ingested in pregnancy as a possible determinant of birth weight: a review of the current epidemiologic evidence. *Epidemiologic Reviews*, **15** (2), 399–413.

Prentice, R. L. (1986). A case-cohort design for epidemiologic cohort studies and disease prevention trials. *Biometrika*, **73**, 1–11.

Prentice, R. L. and Sheppard, L. (1995). Aggregate data studies of disease risk factors. *Biometrika*, **82** (1), 113–25.

Rachootin, P. and Olsen, J. (1983). The risk of infertility and delayed conception associated with exposure in the Danish workplace. *J Occup Med*, **25**, 394–402.

Rothman, K. J. (1976). Causes. *Am J Epidemiol*, **104**, 587–92.

Rothman, K. J. and Greenland, S. (1998). *Modern epidemiology*. Lippincott-Raven, Philadelphia.

Senn, S. J. (1991). Falsificationism and clinical trials. *Stat Med*, **10**, 1679–92.

Steel, D. G. and Holt, D. (1996). Analysing and adjusting aggregation effects: the cological fallacy revisited. *Int Stat Rev* **64** (1), 39–60.

Susser, M. (1991). What is a cause and how do we know one? A grammar for pragmatic epidemiology. *Am J Epidemiol*, **133**, 635–48.

Weinberg, C. R. (1993). Toward a clearer definition of confounding. *Am J Epidemiol*, **137** (1), 1–6.

Chapter 5

Statistics in epidemiology

Per Kragh Andersen

Introduction

Epidemiology deals with assessment of effects of risk factors on disease outcome in human populations, and statistics has played a prominent role in its development over the last decades of the twentieth century. In fact, some authors (Krickeberg, 1992) have claimed that epidemiology is really a part of statistics!

This chapter provides a guide for the 'inexperienced' teacher to teach statistics as a part of a teaching program in epidemiology. By 'inexperienced' I mean that the reader has little or no experience in teaching statistics in an epidemiologic context and not that they know little about statistics. In fact, generally I recommend that statistics be taught by professional statisticians and not by those from an applied field with a more narrow background in statistics. It is, however, crucial that the potential teacher is familiar with the field of epidemiology to motivate the students and to illustrate points with relevant examples. As will be apparent from the following, I think that teaching any statistical topic to students in epidemiology (and from any other field for that matter) should take relevant motivating examples as the starting point. Nevertheless, I would like to emphasize that, in my opinion, statistics is not well suited to problem-based learning. The reason is that the statistical concepts and methods should to a large extent follow a strict logical order which is difficult, if not impossible, to achieve using problem-based learning. Thus the course to be described follows a strict deductive model.

I will assume that a course introducing the standard epidemiologic designs is taught concurrently with the statistics course to be described. It does not make much sense first to give a course describing the designs and not the analysis, and subsequently giving the statistics course. Furthermore, the course to be outlined is intended for undergraduates with no familiarity with statistics. Excellent views on a postgraduate course were presented by David Clayton in Chapter 7 of the first edition (1992) of the text *Teaching Epidemiology*.

Teaching objectives

Since I will assume that this course provides the first teaching in statistics to which the students are exposed the first main objective is to make them

+ understand variation.

Without variation (both interindividual, intraindividual, and sampling variation) there would be no need for statistics whatsoever! Next, the students should

+ understand the concepts of population *versus* sample and parameter *versus* estimate

which naturally leads on to how to

+ understand standard deviations and confidence intervals

by discussing repetition of 'experiments'. (Here I do not think that it is necessary to distinguish between standard deviation and standard error – it is just a question of which experiment to repeat.) After these basics the students should learn how to

+ estimate probabilities ('risks' and 'prevalences') with confidence limits,
+ estimate relative risks (and risk differences) with confidence limits,
+ estimate odds and odds ratios with confidence limits

from cohort studies with common follow-up times for everyone and from cross-sectional studies. Furthermore, the student should learn how to

+ compare two probabilities or odds (among 'exposed' and 'unexposed') using the chi-squared test,
+ understand the concepts of significance level and P value,
+ understand the close connection between significance tests and confidence limits

(in these simple two-sample situations). Next, the students should

+ understand rates and intensities

as useful measures of disease frequency in cohort studies where everyone does not necessarily have the same follow-up time,

+ understand the connection between rates and risks,

learn how to

+ estimate rates and rate ratios with confidence limits,

and how to

+ compare two rates (among 'exposed' and 'unexposed') using a chisquared type test.

The last introductory topic to discuss is case control studies, which are conceptually somewhat more complicated than cohort or cross-sectional studies (involving as they do a sampling of the population generating the cases). The students should

+ understand how a case control study may be thought of as taking place by sampling within a given cohort

(though it is perhaps more natural to discuss this as a part of the concurrent epidemiology course) and how the controls may be selected in various ways. For the sake of simplicity of analysis in a basic course such as that described in this chapter, I would recommend concentrating on the kind of 'case–non-case' design which allows estimation of the odds ratio. (This is also the design for which more advanced regression analyses are most simple.) The student should

+ understand how to analyse the odds ratio based on the same basic two-by-two table as in a cohort study.

At this stage the students are ready to learn how to

♦ understand and estimate a population attributable risk

and see its relevance in a public health context. Exactly where in the later part of the course this topic is taught is probably of minor importance.

The rest of the objectives (and the rest of the course contents, see below) deal with how to

♦ understand and adjust for confounding.

This is a large and complicated task and the teacher's ambition here may be on a number of different levels, ranging from briefly touching upon the topic and discussing stratified (Mantel–Haenszel, cf. their classical 1959 article) analyses to a thorough treatment of, for example, logistic regression. I think that a suitable starting point for the discussion of confounding is that of 'a fair comparison between the exposed and the unexposed group'. That is, if we randomly select an exposed and an unexposed individual, does this then provide a fair comparison? Or do we run the risk that perhaps the exposed individual is older or smokes more than the unexposed? If the latter is the case then some sort of adjustment for age and smoking is required (provided that age and smoking are associated with the disease risk). This way of thinking is very much in line with the discussion of (randomized) experiments given in this context by Clayton (1992), and by Clayton and Hills (1993), and it leads very naturally to the concept of a stratified analysis. A stratified analysis may be performed for all the measures for comparison mentioned above (i.e. relative risks, odds ratios, rate ratios, etc.) and the idea is that the comparison is made between randomly selected exposed and unexposed individuals from the same stratum (e.g. age group) and a common (Mantel–Haenszel) estimate is then obtained by summarizing estimates from the individual strata. The student should be able to

♦ understand the rationale behind stratified analyses

and to

♦ perform a stratified analysis

for each of these measures. This includes

♦ computing the Mantel–Haenszel estimator with confidence limits and the corresponding test statistic

and

♦ examining whether the modeling assumptions behind the analysis are reasonably fulfilled,

i.e. whether the measure is approximately constant over strata. This leads to the requirement that the students should

♦ understand the concept of interaction

and recognize that this is just a formalization of what epidemiologists usually call effect modification. However, students should not necessarily be able to understand the details of, for example the Breslow–Day test for homogeneity of odds ratios across strata, only to interpret the result of such a test.

Last, but not least, the students should

♦ be able to read epidemiological literature which uses and refers to the concepts outlined above.

This poses a dilemma since most modern epidemiologic papers apply some sort of multivariate analysis such as logistic regression or Poisson regression, and these techniques are rather too difficult to be treated thoroughly in an introductory course such as that outlined here (depending, of course, on how much time is available for the teaching). Some compromise is required where the students are introduced to multivariate regression analysis and taken through typical tables from epidemiologic papers, hopefully leading to a basic understanding of the fact that regression coefficients and their associated confidence intervals are just like (log) odds ratios which are mutually adjusted as in a series of stratified analyses. A particular problem to deal with in this connection is effects of quantitative explanatory variables that do not have exact analogues in Mantel–Haenszel analyses.

A topic dealt with in most introductory courses on design and analysis of epidemiologic studies is 'standardized rates'. In textbooks on epidemiology these are frequently introduced as one of the basic measures of disease frequency like a risk or a prevalence. However, as is also the point of view of Clayton and Hills (1993), standardized rates belong much more naturally under the heading of adjustment for confounding. Thus, a directly standardized rate, being just a weighted average of age-specific rates, is computed when age confounding is suspected in a comparison of rates from different groups. Such a comparison, however, can be performed much more directly using stratified analysis (if one wants to compare the mortality rates among carpenters and bricklayers there is really no compelling reason to introduce a world standard age distribution), whereas directly standardized rates may be useful, for example, as a one number graphical summary of each group. The analogous indirectly standardized rate (and the equivalent standardized mortality ratio, SMR) is useful when comparing observed rates with standard (population) rates. Again, some sort of age adjustment is necessary and, under the simplifying assumption that the observed age-specific rates are proportional to the population rates (an assumption which may be checked), the SMR is a suitable measure of the common rate ratio. Thus, the student should

♦ understand the principles and limitations of standardization.

In summary, there are a number of concepts that the student should understand and be familiar:

♦ variation, population *versus* sample, parameter *versus* estimate, standard deviation/confidence limits, risk, prevalence (probability), odds, rate (intensity), control sampling, population attributable risk, confounding, interaction.

There are a number of techniques that the student should be able to apply:

♦ estimate risk, prevalence, odds, rate (and the corresponding ratios for two groups) with confidence limits, test whether ratios are unity using chi-square tests, perform stratified analyses, compute standardized rates.

There are some topics for which the student should understand the principles as applied in the literature:

♦ test for interaction, multivariate analysis (including linear effects).

Teaching contents and format

The teaching format will depend heavily on the availability of computers in the classroom. The ideal situation is one in which students have constant access to a computer (say, at least one for every two students) with a statistical package like SAS, SPSS or STATA installed. This provides the possibility of mixing lectures with exercises in which students try the methods just discussed on real datasets. Alternatively, lectures may take place in a classroom without computers, but the students should then have access to computers elsewhere to work with day-to-day exercises illustrating the methods taught during the lectures. To arrange a basic statistics course without some inclusion of computer exercises is just out of the question nowadays. The lectures to be described in the following are assumed to be supplemented by

♦ an introduction to a statistical computer package

and

♦ a series of computer exercises (in one of the formats just described).

Each lesson should be completed in about three to four 45-minute lectures plus computer exercises.

Lesson 1: variation and confidence intervals

Introduce this lesson by giving the students a general idea about what statistics is about (i.e. drawing inference on scientific problems from data), and turn quickly to a simple introductory example to ease the understanding of population and sample. I have sometimes used the following example but, obviously, any similar simple example would do. Imagine that you want to assess the prevalence of asthma in a well defined geographical region among teenagers using a questionnaire. Based on this example one may discuss population, sample, sampling variation, and interindividual and intraindividual variation. Furthermore, such an example should make the students feel the need for a confidence interval for the true asthma prevalence and they should be taught how to do this from the estimated standard deviation of the proportion in the sample. (However, they need not understand why the standard deviation is computed in the way that it is.) The interpretation of standard deviation, of distribution of prevalence estimates, and of confidence interval through hypothetical repeated sampling should be explained and, if possible, illustrated on a computer. In a similar vein, risk parameter estimates for exposed and unexposed individuals from a cohort study could be discussed with standard deviations, leading to the wish to make a statistical comparison of the two.

Lesson 2: comparing risks and odds

Begin by repeating the highlights of lesson 1, emphasize what the students are supposed to understand and what they have to accept, then go on to introduce the relative risk and associated confidence interval. Repeat the interpretation of a confidence interval and examine whether the 'null value' RR = 1 is inside or outside the confidence limits in your example. Next, based on that example, introduce the concepts from significance testing: null hypothesis, test statistic, distribution of test statistic, P value, significance level, acceptance/rejection of null hypothesis. I would recommend using the Mantel–Haenszel version of the chi-squared test in a two-by-two table because this is the one in which it is seen most easily how the test statistic measures discrepancies from how the data would be expected to look if the null hypothesis were true. Furthermore, it generalizes easily to stratified analysis and to comparison of rates. The students should understand the need for a standard deviation for the difference between observed and expected but they need not understand why the formula looks the way it does. They should understand how a distribution of test statistics under the null may be obtained through repeated sampling and how one then compares the observed value of the test, statistic with this distribution (the chi-squared distribution with one degree of freedom) and obtains the P value using a table of the distribution. Finally, they should understand how one accepts or rejects the hypothesis by comparing the P value with the (arbitrary!) significance level and they should understand the close connection between confidence limits and test statistic (in this simple one degree of freedom situation). The students should also have mention of odds ratio (with confidence interval) and it should be emphasized that the test statistic can just as well be seen as a test for the hypothesis that the odds ratio is unity.

Lesson 3: rates and case control studies

Begin by repeating the highlights of lesson 2, emphasize what the students are supposed to understand and what they have to accept, and promise them that all the concepts introduced in connection with significance tests will be repeated several times later in the course! Next, introduce the rate as a frequency measure useful in cohort studies with unequal follow-up times and explain how to compute confidence intervals for rates and rate ratios. The connection between a rate (i.e. a constant intensity) and a probability (risk) should be explained. Next, discuss the Mantel–Haenszel type test for comparing two rates and repeat the concepts from significance testing. At this stage, case control studies can be discussed, emphasizing how odds ratios may be estimated based on observation of cases and a sample of disease-free controls. One could also mention the alternative design in which cases are compared to a random sample from the whole population ('study base'), enabling estimation of the relative risk but complicating analysis because of lack of independence between cases and 'controls'.

Lesson 4: adjustment for confounding using stratified analysis

Begin by repeating the highlights of lesson 3, emphasize what the students are supposed to understand and what they have to accept, and continue to discuss confounding. This may, for instance, be done by presenting a (perhaps hypothetical) situation in which an exposed and an unexposed group are to be compared and where, for some reason, the exposed group is older than the unexposed. In this case, an individual randomly selected from the exposed group and one randomly selected from the unexposed group will not provide a fair comparison since differences between the risks in the two groups may to some extent be ascribed to effects of age (if age is a risk factor for the disease outcome). Thus, to compare like with like an age stratification of the two groups is needed and this leads very naturally to a discussion of stratified (Mantel–Haenszel) analysis of, for example, the odds ratio. A good real example with confounding is given by Lauritzen (1996). The students should understand that the ingredients of a stratified analysis are just what one would have used for comparisons of exposed and unexposed, stratum by stratum (i.e. observed, expected, and standard deviation of observed), but that, instead of performing several analyses, one for each stratum, the three sufficient statistics are instead added over strata, enabling one to make a single comparison between exposed and unexposed adjusted for the stratification variable (the confounder). Technically, students should learn about the Mantel–Haenszel estimator, its associated confidence interval, and the Mantel–Haenszel chi-squared test. Students should understand that the estimation procedure corresponds to the calculation of a weighted average of the stratum-specific odds ratios and that it therefore only makes sense if all the stratum-specific odds ratios are 'similar', i.e. if there is no effect modification ('interaction'). They should know that tests for no interaction exist but the details could be left out of this introductory course (depending of course on the available time).

Lesson 5: standardization and attributable risks

Begin by repeating the highlights of lesson 4, emphasize what the students are supposed to understand and what they have to accept, and repeat the basic idea of the stratified analysis by showing how a Mantel–Haenszel analysis of rates is performed. At this stage, standardization techniques can be introduced. The idea behind 'direct' standardization (calculation of a weighted average of age-specific rates) is easily explained and the students should understand that, for a comparison of two groups, an external (arbitrary) standard age distribution is not really needed. The principle of 'indirect' standardization should be explained and the way in which this method may be used when comparing rates from the sample with standard ('population') rates. Estimation of the standard deviation of the SMR should be presented. Finally, the population attributable risk should be introduced, including both its calculation and its interpretation.

Lessons 1 to 5 as they have now been described provide the necessary minimum content of a basic course in epidemiological statistics but, to fulfil the requirement that the students be able to read epidemiological articles, some introduction to multivariate analysis (e.g. logistic regression) should be given. Thus, I would recommend that two extra modules be added with this aim.

Lesson 6: introduction to logistic regression

Begin by repeating the highlights of lesson 5, emphasize what the students are supposed to understand and what they have to accept. To introduce logistic regression, begin by considering tables. First, in a two by two table with one outcome variable (diseased *versus* not diseased) and one binary explanatory variable (exposed *versus* not exposed), the odds ratio may be calculated as a measure of the effect of the explanatory variable on the outcome. The log odds ratio may be seen also as the coefficient b in a regression model

$$\ln(odds) = a + bZ$$

where the explanatory variable Z is coded as 0 or 1. Furthermore, in a three by two table, again with a binary disease outcome and with an explanatory variable with three ordered categories, choosing a reference category enables one to calculate two log odds ratios as measures of the effect. These log odds ratios may be seen as coefficients b_1, b_2 in a regression model

$$\ln(odds) = a + b_1Z_1 + b_2Z_2$$

with the explanatory variable coded using indicator variables Z_1, Z_2 for the two levels of the variable not chosen as reference. Next, denoting the three ordered levels by $Z = 0$ (reference), $Z = 1$ and $Z = 2$, the coefficient b in the model

$$\ln(odds) = a + bZ$$

may be seen as a common log odds ratio for 1 *versus* 0 and for 2 *versus* 1, i.e. if the log odds is plotted against Z a straight line is obtained. This latter model is easily extended to one with a truly quantitative covariate. These are the simplest univariate situations with either one binary, one categorical, or one quantitative explanatory variable, and the tables are seen to be equivalent to simple logistic regression models. To introduce multivariate logistic regression, begin by considering two two by two tables where the relation between the exposure Z and the outcome is studied in two strata defined by a third binary explanatory variable X. In this case, the Mantel–Haenszel estimator may be calculated as a measure of the effect of Z adjusted for X. Now, rearrange the tables such that the roles of Z and X are interchanged and the Mantel–Haenszel estimator for the effect of X adjusted for Z may be calculated and the model (finally) can be studied

$$\ln(odds) = a + bZ + cX$$

including both explanatory variables. In this model it is seen that b is the log odds ratio for Z both when $X = 0$ *and* when $X = 1$ and c is the log odds ratio for X both when $Z = 0$ *and* when $Z = 1$. Thus, this model corresponds to performing both Mantel–Haenszel analyses at one go and thereby mutually adjusting the effects of Z and X. Finally, explain briefly how interaction may be modeled within the logistic regression framework.

With these building blocks, any multivariate regression model can be explained by considering one variable at a time and interpreting the corresponding regression coefficients as log odds ratios adjusted for the other variables in the model.

Lesson 7: literature examples using logistic regression

Begin by repeating the highlights of lesson 6, emphasize what the students are supposed to understand and what they just have to accept. The purpose of lesson 7 is to discuss a couple of epidemiologic articles that use logistic regression. The first of these should, preferably, be one where the data are documented in fair detail with tables and where classical Mantel–Haenszel techniques are used as an introduction to the multivariate analyses. If access to the raw data is possible, then reconstructing some of the tables from the article in computer sessions will usually make an important pedagogic point.

A number of simple statistical methods that really do belong in a basic course in statistical epidemiology have not found their way into these lessons. These include: analysis of quantitative outcomes (e.g. t test and linear regression), analysis of survival data (the Kaplan–Meier estimator and the log rank test), analysis of general r by c contingency tables, and analysis of matched data. If time permits then these are all candidates for inclusion in further lessons.

Assessment of students' achievements

To assess the students' achievement I would recommend a written exam where some studies and their key results in tabular form are presented to the students who are then asked to comment and conclude, possibly by doing some computations based on the tables. The latter would be appropriate, especially if computer access at the exam is possible. Otherwise, key results may be given with the tables for comments.

References

It is not easy to find a textbook with a philosophy exactly as the one outlined above. However, books which, in principle, cover the material described include Kahn and Sempos (1989), Sakai and Khurshid (1996), McNeil (1996), and the recent text by Woodward (1999). More comprehensive background material for the statistical teacher may be found in the now classical monographs by Breslow and Day (1980, 1987), in Clayton and Hills' (1993) book, and in Rothman and Greenland (1998) and Woodward (1999). As mentioned, suitable computer packages to be used by the students include SAS, SPSS, and STATA, while EPIINFO is not sufficiently comprehensive for the purposes of the course described.

Breslow, N. E. and Day, N. E. (1980). *Statistical Methods in Cancer Research. Vol. I; The Analysis of Case-Control Studies.* IARC, Lyon.

Breslow, N. E. and Day, N. E. (1987). *Statistical Methods in Cancer Research. Vol. II; The Analysis of Cohort Studies.* IARC, Lyon.

Clayton, D. (1992). Teaching statistical methods in epidemiology. In: *Teaching Epidemiology – What you should know and what you could do.* (J. Olsen and D. Trichopoulos, eds.), Oxford University Press, Oxford: Ch. 7.

Clayton, D. and Hills, M. (1993). *Statistical Models in Epidemiology.* Oxford University Press, Oxford.

EPIINFO (1994). *The Epi Info Manual: A Word Processing, Database and Statistics System for Public Health on IBM-Compatible Microcomputers.* Version 6.02. Brixton Books, London.

Kahn, H. A. and Sempos, C. T. (1989). *Statistical Methods in Epidemiology.* Oxford University Press, New York.

Krickeberg, K. (1992). Moderne Epidemiologie und ihre Anwendungen. *Mitteilungen der Deutschen Akademie der Naturforscher Leopoldina* **35**, 149–60.

Lauritzen, S. L. (1996). *Graphical Models.* Oxford University Press, Oxford: p. 56.

McNeil, D. (1996). *Epidemiological Research Methods.* Wiley, New York.

Mantel, N. and Haenszel, W. (1959). Statistical aspects of the analysis of data from retrospective studies of disease. *J Nat Cancer Inst* **22**, 719–48.

Rothman, K. J. and Greenland, S. (1998). *Modern Epidemiology*, 2nd edn. Lippincott-Raven, Philadelphia.

Sakai, H. and Khurshid, A. (1996). *Statistics in Epidemiology. Methods, Techniques and Applications.* CRC Press, New York.

SAS Institute Inc. (1992). *Master Index to SAS System Documentation*, Version 6, 4th edn. SAS Institute Inc., Cary, NC.

SPSS Inc. (1997). *SPSS Base 7.5 Applications Guide.* SPSS Inc., Chicago, Ill.

STATA Corp. (1997). *Stata Statistical Software: Release 5.0.* Stata Press, College Station, TX.

Woodward, M. (1999). *Epidemiology. Study Design and Data Analysis.* Chapman & Hall/CRC, London.

Chapter 6

A first course in epidemiologic principles and methods

Kenneth J. Rothman

Introduction

The first course in epidemiologic methods occasionally serves as the introduction to epidemiology for a student, but more typically it is preceded by a more general introductory course. Nevertheless, the students taking a first course in epidemiologic methods are still, for the most part, 'babes in the woods' when it comes to first-hand experience with epidemiologic research. More so than courses in language, music appreciation, or mathematics, few students in an epidemiologic methods course will have a clear concept of what constitutes the subject matter of the course. Most, at best, will have a hazy understanding of the goals of epidemiologic research, and little insight into the principles and methods that they are about to confront. Some will not even have read many, if any, epidemiologic papers; others may have had just enough experience in epidemiology to be dangerous.

Lack of epidemiologic experience poses a barrier to effective learning. People learn more effectively by doing things, under guidance, than by simply listening. Rousing students to action, however, is easier for some topics than for others. When the subject matter is an abstract set of ideas, as is the case for epidemiologic methods, it is difficult to avoid the prototypical lecture scene, a classroom engagement in which the instructor spews abstruse and airy concepts at the audience. This approach can have the same effect as spraying the audience with tear gas: the recipients disperse, enraged at the interaction and hardened in clinging to their former ideas. It is no easy task, however, to devise an action syllabus to explain concepts such as confounding or non-differential misclassification.

The challenge is to involve the student in doing something that breathes life into such abstract concepts. In a chemistry or physics class, laboratory exercises can be constructed that simulate chemistry or physics research. Unfortunately, conducting or simulating actual research is more difficult for an epidemiology class. Nevertheless, the teacher must try to impart some familiarity with research problems to the students, using laboratories and exercises to flesh out the abstract ideas.

Some teachers of epidemiologic methods attempt to start students with high-level programming and data analysis even as they flounder in the basic concepts of epidemiologic measurement and study design. Their hope may be that a 'hands-on' approach to the daily activities of computer modeling and other high-tech methods will allow the students to be active and enable them to see the aims of the early part of the research process. I have a low regard for this popular approach. Teaching students to press buttons is no substitute for an ordered elaboration of the principles and methods of epidemiology. Computers are best left out of this teaching, especially in the early stages. All the computation necessary for teaching epidemiologic methods, at least during the first year or so, can be done handily without any computers at all beyond a pocket calculator.

In this chapter, I suggest a sequence of core topics to broach the teaching of epidemiologic principles and methods. They cover the essential principles and the main methods for conducting epidemiologic research. The topics are: causation and causal inference; epidemiologic measures; types of epidemiologic study; principles of good study design; principles of epidemiologic data analysis; stratified analysis; analysis of interaction; multivariate analysis; and analysis of multilevel or continuous exposures. For each topic, I propose my suggestions on what to focus on in the classroom, based on my own trial-and-error experience.

Teaching objectives

Students do not become researchers after a single course, nor is the objective of studying the methods of epidemiology necessarily to transform students into researchers. Many courses pose as the objective in such a course the goal that the student can read and comment intelligently on published studies. This is a reasonable goal. The main obstacle in achieving it is that, after a student has acquired a small amount of exposure to epidemiologic methods, there seems to be no study that can stand up to the criticism that will then be heaped upon it. Finding fault seems easy, but obtaining the wisdom to know which errors are serious and which are inconsequential is much more difficult to teach. My teaching objective would be to have the students able to discuss and criticize the design of epidemiologic studies in a balanced way, and to demonstrate quantitative regard for various sources of error.

Teaching content and format

Causation and causal inference

Many notions of causation abound. It is important, in a course that will attempt to teach students how to evaluate causal hypotheses, to begin with a common understanding of what a cause is. I introduce the sufficient/component cause model (Rothman, 1976) at the beginning of the course, and rely on it repeatedly as the course proceeds. The model explains several important epidemiologic concepts:

1. The causes that we study in epidemiology are components of sufficient causes, not sufficient in themselves. That is why smoking is a cause of lung cancer and yet not every smoker gets lung cancer.

2. Component causes interact with one another to form sufficient causes; this interaction is a biologic interaction involving causal mechanisms (as opposed to statistical interaction, to be discussed later).

3. Factors can interact with one another in a single causal mechanism even if they act at widely differing times.

4. Induction time is the time that represents the accumulation of other, complementary component causes; induction time characterizes a cause—effect pair, not the disease alone.

And so forth. These conceptual issues can all be illustrated with causal 'pies'.

How can students be drawn into this lesson? I start by recounting how concepts of causation develop in infants and toddlers, by early experience and genetic programming. Having a theory of causation is a useful survival skill, so it is not surprising that some version of causal thinking develops early in life. Nevertheless, most causal thinking is predicated on the notion of a 1–1 correspondence between cause and effect, a notion that the sufficient/component model dispels. Notions of cause are rarely taught in classes before the first course in epidemiologic methods, so students will typically still harbor the concepts that derive from their earliest causal thinking. One can show by example how that thinking evolves during early life, and the ways in which our early concepts of causation tend to be naive. The class succeeds by drawing on insights from child development, psychology, evolution, logic, and philosophy, and by demolishing some cherished misconceptions, a process that is often a good motivator. Exercises can include the fabrication of examples of causal mechanisms illustrating the various teaching points, and can be conducted either individually or in groups.

It is also useful to present the philosophy underlying the scientific method under the heading of 'causal inference'. I emphasize Popper's approach, which stresses the value of formulating hypotheses that can be tested by falsifying them (Rothman and Greenland, 1998). The advantage of this approach is that it encourages the design of studies that address the intersection of competing theories where they make differing predictions. Epidemiologic studies that can distinguish between competing theories will accelerate scientific understanding much more rapidly than scattershot approaches that do not tie the studies closely to competing causal mechanisms. Of course, competing theories in epidemiology are often non-causal theories (such as confounding, selection bias or recall bias) that compete with a causal explanation for an observed finding.

This material may seem dry and can be challenging to teach. In a course on epidemiologic methods, however, a basic introduction to the scientific method is indispensable for a strong orientation. It is most helpful if the principles of choosing among competing theories are re-emphasized along with notions of component causes throughout the course. A useful exercise is to offer examples of competing theories to students and have them propose epidemiologic studies that will refute at least one of the competing theories. One such example is the competing theories to explain, in the 1970s, the reports that use of then new highly absorbent tampons were a strong risk factor for toxic shock syndrome: one theory suggested that the tampons acted as a culture medium for pathogenic bacteria, which produced the toxin, while a competing theory proposed that the toxin was a chemical manufactured in the new tampons. The key epidemiologic observation is the trend of risk of toxic shock syndrome according to the length of time a tampon was used before a new tampon was inserted. The two competing theories would predict opposite trends, so an epidemiologic study that examined this trend would be able to refute at least one of these theories.

As stated above, it is useful to challenge cherished misconceptions head on. In the first class I usually take on the misconception that epidemiologic studies should enroll study subjects who are representative of broader target populations (Rothman and Greenland, 1998). Many students arrive with the belief that representativeness is essential for generalization. I challenge this notion in several ways. First, I emphasize that the concept of statistical generalization, from sample to population, is different from scientific generalization, which is better described as the process of formulating and testing hypotheses about nature. Second, I contrast the conduct of survey research to the conduct of laboratory studies on animals. Surveys conducted to take polls, to obtain marketing information, or even to assess health, depend on representativeness for inference, but their findings are not scientific inferences. Rather, the findings are specific to a single time and place. In contrast, laboratory studies on animals such as hamsters, mice, and rats provide scientific inferences that apply to human health and disease despite the fact that the hamsters, mice, and rats in the studies are not even representative of all hamsters, mice, and rats, much less the humans for which the inferences are targeted. Some students will let go of ingrained misconceptions only reluctantly, but whether successful or not, attacking these misconceptions early in the course will ignite interest in the course material.

Epidemiologic measures

Having dealt with the philosophic building blocks, one can turn to epidemiology itself, beginning with epidemiologic measures. The basic presentation comprises measures of disease frequency and measures of effect. For disease frequency, the crucial distinction is between risk and rate (Morgenstern et al., 1980). The way in which time is handled for both these measures must be understood by students. There should also be a clear idea of the meaning of competing risks. Again, these concepts may seem dry. The teacher needs to liven it up with examples and by engaging students in dealing with the problems that each measure presents. Have students compute the risk of dying for members of a small fixed population. Show them how the risk is near zero over a short period, climbs with time, and how it always reaches 100% given enough time. I usually give students an exercise in which they calculate rates with a hand tabulation of person–time because I believe that every epidemiology student should have to go through the mental exercise of classifying person–time and events for a set of individuals. Doing so will crystallize the process that underlies an ubiquitous epidemiologic concept. As for competing risks, students should be able to explain why a battlefield is not the right spot to conduct a campaign against smoking, and they should be able to explain why risk of death from specific causes is not a directly observable measure.

The teaching of epidemiologic measures may evoke dreary memories of the fuzzy distinctions between force and acceleration or other physical measures that stymied students earlier in their education. Epidemiology teachers face an even greater challenge, because epidemiologic measurements are so hard to come by; it is usually easier to measure a force or a mass than to measure the rate of disease. Presenting students with raw data on individuals and asking them to derive measures from them will reduce the level of abstraction. Giving them exercises in which the conclusions depend entirely on a correct understanding of epidemiologic measures will engage them even further (Horwitz *et al.*, 1981; Crombie and Tomenson, 1981; Merletti and Cole, 1981; Hulka *et al.*, 1981).

Types of epidemiologic study

There are many taxonomies for epidemiologic studies, and newer study types only sow the seeds of confusion into an already confusing arena. I opt for simplicity over complexity, emphasizing the main dichotomy, cohort studies *versus* case-control studies. The prototype for a cohort study is the randomized controlled trial, which is valuable to present both as a paradigm and because it is an important and popular type of study. Nevertheless, one can argue that the conceptual understanding of the case-control study is the greatest achievement of epidemiologic methods. Traditionally, case-control studies have been taught as a type of logically inverted cohort study, where the scientist, rather than looking forward from cause to effect, looks backward from effect to cause. A more enlightened view is that a case control study is a cohort study with an efficiency gain that comes from taking a sample of the denominator experience rather than having to observe the entire denominator experience. The connection between cohort studies and case-control studies can be illuminated by characterizing every case-control study as being nested within a cohort. The definition of the cohort is implied by the definition of the cases in the case-control study; ideally, the controls are sampled from the same people who could have become cases in the study, and during the same time that they could have developed the disease. In practice, controls may be sampled from outside this population, but the study can nevertheless be valid as long as the proxy population gives the same exposure distribution as the actual source population for cases. By emphasizing such parallels between a cohort study and a case-control study, the teacher can provide a conceptual basis for the most perplexing of design issues, namely the suitability of a given type of individual as a control in a case-control study.

If cohort studies always measured risks rather than rates, then the corresponding case-control study would be easy enough to comprehend, except for the stumbling block that controls, being sampled from the denominators of the risk measures in a cohort study, would include some individuals who developed disease. The teaching trick here is to make clear that the sampling represents sampling from the cohort at the start of its follow-up, when everyone in the cohort was free of disease. Thus, at the time of the sampling, the sampled controls were free of disease, despite the fact that some may have gone on to become cases. It is essential when presenting these concepts to emphasize that the cases in a case-control study correspond to the numerator of a risk or rate, and the controls correspond to the denominator. In every cohort in which risk is estimated, any case in the numerator of the risk proportion is also represented in the denominator; by analogy, the corresponding case-control study should not aim to exclude future cases from a control series.

Cohort studies often measure rates, however, rather than risks. The parallel with case-control studies then becomes more difficult to explain, because each control now represents not a sample from a number of people but a sample from an amount of person–time. The teaching issue is the concept of density-based sampling in case-control studies and the related topic of risk-set sampling. I find it useful to consider as a teaching example a case-control study of the relation of bicycle helmets to head injuries among cyclists (Thompson *et al.*, 1989). I ask the students to consider what cohort study they would design to evaluate the problem. The question devolves to a consideration of the time at risk, which for helmet-wearing is clearly only the time spent wearing the helmet while riding the bicycle. (Some would restrict the study base even further, to include only the time of an accident, on the theory that a helmet could only prevent an injury during an accident. This restriction, however, ignores the possible effect of a helmet on the risk of an accident, such as by restricting visibility while riding or by emboldening the rider.) In a cohort study one would ideally calculate rates based on time spent cycling with or without helmets. The class can then focus on how to design a case-control study in which controls can be sampled to give an estimate of the distribution of time spent by riders on a bicycle with and without a helmet. The range of possible designs and the inferences that they allow offer considerable insight into the conceptual underpinnings of the case-control study.

Principles of good study design

A theme I find indispensable throughout the course is the theme of measurement. It is lamentable that much of data analysis is devoted to statistical significance testing, which is not measurement at all, but flawed decision analysis. To elaborate the principles of study design, I start from the premise that the aim of the research is to obtain an estimate of an epidemiologic measure. The principles of good study design then become synonymous with obtaining an accurate measure. In measurement, and in epidemiologic studies, one aims to reduce both random and systematic errors.

Too much emphasis is put on random error, primarily through significance testing in data analysis, but also in planning study sizes by performing power calculations. The usefulness of power calculations is overrated. The most important message is often obscured in discussions of power or study size, which imply that studies are either large enough or not large enough. A better concept is simply that larger studies provide more precise measurements than smaller ones, along a continuous curve. Some study designs are more efficient than others, but size is usually the main determinant of the amount of information that a study will provide.

The core discussion with respect to the principles of good study design relates to systematic error, or bias. Most texts take the approach of dividing bias into three broad types: selection bias, information bias, and confounding. These are useful distinctions to maintain. Students often exhibit an intuitive feel for selection bias. Confounding too, while having its measure of subtlety, can be digested readily by most students.

Clear-cut examples are a boon: I introduce confounding with an illustration of a strong effect of birth order on Down syndrome prevalence, and then a stronger effect for mother's age that accounts entirely for the birth order effect. I then emphasize that, because mother's age is just a marker for the occurrence of other biological processes that occur while the mother is aging, it must therefore also be confounded by an as yet unidentified factor or factors. This presentation casts the research process as a gradual peeling off of layers as each apparent effect is explained by another. The lesson is that, while confounding is considered a bias and therefore something to be avoided or removed, it is also rampant and to some extent inevitable. Nearly every causal mechanism raises possibilities for confounding that ought to be considered. It may also be useful to present an example of Simpson's paradox, in which confounding is strong enough to reverse the direction of an association (Reintjes *et al.*, 2000).

The effects of non-differential misclassification are often the least intuitive of the principles in this section of the course. I emphasize that bias resulting from non-differential misclassification is, if anything, more ubiquitous than confounding and, like gravity, is always tugging in the same direction, at least for dichotomous exposures. Even inexperienced students can readily name myriad sources of non-differential misclassification. An important one that they might not offer is mis-specification of the induction time in the study hypothesis. Many students might believe that, since most studies do not specify any induction time hypothesis, the study cannot have mis-specified the induction time. The teaching goal here is to lead students to the point at which they appreciate that every analysis implicitly rests on some induction time hypothesis, even if it is unstated. To the extent that the hypothesis is wrong, for example, asking about ever-use of aspirin when aspirin affects disease risk only for 24 hours after ingestion, the results can be extremely biased. It is equally important as a teaching goal to help students appreciate that even serious non-differential misclassification cannot explain a strong non-null finding (again, assuming a dichotomous exposure). A good teaching example is the criticism of studies showing a strong relation between spermicides and birth defects; a major criticism was that the underlying data on spermicide use, based on prescriptions rather than on actual use, were a poor proxy for exposure. A clear understanding of the principles of study design should lead the students to understand why the criticism is wrong, but why it would have been important if the study had found no effect.

Principles of epidemiologic data analysis

The one principle that I emphasize most strongly in the course is that we should use estimation rather than significance testing. Examples of mistakes stemming from mindless applications of statistical significance testing are legion, and are useful. Many teachers seem to urge students simply not to repeat the same mistakes, but just to be 'more careful' in their significance testing. I teach that there is no use at all for statistical significance testing in epidemiologic analysis. It is perfectly possible to write excellent papers, which will be acceptable to the best journals, without a single test of significance nor a single *P*-value. Estimation methods not only convey more information than *P*-values or significance testing, but they also help avoid the pitfalls that come with testing.

Despite emphasis, the key conceptual point is sometimes lost on students. Many defenders of significance testing point out that a confidence interval and a *P*-value have mathematical links, implying some sort of equivalence. True enough: one can use confidence intervals as surrogate tests, and lose nearly all the value in having obtained the estimate. The real distinction is in how the estimate is interpreted, which should be quantitatively rather than qualitatively. If a confidence interval is used as a test to assess whether the null value lies within the interval or not, the interpretation is qualitative. Instead I present the confidence interval function as a tool for visualizing a quantitative interpretation for the estimate. With a quantitative interpretation, the exact location of the boundary of the interval or the exact level of confidence does not matter. It may seem less precise, but it is more quantitative than testing, because it is gradual rather than all or none (Poole, 1987; Lang *et al.*, 1998).

From this point on in the course, as we delve more deeply into analytic topics, I continue to emphasize quantitative interpretations. Typically it is only with the greatest reluctance that students overcome their reliance on statistical significance testing. I believe that there are three components to the enduring fondness with which students embrace statistical significance testing:

1. Before one learns anything at all about statistics or science, one hears about results that are 'statistically significant'. The phrase has such an authoritative ring that it must encourage students to covet work that would likewise be 'statistically significant'. It has marketing appeal.

2. Interpreting data, which can be hard work, seems much easier when one relies on labels such as 'statistically significant' or 'not significant'. The reason, of course, is because one is no longer going through the effort to interpret the data, so of course it is much easier.

3. Finally, everywhere they turn, including statistics courses, other epidemiology courses, and most published work in the health field, students will see a conventional reliance on statistical significance testing being reinforced.

To swim against the tide with regard to significance testing is not easy, and few teachers attempt it. Nevertheless, if the teacher succeeds, it could be the most important advantage that they bestow on the students in their course. Perhaps the biggest didactic obstacle is the third point in the above list. Many students object to dissonance between courses. It is helpful to stress that there is little reason for different courses to be harmonious when the world at large is not: students must learn to evaluate divergent views on their own and on their merits. Students may be shy about challenging the teaching despite lingering objections relating to the list above. To stimulate discussion, it helps to bring up relevant arguments in a simulated debate and address them without waiting for the questions to be raised by students. Another approach is a real debate between faculty members. I do not favor it because the goal is not to confront or to teach the other faculty but to teach the students on your course, and it is too easy to become diverted in a different direction when your teaching principle becomes a debate topic. On the other hand, it is useful for students to understand that there is divided opinion about many issues. I emphasize to students that it is their responsibility to challenge their teachers vigorously to defend the principles that they teach, so that students will be equipped to make up their own minds about controversial issues.

Stratified analysis

After elaborating the basics of calculating point and interval estimates, the core of epidemiologic analytic thinking can be conveyed in a thorough discussion of stratified analysis. This is the time that I introduce the concept of 'effect–measure modification'. Stratified analysis is the primary tool (or, more accurately, should be the primary tool) for evaluating and controlling confounding, as well as for describing effect–measure modification. These two issues are occasionally confused by students, who often ask whether a third variable can be both a confounder and an effect–measure modifier at the same time.

My approach to stratified analysis is to keep the evaluation and control of confounding as separate as possible from the description of effect–measure modification. To begin with, emphasize that when confounding occurs, it is the crude effect estimate, obtained without stratification, that is confounded. Stratified analysis to control confounding aims to replace that crude estimate with an unconfounded replacement. The Mantel–Haenszel version of a pooled estimate is simple and statistically well behaved, and should suffice in a first course on methods as the only pooled estimate to consider. The Mantel–Haenszel estimate becomes a replacement for the crude estimate, and the difference between (or ratio of) the two estimates is a measure of the amount of confounding. A discussion of standardization, which does not require a uniform effect over strata to obtain an unconfounded summary estimate, should also be included.

Where does effect–measure modification figure in an analysis? Pooling assumes that the effect parameter is uniform over the strata. If it is not, then the primary interest in the analysis may shift to the description of how the effect changes by level of the stratification variable. In this case the results may be reported separately by each stratum. Doing so precludes confounding (except within strata) because the crude estimate, which is where the confounding occurs, is not presented. Thus a stratified analysis typically aims either to evaluate and control confounding or to describe effect–measure modification, which, if present, precludes confounding from being a problem. Describing effect–measure modification dispatches the question of confounding, which does not arise when looking at stratum-specific results.

With analytic issues such as these, exercises provide excellent reinforcement. These exercises can be carried out with paper, pencil, and pocket calculator, the latter being optional. One of the subtle teaching points relates to the ambiguity of effect–measure modification. One cannot say that age either is or is not an effect modifier (this is the reason to avoid the shorter term 'effect modification'), because the answer will depend on which measure of effect is under discussion. The ambiguity of effect–measure modification comes from the choice of effect measures with which we can describe an effect. It is critical to explain how there can be effect–measure modification with respect to, say, rate difference, but not with respect to rate ratio or vice versa. Despite the ambiguity, effect–measure modification, unlike confounding, is not something that an investigator can influence. That is why we aim to eliminate confounding (if we have not already prevented it in the study design), but we aim to describe effect–measure modification. With these distinctions carefully drawn, students will be on their way to a clear understanding of how to cope with a stratified analysis. As usual, it is the conceptual approach and not the application of statistical formulas that needs to be emphasized in the teaching.

A straightforward extension of stratified analysis is the analysis of case control studies in which matching has been employed in subject selection. Indeed, the major teaching point is simply that an analysis of matched data amounts to nothing more than a stratified analysis, in which one stratifies by the matching factors. This lesson tends to get lost now that conditional logistic regression is used routinely to analyze case control studies with individual matching. Using stratified analysis is an effective way to teach students how matching biases results in case control studies, by selecting controls according to one or more factors that are related to exposure. Surprisingly, this selection bias can be removed in the analysis. Although it involves no new principle, matching in case control studies is so counterintuitive that its teaching is nevertheless challenging. An unparalleled teaching example is the classic paper by Johnson and Johnson (1972), which presents data from which students can calculate effect estimates from matched data as well as from the source population from which the matched subjects were drawn. It illustrates nicely the effect of matching.

Analysis of interaction

The evaluation of interaction is complicated by the fact that it is often considered a statistical issue and treated in statistics classes. The treatment is invariably an analysis of departure from some basic model structure, usually by examining product terms in a general linear model. I refer to this interaction as statistical interaction, which has the same ambiguity as the nearly identical concept of effect–measure modification. As a biologist (an identification worthy of emphasis in an epidemiology course), an epidemiologist ought to be more focused on a different type of interaction, which I refer to as biologic interaction. This interaction corresponds to the joint participation of component causes in a causal mechanism (see above).

The main teaching point is that biologic interaction, being a description of nature, cannot have the kind of ambiguity that depends on a choice of scale or choice of effect measure. Thus, statistical interaction is ambiguous, but biologic interaction is not. One can use the causal pies to derive expressions to evaluate interaction. These expressions show the fundamental role of additivity of effects as a baseline from which interaction should be measured.

Several important teaching points emerge:

1. The usual evaluation of statistical interaction, which examines departures from additivity within a logarithmic model such as a logistic model, corresponds to evaluating departures from a multiplicative relation. Thus, the usual approach taught in statistics classes does not apply to the evaluation of biologic interaction.

2. Instead, inferences should be tied to departures from additivity of effects, additivity being the relation (with some qualifications) that one would expect for biologically independent causes. With proper handling, logistic models and other models that involve logarithmic transformations can yield straightforward evaluations of interaction based on departures from additivity of effects.

3. Statisticians have sometimes argued that both 'additivity' and 'multiplicativity' are reasonable models, each with its areas of application: for example, in multistage models factors acting at different stages would be expected to have a multiplicative relation (Siemiatycki and Thomas, 1981). The flaw in the argument is that in the evaluation of interaction additivity is not used as a model to describe what occurs, it is used as a definition of independence from which interactive effects are measured. In the multistage model, although a multiplicative relation is expected for factors acting at distinct stages, it is the departure from additivity of these effects that we use to measure the interaction.

4. In stratified analysis of ratio measures of effect that rely on pooling, one assumes that the ratio is constant over strata. This assumption is equivalent to assuming a multiplicative relation between exposure and the stratification variable. Thus, the assumption underlying a pooled analysis is one of interaction between the exposure and the stratification variable.

The key concept to grasp in the evaluation of interaction is the importance of using a common referent category for all effect estimates, defined on the basis of joint combinations of the two exposure categories. This concept can be taught effectively using examples of stratified data. The trend toward conducting multivariate analyses in lieu of stratification has often obscured the problems of an interaction evaluation.

In theory, as more is learned about causes of disease, there will be a greater emphasis on learning about interactions. In practice, this theory seems to have been borne out, as more interaction evaluations see the light of day. No doubt we can look forward to learning about many gene–environment interactions in years to come. Nevertheless, a precise evaluation of interaction requires so much more data than an evaluation of a single effect that most interaction evaluations are doomed to remain uninformative. As a result good teaching examples are hard to find.

Multivariate analysis

Students will face entire courses on multivariate analysis. I suggest offering some counterweight. Multivariate analysis is helpful to achieve various analytic ends, but its problems are often underestimated. Furthermore, there are multiple purposes for multivariate modeling, and the methods for model construction and inference differ depending on the purpose. These issues are glossed over surprisingly often in courses that deal with multivariate modeling.

To balance these influences, I suggest emphasizing the importance of conducting stratified analysis as a primary analysis. Even in the face of many confounders, the inferences drawn from a well conducted stratified analysis will usually seldom be modified by a multivariate analysis. The approach to multivariate analysis is conceptually similar to that of stratified analysis, from the evaluation of confounding to the evaluation of interaction. My teaching emphasizes caution in respect to multivariate models, which have more pitfalls than stratified analysis but have become fashionable, presumably because the technology allows such analyses to be conducted more readily.

Many teachers employ computer labs and give students datasets to conduct logistic regression analyses, or Poisson regression or other sophisticated analyses. Conducting these analyses will not make the students into sophisticated analysts. On the contrary, I suggest that the epidemiology teacher leave these computer labs to the statistics courses and place the emphasis instead on pencil and paper analyses. The power of thought is much more potent an analytic tool than the power of computation.

Analysis of multi-level or continuous exposures

The evaluation of trend in epidemiologic data analysis is an analytic area that has been extremely weak. For decades the only trend evaluation in a typical paper has been a declaration of the presence or absence of a 'statistically significant' trend. This reversion to qualitative thinking occurred even in papers that were much more careful to quantify effects in the analyses based on dichotomized exposures.

The main teaching point is to maintain the quantitative outlook in the evaluation of trend. One approach is simply to estimate trend rather than to evaluate it by significance tests. Reporting slope coefficients can accomplish this goal. The drawback of this approach is that the shape of the trend curve is determined by the parametric form of the statistical model used. Therefore it is worth considering less restrictive alternatives. These alternatives are typically graphical presentations, such as spline regression or other smoothing methods that depict trend curves that follow the pattern of the actual data-points, rather than a fully parametric model (Greenland, 1995). These points are easily conveyed by appropriate illustrations and some teaching examples.

Assessing students' achievements

Assessing performance in a course serves both the students and the teacher, by allowing both to gauge progress toward the course goal. In a formal course I suggest frequent quizzes so that both professor and student can adapt their activity as needed during the course, a process that we might aptly call 'course corrections'. Psychologists tell us that feedback should be prompt if it is to be effective. I give short quizzes and go over the answers to all questions in class immediately after each quiz, to give the students prompt feedback. I grade the quizzes right after class to get my own prompt feedback. My preference for quizzes is to ask short multiple choice questions about major points covered. A good question is one that the student would have no idea about without the class and which is easy to answer after the class. Among the choices for each question I always include an option that indicates that the student does not know the answer. If a student chooses that option, he or she gets half credit for the question, which is considerably better than a wrong answer. This device is intended to simulate the real-world situation in which offering a wrong answer is much worse than indicating lack of knowledge.

Conclusion

The above discussion is merely an outline of the main teaching points and methods for a first course in epidemiologic methods. The choice and construction of the exercises and teaching examples, as well as choices about specific didactic methods such as seminars, laboratories, class discussions, and so forth, will bear heavily on the success or failure of the course. I hope that these suggestions serve to point the teacher who faces this daunting task in a promising direction.

References

Crombie, I. K., Tomenson, J. Detection bias in endometrial cancer. *Lancet* 1981; **2**, 308–9.

Greenland, S. Dose-response and trend analysis in epidemiology: alternatives to categorical analysis. *Epidemiology* 1995; **6**, 356–65.

Horwitz, R. I., Feinstein, A. R., Horwitz, S. W., Robboy, S. J. Necropsy diagnosis of endometrial cancer and detection-bias in case-control studies. *Lancet* 1981; **2**, 66–8.

Hulka, B. S, Grimson, R. C., Greenberg, B. G. Endometrial cancer and detection bias. *Lancet* 1981; **2**, 817.

Johnson, S. K., Johnson, R. E. Tonsillectomy history in Hodgkin's disease. *N Engl J Med* 1972; **287**, 1122–5.

Lang, J., Rothman, K. J., Cann, C. I. That confounded *P*-value. *Epidemiology* 1998; **XX**: 7–8.

Merletti, F., Cole, P. Detection bias and endometrial cancer. *Lancet* 1981; **2**, 579–80.

Morgenstern, H., Kleinbaum, D. G., Kupper, L. L. Measures of disease incidence used in epidemiologic research. *Int J Epidemiol* 1980; **9**, 97–104.

Poole, C. Beyond the confidence interval. *Am J Public Health* 1987; **77**, 195–9.

Reintjes, R., de Boer, A., van Pelt, W., Mintjes-de Groot, J. Simpson's paradox: an example from hospital epidemiology. *Epidemiology* 2000; **11**, 81–3.

Rothman, K. J. Causes. *Am J Epidemiol* 1976; **104**, 587–92.

Rothman, K. J., Greenland, S. *Modern epidemiology*, 2nd edn. Lippincott–Raven, Philadelphia, 1998: Chapters 2 and 8.

Siemiatycki, J., Thomas, D. C. Biological models and statistical interactions: an example from multistage carcinogenesis. *Int J Epidemiol* 1981; **10**, 383–7.

Thompson, R. S., Rivara, F. P., Thompson, DC. A case-control study of the effectiveness of bicycle safety helmets. *N Engl J Med* 1989; **320**, 1361–7.

Exposure oriented epidemiology

Chapter 7

Biomarkers

Paolo Boffetta and Nathaniel Rothman

Introduction

A biomarker is commonly defined as any substance, structure, or process that can be measured in the human body or in its products and which may influence or predict the occurrence or outcome of disease (Toniolo *et al.*, 1997). Biomarkers are classified into markers of exposure, effect, susceptibility, and disease. In this chapter, exposure biomarkers will be discussed primarily; most teaching activities, however, encompass all types of biomarkers, with an increasing emphasis on genetic markers.

The application of biomarkers to epidemiology is not a new approach (for review see Schulte, 1993). In particular, the epidemiology of cardiovascular and infectious diseases has long included in its armamentarium a number of approaches which today would be included under the umbrella of biomarkers.

In recent years, however, the interest of epidemiologists in measurement of markers of exposure, effect, and susceptibility in biological media has grown substantially in essentially all branches of the field. This is due to several factors:

1. Greater understanding of the clinical pathogenesis of many diseases, leading to new hypotheses that can be tested in observational and intervention epidemiological studies.

2. Advances in chemical, physical, immunological, and molecular methods to measure exogenous and endogenous exposures.

3. Advances in molecular biology and genetics to evaluate a wide range of inherited risk factors.

4. A trend towards logistic ease and cost-effectiveness in the collection, processing, and, increasingly, automated analysis of biomarkers.

5. A sense that the standard tools of epidemiology must be enhanced to evaluate low level risks, risks associated with complex exposures, and risks that are extensively modified by other (e.g. genetic) factors.

These trends have given rise to the creation of a new discipline, often termed 'molecular epidemiology' (Schulte and Perera, 1993a).

Given the rapidly evolving nature and importance of the application of biomarkers in epidemiology, courses are required for students and practitioners at all levels. These include:

1. Practising epidemiologists and laboratory scientists who seek intensive, short-term courses to cover basic issues.

2. Students in a general epidemiology or laboratory-based graduate program who need either a few lectures on basic principles or who might benefit from one or two full-length courses that develop the issues more extensively.

3. Students seeking training at doctoral level in an epidemiology program who have a major interest in laboratory-based methods, or doctoral students in a laboratory-based program interested in the application of biological methods to epidemiological studies.

4. Postdoctoral fellows carrying out molecular epidemiology studies.

We begin with a description of the teaching objectives and format for an intensive, week-long course in molecular epidemiology targeted at both practising epidemiologists and laboratory scientists which is based on recent experience offering such a course. Clearly, even briefer (e.g. 1-day) courses can be presented to epidemiologists or laboratory scientists on these topics. We then discuss how the general approach and goals of this type of course can be applied and expanded for the scenarios described above.

Teaching objectives

Given the heterogeneity of the students of a typical course in molecular-based epidemiology targeted at professionals in the field, it is useful to set different teaching objectives according to the background of the participants (Table 7.1). In case of a training course for graduate students in 'molecular epidemiology', both sets of objectives listed in Table 7.1 should be met at a greater level of detail. In other words, the general objectives of a course for professional epidemiologists and laboratory scientists are, on the one hand, to enhance the efficacy of a collaboration between disciplines, helping mutual understanding but without the need for a full acquisition of the techniques of each other's discipline (similar objectives are set for a course in biomarker-based epidemiology included in a traditional program in epidemiology). On the other hand, students in a program of molecular epidemiology should be able to design and conduct a proper epidemiologic study as well as measure the relevant biomarkers in the laboratory.

Teaching contents

Training activities in molecular epidemiology encompass three sets of issues:

1. Epidemiologic study design and analysis.
2. Laboratory techniques and their applications.
3. Those specific to biomarker-based studies.

Emphasis on one or the other group of issues depends mainly on the needs and knowledge of the participants.

Table 7.1 Teaching objectives in biomarker-based epidemiology (advanced course for professionals in the field)

Background	Objective	Examples of what participants should be able to do
Epidemiologists	To learn the foundations of modern techniques in molecular biology, biochemistry, analytic chemistry, immunologic methods, etc.	To understand the basics of molecular methods used in a molecular epidemiology study
	To understand the application of these methods to measuring specific classes of exposure, effect, susceptibility, and disease biomarkers	To discuss with molecular biologists the advantages and disadvantages of using alternative approaches in collaborative studies
	To learn specific methodologic issues in the use of biomarkers in epidemiologic studies, including biomarker selection; biologic sample collection, processing and storage; assay quality control and measurement error; potential biases; statistical analysis; ethical issues	To assess potential sources of bias in molecular epidemiology studies (e.g. influence of sample processing and storage, validity and r eproducibility of assays
	To understand the biologic significance of biomarker-based measurements and incorporate this information into further understanding the disease of interest	To address these issues in the discussion of results of molecular epidemiology studies
Laboratory scientists	To learn the basic concepts of epidemiology (study base, bias, confounding, random error, and effect modification)	To understand the basics of the epidemiologic methods used in a molecular epidemiology study
	To learn specific issues in biomarker-based epidemiology (transitional studies, ethical issues, etc.)	To contribute to the epidemiologic aspects in the preparation of a protocol of a molecular epidemiology study
	To identify the potential applications of biomarkers (in particular those of their particular expertise) to epidemiology	To discuss with epidemiologists the advantages and disadvantages of using alternative approaches in collaborative studies

Issues in design and analysis of biomarker-based epidemiologic studies

It is important to present and discuss the fundamentals of epidemiologic methods, including aspects such as:

- study base
- types of study design
- selection and information bias, with emphasis on measurement error
- confounding
- measures of occurrence and association
- univariate and multivariate statistical analysis
- interaction
- power, study size.

The reader is referred to the specific chapters of the book for a detailed discussion of these general methodological issues in epidemiology. It is obvious that, even when discussing general epidemiological methods, examples should be selected preferably from biomarker-based studies.

The presentation of basic topics of epidemiologic methodology is particularly important if some of the participants have no epidemiologic background and experience. The most important concepts, if the brevity of the training program imposes severe choices are, in our view, bias, confounding, and sample size. The goal of such a brief introduction to epidemiology for laboratory scientists is mainly to enable the participants to interact with epidemiologists in the planning, conduct, and interpretation of biomarker-based studies. In this instance, the discussion of possible reasons for false-negative and false-positive results is often the main point of disagreement between researchers from the two different fields. In this chapter, we denote as 'laboratory sciences' the ensemble of experimental disciplines which may contribute to biomarker-based epidemiology, including among others molecular biology, molecular genetics, molecular toxicology, biochemistry, microbiology (and virology in particular), and molecular pathology.

It is particularly important to stress the importance of validation research needed before a new biomarker can be effectively applied in an epidemiologic study. Although the validation of any new instrument in epidemiologic research is a common need, there are particular aspects that apply uniquely to biologic markers. To emphasize the importance of this area of research, Barbara Hulka introduced the term 'transitional studies', which bridges the gap between laboratory methods and their application in epidemiologic studies (Hulka, 1991). Other authors (Schulte, 1992; Schulte *et al.*, 1993; Rothman *et al.*, 1995; Schulte and Perera, 1997) have extended the concept and provided a more general theoretical framework for these types of studies.

It is useful to distinguish transitional studies into three functional groups: developmental, characterization, and applied studies (Rothman *et al.*, 1995; Schulte and Perera, 1997) (Table 7.2). These portray the sequence of research questions that generally need to be addressed to use a promising biomarker effectively in epidemiologic

Table 7.2 Types of transitional studies for exposure biomarkers

Type of study	Aims	Characteristics
Developmental	Development of biomarkers	Builds on experimental studies
		Test assay in human samples
		Evaluate biologic sample collection, processing, and storage
		Evaluate assay accuracy, precision
Characterization	Validation of biomakers	Assessment of biomarker range in representative human populations
		Evaluation of external (or internal) exposure-biomarker relationship, biomarker kinetics, and potential confounders and effect modifiers
Applied	Use in cross-sectional, metabolic, panel studies	Evaluation of exposure status of various populations and further validation of the biomarker

studies. The distinctions between these study categories are less important than conveying to students the overall study goals. Often, aspects of all three study types are combined into the same research project. In the case of exposure biomarkers, these studies evaluate the following:

– assay precision and accuracy
– optimal protocols for collection, processing, and storage
– analyte stability
– biomarker kinetics
– distribution in representative populations
– intra-subject *versus* inter-subject variation over relevant time period
– exogenous and endogenous factors that influence the biomarker.

Special attention should be given to introducing and discussing the concepts of sensitivity, specificity, and predictive value of biomarkers. While these concepts apply to all areas of epidemiology, they are particularly relevant to biomarker-based studies, since the sources of variability in measurements based on biomarkers are usually more numerous than those acting on other types of measurement used in epidemiology. The validity issues should in particular be presented and discussed within the framework of the technical sources of variability, which depend on the laboratory methods used to measure the biomarker. While it is difficult to cover the sources of technical variability of all possible biomarkers, the following concepts should be included:

– random and systematic error
– sensitivity, specificity, and predictive value of a test

- reliability, reproducibility, and repeatability
- laboratory drift
- internal and external validity
- statistical approaches to assess validity.

Three references that might be used in this context are the papers by Vineis *et al.* (1993), Schulte and Perera (1993b), and Schulte and Mazzuckelli (1991).

Sometimes an exposure biomarker may have utility only to evaluate exposure status in cross-sectional or metabolic studies. In other instances, the biomarker may have application in the direct evaluation of disease risk in prospective cohort studies (and less often in case control studies because of a potential disease and other sources of bias). Here, transitional studies provide the critical data needed to determine if and how a biomarker should be used.

Issues in application of laboratory techniques

We assume that non-laboratory scientists participating in an intensive course on molecular epidemiology will have a basic background in molecular biology and toxicology, and possess some understanding of the underlying pathogenesis of the disease on which they and the course focus. If that is not the case, some basic introductory material may need to be covered.

A basic introduction to laboratory techniques used to measure biomarkers is usually needed, in particular when the students have limited or no experience of laboratory work. Given the variety of molecular biology approaches that can be used, it is useful to direct the training toward generally used methods, unless the course is focused on particular exposures (e.g. nutrition, environment, infectious agents, etc.) or diseases (e.g. cancer, cardiovascular disease, etc.). General analytic methods in common use include HPLC, GC/MS, and immunological methods (e.g. ELISA, RIA). General molecular methods focus on the isolation and analysis of DNA and RNA. Basic techniques should be covered (e.g. PCR with detection by restriction enzyme digestion, DNA sequencing), but it should also be made clear that this area is undergoing rapid change (e.g. chip technology). Clearly, any course needs to be updated with regard to current and foreseeable technologies.

The primary approach to teaching laboratory methods in a short course is often, out of necessity, at the theoretical level. In general, however, it is useful to organize (even in short courses) at least one session in a laboratory, where inexperienced participants are exposed to a very basic component of the laboratory work (e.g. part of a PCR or one step in a robot-based DNA extraction), including safety issues. Direct exposure to the reading and scoring of outputs of laboratory measurements (gels, chromatograms, pathology images, etc.) is also very helpful. Apart from learning, admittedly at a superficial level, key aspects of important technologies, it is even more important to develop the ability to assess possible sources of error in biomarker measurement. A general introduction to the principles of measurement error should be presented, with a focus on how to evaluate it, how to identify its sources, how to control it in the laboratory, and how to account for it statistically.

Issues specific to epidemiologic studies involving the use of biomarkers

Occasionally, training activities can be organized on issues that are specific to bio-marker-based epidemiologic studies. Table 7.3 provides a list of issues which may fall into this category. These training activities tend to be quite specialized, and are typically targeted at professionals in the field. For these reasons they tend to be rather brief (typically one or a few days, in the form of a workshop or a short course).

Teaching methods and format

We have described above three possible target audiences for training in biomarker-based epidemiology: practising epidemiologists and laboratory scientists, students in a general epidemiology program, and students in a molecular epidemiology program. In the first two cases, the teaching format consists of a relatively short course, typically a 1-week intensive course or a one-semester course with weekly sessions of 2–3 hours. The total duration of the lectures and practical sessions is therefore of the order of 20–40 hours. A discussion of biomarker-based methods may be introduced in a course of general epidemiology in the form of one or a few specific lectures. Doctoral programs in molecular epidemiology have also recently been introduced in American universities.

Short course for professionals

The choice of topics to be covered in a short course on biomarker-based epidemiology for professionals in the field obviously depends on the outcome of interest (cancer, cardiovascular diseases, infectious diseases, etc.). However, it is possible to identify some general characteristics, which are included in the proposed outline of the course in molecular cancer epidemiology presented in Table 7.3.

It is useful to visit a molecular biology laboratory during the introductory session (see below). However, the inclusion of a full experiment (e.g. measure of DNA adducts in a biological sample) is not recommended, because most experiments require repeated steps of little educational value and it is difficult to guarantee the access of a relatively large group of students to the details of the key aspects of the technique (e.g. electrophoresis).

One important aspect is the splitting of participants early in the course into parallel sessions on basic epidemiology and on molecular biology, each targeted at professionals of the other discipline. This approach might be criticized since it does not favor interaction among participants with different backgrounds (which is, after all, one of the objectives of the course). However, in practice it has proven to be an efficient way to improve the access of participants to intermediate and advanced concepts and methods of unfamiliar disciplines. The typical duration of the introductory sessions is 1–1.5 days. It is useful that the introductory session on molecular biology techniques includes a visit to a laboratory. A practical demonstration of a PCR amplification may be organized during the visit, given the importance of this technique in many biomarker-based methods and its accessibility for a group of students in a relatively short time.

Table 7.3 Outline of a course in molecular cancer epidemiology

Opening session
Keynote lecture: historical overview of molecular epidemiology
Session 1 – Basic techniques
Session 1A – Primer of epidemiology for laboratory scientists
study design
bias and confounding
explorative and univariate data analysis
Session 1B – Primer of laboratory techniques for epidemiologists
genotyping by PCR
search for mutations
technology of DNA and protein adducts
HPLC, GC/MS
laboratory quality control
Session 2 – Molecular dosimetry: techniques and methods
DNA adducts and protein adducts
From adduction to DNA damage
Application of DNA and protein adducts to epidemiologic studies*
Session 3 – Genetic susceptibility
High penetrance cancer genes
Low penetrance genes (metabolic polymorphisms)
DNA repair
Epidemiologic studies of metabolic polymorphisms and DNA repair*
Session 4 – Genetic damage
Acquired mutations and mutational spectra: oncogenes
Acquired mutations and mutational spectra: tumor suppressor genes
Cytogenetic damage
Epidemiologic studies of acquired mutations*
Session 5 – Epidemiologic methods
Transitional studies*
Case control and cohort studies*
Bias and confounding
Misclassification
Interaction and effect modification
Stratified and multivariate statistical analysis
Session 6 – Issues in molecular epidemiology
Ethical aspects of biomarker-based studies
The future of molecular epidemiology
Course overview and evaluation

* This includes critical reading of papers of relevant studies and presentation of ongoing studies by participants.

Experience has shown that it is preferable to concentrate the presentation and discussion of biomarker-based techniques by subject matter (for cancer research these would be: interaction with DNA, host response, acquired alterations, etc.) and to discuss epidemiological issues common to different types of biomarker-based studies in a separate session.

Each session of the course presented in Table 7.3 (except the first one) lasts between 0.5 and 1 day. The practical exercises consist mainly of critical reading of reports of relevant studies and of the discussion of planned or ongoing projects by participants.

One important aspect of any short course in molecular epidemiology is the heterogeneity of the laboratory methods to be reviewed. This requires a relatively large number of lecturers, each an expert in a particular technique. For example, the course outlined in Table 7.3 requires separate lecturers for DNA adduction, high penetrance genes, low penetrance genes, DNA repair, and acquired mutations. Additional lecturers with an epidemiologic background are required, who should guarantee the continuity among the technical sessions.

A short course in molecular epidemiology can be complemented by a more technical course on molecular biology for epidemiologists. In this case, the course in molecular epidemiology emphasizes the methodologic issues in the application of biomarkers, including validation, transitional studies, and interaction analysis, without the need to address the technical aspects of the assays used to measure the biomarkers. This approach is best suited for summer schools of epidemiology, where the two courses can be offered in parallel or during subsequent weeks or as full semester courses.

The available textbooks on biomarker-based epidemiology (Hulka *et al.*, 1990; Schulte and Perera, 1993a; Toniolo *et al.*, 1997) have not been specifically designed for teaching purposes. The recent textbooks on general epidemiologic methods (Kelsey *et al.*, 1996; Rothman and Greenland, 1998; Dos Santos Silva, 1999) do not include a separate discussion of biomarker-based epidemiologic studies, which probably reflects the perception of their authors that there are no major methodologic issues specific to this type of study.

Specific lectures in a general epidemiology course

For students in general epidemiology graduate programs, a discussion of key biomarker-based methods described previously might be introduced in a course of general epidemiology in the form of one or a few specific lectures. Obviously, this approach only allows a superficial overview of the advantages and problems of molecular epidemiology. In our view, the following topics should receive priority in the selection of topics: rationale for the use of biomarkers, transitional studies with focus on precision, accuracy, and validation of biomarkers, and ethical issues in the application of biomarkers to epidemiology. A useful tool for a general lecture is the consensus report included in the book by Toniolo and colleagues (Workshop report, 1997).

For students who wish to gain a broader background in biomarker-based epidemiology, it is probably optimal to establish two full semester courses; one that covers relevant analytic methods and a subsequent course that covers the design, conduct, analysis, and interpretation of molecular epidemiology studies discussed previously. Both could be integrated into one course, but this may not be preferable.

For students in laboratory based programs that are within or in close proximity to schools of public health or departments that teach related courses, a basic background in epidemiology can be obtained by taking an introductory course in epidemiology. Students interested in the direct application of biomarkers to human populations could then take the course described above on the design and conduct of molecular epidemiology studies. As with short-term courses in molecular epidemiology, it has been our experience that longer duration classes benefit substantially by having students from both general disciplines represented. This helps particularly during discussions of how to establish effective and respectful collaborations between epidemiologists and laboratory investigators. Further, students can be formed into 'interdisciplinary' groups and asked to develop a research proposal, which can be the main approach to evaluation.

Doctoral training in molecular epidemiology

There are several US programs that offer doctoral training in molecular epidemiology. Some are essentially genetics programs while others are based more broadly. Fundamentally, we believe that the vast majority of practitioners of biologically based epidemiology will spend essentially all of their time, after training, either in the laboratory or designing, carrying out, and analysing epidemiologic studies. As such, we believe that one needs to be a fully trained epidemiologist or laboratory scientist to be a successful practitioner. That said, there is a rationale and a need for doctoral programs in molecular epidemiology, as long as a student has a primary department and obtains the same quality training as other students in that department. Such programs would provide the infrastructure and support to allow epidemiology graduate students to take basic coursework in relevant laboratory based areas and to spend time obtaining pertinent laboratory experience. This is particularly important for students who do not have an undergraduate background in biology, chemistry, or a related discipline, or previous laboratory experience. The actual methods students learn will inevitably become obsolete; more importantly, obtaining an in-depth laboratory experience will provide them with a better understanding of the nature and dynamics of the laboratory environment. This will help in analysing data from future laboratory collaborators and should enhance their ability to develop successful collaborations. Similarly, doctoral students in the laboratory sciences could take basic courses in epidemiology and biostatistics, perhaps leading to a degree of master in public health, as well as participate in biomarker-based research in collaboration with the epidemiology faculty.

Postdoctoral fellowships in molecular epidemiology

There are an increasing number of postdoctoral fellowships in molecular epidemiology being offered at schools of public health and government research institutes, primarily in the USA and the UK. This reflects the rapidly expanding need for investigators in this area. These programs vary, but often include a didactic component and experience in both laboratory and epidemiologic aspects of research. The exact mixture of activities depends on the goals of the program, available faculty, and background and interests of the fellows. Again, an important theme is that after training, a researcher needs to be fully qualified to function as either an epidemiologist or as a laboratory investigator, regardless of the term used to describe their position. This should be a guiding principle for students seeking to work in this exciting and expanding research field.

Assessing students' achievements

The short-term achievements of participants in molecular epidemiology training can be assessed with projects or exams. Students' views of the immediate success of a training program can be assessed with course/program evaluations. Formal longer term assessment is of great importance. Surveying students at some time in the future about the impact that a given course or program had on their career, as well as obtaining suggestions for course improvements, would be beneficial given that there is very little experience in teaching molecular epidemiology. Obtaining data on new interdisciplinary projects started by trainees and relevant publications would also be helpful.

References

Dos Santos Silva, I. (1999). *Cancer epidemiology: principles and methods.* International Agency for Research on Cancer, Lyon.

Hulka, B. S. (1991). Epidemiologic studies using biological markers: issues for epidemiologists. *Cancer Epidemiol Biomarkers Prev,* **1**, 13–19.

Hulka, B. S., Wilcosky, T. C., and Griffith, J. D., eds (1990). *Biological markers in epidemiology.* Oxford University Press, New York.

Kelsey, J. L., Whittemore, A. S., Evans, A. S., and Thompson, W. D. (1996). *Methods in observational epidemiology,* 2nd edn. Monographs in Epidemiology and Biostatistics, Vol. 26. Oxford University Press, New York.

Rothman, K. J. and Greenland, S., eds (1998) *Modern epidemiology,* 2nd edn. Lippincott-Raven Publishers, Philadelphia.

Rothman, N., Stewart, W. F., and Schulte, P. A. (1995). Incorporating biomarkers into cancer epidemiology: a matrix of biomarker and study design categories. *Cancer Epidemiol Biomarkers Prev,* **4**, 301–11.

Schulte, P. A. (1992). The use of biological markers in occupational health research and practice. *J Toxicol Env Health,* **40**, 359–66.

Schulte, P. A. (1993). A conceptual and historical framework for molecular epidemiology. In: *Molecular epidemiology: principles and practices* (eds P. A. Schulte and F. P. Perera), pp. 3–44. Academic Press, San Diego.

Schulte, P. and Mazzuckelli, L. P. (1991). Validation of biological markers for quantitative risk assessment. *Environ Health Perspect,* **90**, 239–46.

Schulte, P. A. and Perera, F. P., eds (1993a). *Molecular epidemiology: principles and practices.* Academic Press, San Diego.

Schulte, P. A. and Perera, F. P. (1993b) Validation. In: *Molecular epidemiology: principles and practices* (eds P. A. Schulte and F. P. Perera), pp. 79–107. Academic Press, San Diego.

Schulte, P. A. and Perera, F. P. (1997) Transitional studies. In: *Application of biomarkers in cancer epidemiology,* IARC Scientific Publications No. 142 (eds P. Toniolo, P. Boffetta, D. E. G. Shuker, N. Rothman, B. Hulka, and N. Pearce), pp. 19–29. International Agency for Research on Cancer, Lyon.

Schulte, P. A., Rothman, N., and Schottenfeld, D. (1993). Design considerations in molecular epidemiology. In: *Molecular epidemiology: principles and practices* (eds P. A. Schulte and F. P. Perera), pp. 159–98. Academic Press, San Diego.

Toniolo, P., Boffetta, P., Shuker, D. E. G., Rothman, N., Hulka, B., and Pearce, N., eds (1997). *Application of biomarkers in cancer epidemiology*, IARC Scientific Publications No. 142. International Agency for Research on Cancer, Lyon.

Vineis, P., Schulte, P. A., Vogt, R. F., Jr (1993) Technical variability in laboratory data. In: *Molecular epidemiology: principles and practices* (eds P. A. Schulte and F. P. Perera), pp. 109–35. Academic Press, San Diego.

Workshop report (1997) Application of biomarkers in cancer epidemiology. In: *Application of biomarkers in cancer epidemiology*, IARC Scientific Publications No. 142 (eds P. Toniolo, P. Boffetta, D. E. G. Shuker, N. Rothman, B. Hulka, and N. Pearce), pp. 1–18. International Agency for Research on Cancer, Lyon.

Chapter 8

Questionnaires in epidemiology

Jakob Bue Bjørner and Jørn Olsen

Introduction

The use of questionnaires is an essential epidemiologic tool. Epidemiologic findings are often based on responses to questionnaires, which are used extensively for collecting information on exposures, outcomes, modifiers, and confounders. In such studies, high quality questionnaire data are a prerequisite for drawing valid conclusions. Questionnaires should be designed and used so that they are acceptable to all participants, the response rates are high, and the responses have maximal validity (absence of systematic error/information bias) and reliability (minimal random error).

The design and use of questionnaires requires language skills (e.g. in writing questions that are easy to understand and unambiguously phrased) and some theory (e.g. a basic understanding of the cognitive processes of a person who responds to questionnaire items). Teaching must therefore combine practical training and theoretical topics. The use of questionnaires requires relevant study design, data collection, data processing, statistical analysis, ethics, and privacy. No single step can be understood fully without some knowledge of the other steps. We recommend providing an initial broad overview of the topics pertaining to questionnaires to provide background and perspective, and thereafter giving a step by step introduction to each of the practical tasks of questionnaire development, validation, and use.

Question writing is particularly suited to practical training during a course. Students should first be shown examples of good and poor questionnaires (for sources of questionnaires, see below). They should then write a short questionnaire (on simple issues like smoking, visits to the GP, etc.) and they should comment on each others' drafts.

Students should exercise their question writing skills to experience how difficult it is to ask good questions and to learn to recognize good questions. However, it is very important that they do not reinvent the wheel. Standard questions and standard questionnaires should be used whenever possible, but only after pilot testing in the study population in question. Validity and reliability are not fixed properties of a questionnaire but depend on the match between the questionnaire, the study purpose, and the respondent. Students should recognize that questionnaires used for self-administration need to be simpler than questionnaires used in an interview. As a principle, questionnaires for self-administration need to be short and without complicated branching. They must be easy to fill out and appear well designed, with a professional finish.

Teaching objectives

1. Students should know the basics of questionnaire design (specifying a variable list, writing questions, designing response choices, and planning the coding of the answers), and they should be able to apply these principles in writing simple questionnaires on their own. They should be aware of the need for testing and revising the questionnaire several times.

2. Students should know the main data collecting methods that use questionnaires (e.g. postal surveys, phone interviews, face-to-face interviews), they should be able to evaluate the strengths and weaknesses of each data collection method for a particular study, and they should be able to design the questionnaire taking the chosen data collection method into account.

3. The students should know important sources for standard questionnaires and be able to perform an effective search for standard questionnaires for a given research topic.

4. Students should know basic approaches to pilot testing a questionnaire and be able to perform such a pilot test.

5. Students should know how questionnaire data are to be processed (e.g. coding, keypunching, data cleaning) and be able to design the questionnaire and the data collection to enable data processing.

6. The students should be aware that crosscultural issues may play a role in questionnaire administration and data interpretation.

7. Finally, students need an understanding of basic psychometric concepts (e.g. reliability, validity, discrimination, sensitivity, and specificity) and how such measurement properties may be affected by questionnaire and study design (e.g. differential recall bias in case control studies).

Students should also realize that designing questionnaires covering new ground is a job that requires experience and skills that go beyond what they learn in a single course. Besides using validated questionnaires as much as possible they should also seek professional advice.

Teaching contents

Overview

Initially, examples could be given to illustrate different formats, show examples of good questionnaires, define the concept of an item (a question and its response options), and introduce the different data collection methods that make use of questionnaires (e.g. paper-and-pencil survey, personal interviews, phone interviews, computerized surveys). Examples of questionnaires could come from well known epidemiologic studies or from other work with which the teacher is familiar. Some sources of general surveys are the US National Center for Health Statistics (current www-address www.cdc.gov.nchs), the Inter-University Consortium for Political and Social Research located at the University of Michigan (current www-address www.icpsr.umich.edu), and the Center for Applied Social Surveys in the UK (current www-address www.scpr.ac.uk/class). Further, a variety of sources exists for question-naires about health status (McDowell and Newell, 1996; Ware *et al.*, 1993). The latter source (the manual of the SF-36 questionnaire (Ware *et al.*, 1993)) also illustrates how the same items can be changed in layout to suit different data collection methods.

A general introduction to the methods of questionnaire research could cover the fol-lowing topics: questionnaire design and the properties of high quality questionnaires, methods of data collection, important sources of random and systematic error (and the concepts of reliability and validity), data processing, and issues in data analysis.

Properties of good questionnaires

The fields of questionnaire research and psychometrics use a bewildering number of terms to describe the properties of good questionnaires. Although students need not know this terminology, it is best to focus on the relations between a moderate number of well defined concepts that are introduced gradually (see Ware *et al.*, 1993 for short definitions of psychometric concepts). Basically, the concepts deal with general meas-urement properties: that you measure what you intend to measure and that your measuring instrument is as independent as possible of the situation in which it is used. The initial discussion should focus on criteria that can be evaluated by looking at the questionnaire. The concept of content validity could be introduced with a dis-cussion of whether the items in a questionnaire match the variables we want to meas-ure. Further, standard criteria for good item writing should be discussed. The items should be (Stone, 1993; Streiner and Norman, 1989):

1. Appropriate for the group to be studied.

2. Intelligible (this implies using a reading level that all respondents can understand, avoiding double negatives, using common language, and avoiding jargon).

3. Concerned with only one topic for each item.

4. Unambiguous (i.e. the researcher and all the respondents should understand the questions the same way regardless of their age, sex., ethnic, or social background).

5. Without value-laden words.

6. Omnicompetent (i.e. capable of coping with all possible experiences of the respondents regarding the topic) and, in case closed-form response choices are used, the response choices should be mutually exclusive and exhaustive. The respondent should always be able to find an appropriate answer (options such as 'don't know', 'not relevant' have their (limited) use).

7. Paper-and-pencil questionnaires should have appropriate visual design (large enough fonts, simple and not too compact visual form, the appearance should be professional and serious, and all response options placed horizontally or all response options placed vertically).

Questionnaire design

The process of designing a questionnaire could be taught in a step-by-step manner. Item development should be guided by a *variable list*, which should by kept as short as possible by excluding the items for which no clear use in the data analysis is foreseen. It should be emphasized that the reuse of relevant items from previous studies is preferable to developing items anew, but in some cases writing new items is necessary.

General survey research distinguishes between measurement of *attitudes* and measurement of *behavior* (see, for example, Sudman and Bradburn, 1982). In epidemiology, *attitudes* are all the things that can only be assessed through information from the respondent (symptoms, self-rated health, personality traits, etc.), while *behavior* could also be assessed by somebody else (number of cigarettes smoked, occupational exposures, etc.). The distinction has implications for the ways the question can be phrased, the possible response options, and the methods that can be used to evaluate the validity of the answers.

Although the response options are an integral part of the item, the topic warrants special discussion. For questions about quantities, the researcher can choose to have the respondent write the specific number or amount (e.g. *When were you born? (Date/Month/Year)* _/_/_) or offer a limited number of response choices. Although there is an advantage in obtaining data which is as precise as possible (information can always be collapsed in the analysis, but not expanded), it is not advisable to require the respondent to provide greater precision than that of which he is capable. If this is done the respondent will make his own guess since there is a tendency to respond even if the answer is unknown. Such guessing produces an unknown source of measurement error. For some pieces of information, where exact quantification is difficult, it is far easier for the respondent to choose between a limited number of response options. For the 'behavior' type of items, typical response options are: confirmation (*yes/no*), nominal categories (e.g. different types of jobs), amount, time, or frequency. For the 'attitude' kind of items, additional response types are: true–false (e.g. with four categories: *definitely true, mostly true, mostly false, definitely false*), agree–disagree, evaluation (e.g. *in excellent health–in poor health,* or *to a large extent–to a small extent*). For yes or no and true or false type questions, double negatives between the question and the response options should be avoided, since this often leads to confusion. This implies phrasing the question without negatives.

Another important issue is the order of items. Start with neutral questions and place sensitive questions at the end of the questionnaire. If the questionnaire has global questions (e.g. *How would you rate your health in general?*) and very specific questions (e.g. *How much bodily pain have you had during the past 4 weeks?*) about the same topic, it is advisable to put the global questions first to avoid framing effects (undue influence of the specific items on the global items).

Finally, teaching should address how best to enable the coding of responses and the data processing.

A number of papers and textbooks have dealt with questionnaire design. This ranges from papers in medical journals (Stone, 1993) to short textbooks (Converse and Presser, 1986; Kelsey *et al.,* 1996) and elaborate textbooks (Streiner and Norman, 1989; American Educational Research Association, 2000). We recommend the short paper by Stone (1993), which could be supplemented by one or more of the textbooks depending on the length of the course. A useful comparison of advantages and disadvantages in using self-administered questionnaires *versus* interviews is given in Armstrong *et al.* (1992).

At this point, it is helpful to introduce an individual exercise in item writing to be discussed thereafter in small groups.

Sources for standard questionnaires

Since the use of standardized items should be strongly encouraged (Olsen, 1998), it is important to locate sources for items. For measurement of health status (e.g. symptom of disease) handbooks incorporating a large number of questionnaires are available (McDowell and Newell, 1996; Bowling 1991; 1995); however, often the search is less straightforward. A typical strategy is to locate the most important studies for the given topic and then contact the authors. Some www sources are available (see above). For Europe, a WHO collaborating project (EUROHIS) (DeBruin *et al.*, 1996) is currently (year 2000) aiming at proposing guidelines for standardized Health Interview Surveys for a number of important topics in epidemiologic research. Most standard questionnaires are free to use but some are restricted.

Cognitive and linguistic research on questionnaires

During the past 20 years, psychologists have studied the cognitive processes involved in answering questionnaires. Items in a questionnaire are not simply answered by retrieving the relevant information from memory. More complex processes are involved, such as question interpretation, retrieval of partial information from memory, and construction of answers based on inference from this partial information (Bradburn *et al.*, 1987). During this process the present situation affects what is being 'remembered' about the past, which is one reason for recall bias. In a study of the risk of spontaneous abortion among hospital personnel, researchers compared questionnaire data and hospital records and showed that, among women exposed to anesthetic gases, 100% of all miscarriages were reported, while among unexposed women only 70% of all miscarriages were reported (Axelsson and Rylander, 1982; see also Hennekens and Buring, 1987).

Some results from cognitive research have direct rule-of-thumb implications for item writing (see, for example, Bradburn *et al.*, 1987, and Converse and Presser, 1986), and suggest new methods for pilot testing (Jobe and Mingay, 1990; see below).

Pretesting and pilot testing of questionnaires

It is important to stress that questionnaire development involves extensive testing and revisions. The first rounds of testing should be performed by the researcher himself (trying to answer your own questionnaire can be a disturbing and very revealing experience), by colleagues, and by supervisors. Translation of the questionnaire to a different language followed by independent back translation may help to spot ambiguous phrasings. When the researcher considers the questionnaire to be without obvious flaws, the time has come for real pilot testing (Converse and Presser, 1986; DeMaio and Rothgeb, 1996). A simple scheme is to have respondents answer the questionnaire and then interview them about the answering process: were the questions appropriate? were they understandable? was the questionnaire too long? The understanding of a sample of items should be checked and, for a few items, one should ask directly about the reasons for giving the specific answer (e.g. *What went through your head when you saw that question?* or *When you gave this answer, what did you think of?*). Although such interviews provide important knowledge, results and statements should be interpreted cautiously. Respondents can be fairly uncritical (Converse and Presser, 1986), and the items preferred by the respondents are not always the items that give the most correct and useful information (Bradburn *et al.*, 1987).

More elaborate techniques involve, for example, think-aloud sessions where the respondent verbalizes his thought process (Jobe and Mingay, 1990; DeMaio and Rothgeb, 1996). At this point, students could try to conduct interviews or think-aloud sessions in small groups.

If a sufficient number of people have answered the questionnaire during pilot testing, preliminary quantitative studies can be performed. Such analyses should focus on the magnitude of non-response, on items where all (or nearly all) responses are in one category (indicating that the response options are not targeted at the population of interest), and on obvious response errors.

Data collection

Students should learn about the main methods of data collection (postal surveys, phone interviews, face-to-face interviews), the advantages and disadvantages of each method, and the implications of the data collection method for questionnaire design (for a good review see Kelsey *et al.*, 1996).

General rules for conducting structured interviews should be outlined. The ways to conduct follow-up to enhance response rates should be discussed as well as the problems related to non-responders and non-responses for part of the questionnaire. Discuss also the possibilities of characterizing non-responders on a few important variables to evaluate the likely effects of non-response. When the data collection involves collaboration with others (perhaps in distributing questionnaires), it is important to stress that their collaboration and enthusiasm are essential for the success of the study.

Data processing

Data processing involves the coding of responses, keypunching or scanning, quality control, and data cleaning. It is important to discuss principles for coding (Ware *et al.*, 1993). It should be emphasized that the coding strategy must be established before data are collected.

When conducting phone interviews or computerized assessment, data processing may be performed simultaneously using computer programs with preprogrammed data entry screens and built-in quality controls (e.g. out of range responses not allowed).

The freeware program Epi-Info (available from WHO and CDC www-servers) has nice data entry facilities. If response codes are keypunched from coded questionnaires directly into ASCII files, it is advisable to conduct the keypunching twice and recheck all cases of discrepancy.

At this point, the students should carry out short exercises in data processing.

Crosscultural issues

Crosscultural issues are of increasing importance in questionnaire research. Most standard questionnaires have been written in English, and the questionnaire has to be translated and adapted when used for respondents with other native languages. A number of steps have to be taken to ensure comparability between the different versions if results are to be generalized across countries (Guillemin *et al.*, 1993; Bullinger *et al.*, 1998). In general, questions should be phrased in the respondents' native language and interviewers should never be asked to translate from a questionnaire written in a different language.

Students at the postgraduate level should have some knowledge of basic methods for testing cross-language equivalence: independent ratings, forwards–backwards translation, and psychometric methods (see below). It should be stressed that sometimes institutional or cultural differences can make it impossible to construct questionnaires that are exactly equivalent (for example, different ways of organizing the educational system makes it difficult to compare education across some countries, pregnancy planning may mean something different in different cultures, a word like wheezing does not exist in all languages).

Basic psychometric concepts

The field of psychometrics is complex and we recommend starting with simple concepts and the use of examples. Initially, issues like data completeness (low frequency of non-response to each item), item discrimination, and floor and ceiling effects should be discussed (Ware *et al.*, 1993; Streiner and Norman, 1989).

In further discussions, we advise focusing on two main unifying concepts: first, random measurement error and, second, systematic (non-random) measurement error. It is convenient to introduce the concept of a latent variable as the measurement which would have been achieved if we had been able to measure without error at all ('true measure').

In epidemiology, items often have yes or no type responses and the latent variable (or the effects of the latent variable) is also conceptualized as taking two values. In this situation, random measurement error of the items is assessed by their specificity and sensitivity. Systematic measurement error involves information bias and differential misclassification.

When the item responses are on a continuous scale (or can at least take a large number of ordered values) and the latent variable is also conceptualized as continuous, the concept of reliability can be introduced in the discussion of random measurement error and that of validity in the discussion of systematic measurement error. Assessment of random and systematic measurement errors in the situations above requires the availability of a gold standard measure (i.e. very close to the true measure).

A common way to deal with random measurement error, and floor and ceiling problems of individual items is to ask several questions about the same topic and combine the answers to these questions (for example, by taking the average of the item responses or using the simple sum of item responses). Such combination of items into a scale assumes unidimensionality, that all items measure the same thing. In principle (ignoring problems of random error, floor, and ceiling) we should reach the same conclusion using any single item or subsample of items in the scale. The statistician Georg Rasch has developed the statistical model implicit in this basic requirement (Rasch, 1966; Andrich, 1988; Fischer and Molenaar, 1995).

The analysis of this type of data is termed latent structure analysis and uses techniques such as factor analysis, structural equation modelling, item response analysis, and latent class analysis. Often, the goal is simply to test the appropriateness of the scale construction, which will be used in a standard statistical analysis. Any of these techniques requires a course by itself and should be restricted to postgraduate teaching in epidemiology, but a few basic concepts and problems may be mentioned. One such concept is the distinction between effect indicator models and cause indicator models (Bollen and Lennox, 1991). Latent structure analysis has been developed in areas where the items are naturally conceptualized as effects of a latent cause (like intelligence, anxiety, and depression). We often encounter concepts where the items must be seen as causes of the latent variable (e.g. education is the cause of being in a certain social class). While data that conform to the effect indicator model can be analyzed by straightforward application of latent structure analysis (and the reliability of the composite scale can be assessed with techniques such as Cronbach's alpha; Carmines and Zeller, 1979), standard application of these techniques is wrong when the items are causal indicators (Bollen and Lennox, 1991). The important requirement for causal indicators is that they have effects on the outcomes of interest that are in the same direction and have approximately the same strength (for discussion of how to test such assumptions see Bollen and Lennox, 1991, and Kreiner, 1993).

Another problem is that the items in multi-item scales are often discrete, while the latent variable is conceptualized as continuous. This discrepancy has traditionally been solved by ignoring the discrete nature of the items (in so-called classical psychometric methods, see Carmines and Zeller, 1979) but, if the items are skewed or have few response categories, treating them as continuous may cause errors. In such situations item-response theory methodology (Andrich, 1988; Fischer and Molenaar, 1995; Kreiner, 1993; Hambleton et al., 1991; van der Linden and Hambleton, 1997) or structural equation modelling of categoric data (Muthen and Muthen, 1998; Browne and Arminger, 1995) should be used.

We do not encourage teaching latent structure analysis in a basic questionnaire course, but suggest providing two cautions in the application of techniques such as exploratory factor analysis and reliability analysis using Cronbach's alpha. These standard techniques assume that data conform to an effect indicator model and that they are measured on a continuous scale.

Teaching method and format

We suggest that undergraduate students are taught the basic principles in at least two lectures. At the postgraduate level, in PhD courses, it is our experience that much more time should be spent on the topic. A 1–2-day course is the minimum and students who work with measuring latent concepts need at least a 1-week course.

For a relatively short course (2–4 lectures), classroom teaching with some individual and group exercises is preferable. For a longer course, students could be assigned to do a small questionnaire study in groups of between three and five. Such a study should take them through all the steps of variable list construction, reviews of existing questionnaires, questionnaire design, data collection, data processing, analysis, and presentation.

Assessing students' achievements

Since the questionnaire topic requires both practical skills and theoretical knowledge, students are best assessed through a combination of item writing and examination.

References

American Educational Research Association (2000). *Standards for educational and psychological testing 1999.* American Psychological Association, Washington DC.

Andrich, D. (1988). *Rasch models for measurement.* Sage Publications, Beverly Hills.

Armstrong, B., White, E., and Saracci, R. (1992). *Principles of exposure measurement in epidemiology.* Oxford University Press, Oxford.

Axelsson, G. and Rylander, R. (1982). Exposure to anaesthetic gases and spontaneous abortion: response bias in a postal questionnaire study. *International Journal of Epidemiology,* 11, 250–6.

Bollen, K. A. and Lennox, R. (1991). Conventional wisdom on measurement: a structural equation perspective. *Psychological Bulletin,* 110, 305–14.

Bowling, A. (1991). *Measuring health—a review of quality of life measurement scales.* Open University Press, Buckingham.

Bowling, A. (1995). *Measuring disease—a review of disease-specific quality of life measurement scales.* Open University Press, Buckingham.

Bradburn, N. M., Rips, L. J., and Shevell, S. K. (1987). Answering autobiographical questions: the impact of memory and inference on surveys. *Science,* 236, 157–61.

Browne, M. W. and Arminger, G. (1995). Specification and estimation of mean- and covariance-structure models. In: *Handbook of statistical modeling for the social and behavioral sciences* (eds G.Arminger, C. Clogg, and M. E. Sobel), pp. 185–250: Plenum Press, New York.

Bullinger, M., Alonso, J., Appolone, G. *et al.* (1998). Translating health status questionnaires and evaluating their quality: the IQOLA project approach. *Journal of Clinical Epidemiology,* 51, 913–23.

Carmines, E. G. and Zeller, R. A. (1979). *Reliability and validity assessment.* Sage Publications, Beverly Hills.

Converse, J. M. and Presser, S. (1986). *Survey questions—handcrafting the standardized questionnaire.* Sage Publications, London.

DeBruin, A., Picavet, H. S. J., and Nossikov, A. (1996). *Health interview surveys. Towards international harmonization of methods and instruments.* WHO Regional Office for Europe, Copenhagen.

DeMaio, T. J. and Rothgeb, J. M. (1996). Cognitive interviewing techniques: in the lab and in the field. In: *Answering questions. Methodology for determining cognitive and communicative processes in survey research* (eds N.Schwarz and S. Sudman), pp. 177–98). Jossey-Bass, San Francisco.

Fischer, G. H. and Molenaar, I. W. (1995). *Rasch models—foundations, recent developments, and applications.* Springer–Verlag, Berlin.

Guillemin, F., Bombardier, C., and Beaton, D. (1993). Cross-cultural adaptation of health-related quality of life measures: literature review and proposed guidelines. *Journal of Clinical Epidemiology,* **46**, 1417–32.

Hambleton, R. K., Swaminathan, H., and Rogers, H. J. (1991). *Fundamentals of item response theory.* Sage Publications, London.

Hennekens, C. H. and Buring, J. E. (1987). *Epidemiology in medicine.* Little, Brown, and Company, Boston.

Jobe, J. B. and Mingay, D. J. (1990). Cognitive laboratory approach to designing questionnaires for surveys of the elderly. *Public Health Reports,* **105**, 518–24.

Kelsey, J. L., Whittemore, A. S., Evans, A. S., and Thompson, W. D. (1996). Measurement I: questionnaires. In: *Methods in observational epidemiology,* pp. 364–90. Oxford University Press, Oxford.

Kreiner, S. (1993). Validation of index scales for analysis of survey data – the symptom index. In: *Population health research – linking theory and methods* (ed. K. Dean), pp. 116–44. Sage Publications, Beverly Hills.

McDowell, I. and Newell, C. (1996). *Measuring health: a guide to rating scales and questionnaires.* Oxford University Press, Oxford.

Muthen, B. O. and Muthen, L. (1998). *Mplus user's guide* [Computer software]. Muthén & Muthén, Los Angeles.

Olsen, J. (1998). Epidemiology deserves better questionnaires. IEA European Questionnaire Group. International Epidemiological Association. *International Journal of Epidemiology,* **27**, 935.

Rasch, G. (1966). An item analysis which takes individual differences into account. *British Journal of Mathematical and Statistical Psychology,* **19**, 49–57.

Stone, D. H. (1993). Design a questionnaire. *British Medical Journal,* **307**, 1264–6.

Streiner, D. L. and Norman, G. R. (1989). *Health measurement scales: a practical guide to their development and use.* Oxford University Press, Oxford.

Sudman, S. and Bradburn, N. M. (1982). *Asking questions. A practical guide to questionnaire design.* Jossey-bass Publishers, San Francisco.

van der Linden, W. J. and Hambleton, R. K. (1997). *Handbook of modern item response theory.* Springer, Berlin.

Ware, J. E., Jr., Snow, K. K., Kosinski, M., and Gandek, B. (1993). *SF-36 health survey. Manual and interpretation guide.* The Health Institute, New England Medical Center, Boston.

Chapter 9

Routine registries

Henrik Toft Sørensen

Introduction

In *Last's Dictionary* a registry is defined as follows:

> In epidemiology, the term 'register' is applied to the file of data concerning all cases of a particular disease or other health-relevant condition in a defined population such that the case can be related to a population base.

The register is the actual document, and the registry is the system of ongoing registration (Last, 1995). This definition only covers disease registries but is too narrow for current epidemiology, since many registry-based studies are based also on exposure registration.

Disease registries have existed in the Nordic countries for many years. The first disease registry was established as early as 1856, with the Leprosy Registry in Norway (Hansen and Looft, 1973). At the beginning of this century, causes of death and cancer registries sprouted in Scandinavia and the UK, and later in other countries.

However, technological development during the last decades has led to a considerable increase in the number of other individual-based data sources such as administrative registries, databases, and information systems that may be of value in epidemiologic research, and the number of studies that are based on registries may be expected to increase.

Teaching objectives

When I teach about the use of routine registries, the basic goals are to give the students insight into:

1. Registries available for research.
2. The strengths and limitations of registry-based research and that registries are a data collection method like other methods, e.g. interview, questionnaires, etc. to obtain an epidemiologic measure.
3. The relation between the research question and the demand for data quality.
4. The basic principles for and terminology about validation of a registry with respect to research.
5. The factors affecting the quality of registry data.

Teaching contents

Registries available for research

Within epidemiology the classic registry is a case registry in which information about a relevant disease or group of diseases (e.g. cancer) is collected: this is often based on notifications. These registries are mainly used for the purpose of surveillance or research. However, many other registries are now available for research and such registry data (Sørensen et al., 1996) are often collected for:

♦ Management, claims, administration, and planning

♦ Evaluation of activities within health care

♦ Control functions.

Regardless of the purpose of the registry, the methodologic problems are the same (Sørensen et al., 1996).

Registries can be used as a sampling frame to select study populations, and to collect information on exposure, diseases, and sometimes confounders (Sørensen et al., 1996; Mortensen, 1995). Registry and primary data are increasingly being combined, for example in Scandinavia, where several cohort studies based on baseline data obtained by interviews or questionnaires are combined with follow-up data from the disease registries.

Strengths and limitations

The student must be clear that the concepts of originality and credibility are essential in all medical research, whether registry-based or not. As in all research matters, planning a study should aim at reducing both systematic and random errors (Mortensen, 1995; Sørensen, 1997). Any study based on registry data should be designed with the same critical approach as studies based on primary data, i.e. specifying hypotheses. Students are often under the mistaken belief that registry-based research is quick and easy. It is also important to emphasize that there is a demand for optimal use and extraction of as much information as possible within the framework of the existing resources, since large data analyses can be very demanding on time and money. In this way, registry-based research is no different from other types of research.

The student must be aware that the use of existing registries in epidemiologic research is because of their many advantages (Sørensen et al., 1996), primarily because the registries already exist; the time spent on the study is therefore likely to be considerably less than that spent on studies using primary data collection. Furthermore, compared with collection of primary data, the costs of the project, and the waste of data, are reduced considerably. There are other advantages of registries:

1. Their large size, which allows for great precision of estimates and makes it possible to study rare exposures, diseases, and outcomes.

2. The completeness of the registries with respect to the people in the target population, which ensures representativeness.

3. The collection of the registry data independently of the research project, which leaves less room for certain types of bias (e.g. recall, non-response, and diagnostic).

4. A number of health factors will appear many years after the exposures.

Existing registries are often suitable (and sometimes the only source) for examination of health conditions when there is a long period between exposure and manifestation of overt disease.

The limitations in using registries are numerous, though they are often ignored and not recognized by students. On the other hand, several students are paralysed by the misclassification that exists in all registry data. The limitations are related to data selection and quality since the methods of data collection are predetermined, not controlled by the researcher, and sometimes impossible to validate. The data required for the research question may not have been collected at all (Sørensen, 1997). Often, it is only the number of cases in an exposed cohort (e.g. number of cancer cases in patients with venous thromboembolism; Sørensen *et al.*, 1998) and the total number of cases in the population that are known. A comparison with the disease incidence in the general population can then be made. The basic problem with methods that use the registries is the degree of completeness and validity of the information, and the possible lack of information on potential confounders. Poor data quality can constitute a permanent obstacle to registry-based research. Another problem is the risk that the relatively large number of available data may lead to data dredging and misleading *post hoc* analysis. How good registry data need to be depends of course on the research question and study design in mind (Sørensen *et al.*, 1996). Lack of experience with programming or lack of collaboration with a programmer may cause potential errors in preparing registry data for analysis or in the analysis.

Factors affecting the quality of registry data and terminology

In basic courses I recommend dividing the factors affecting the quality of registry data into seven sections.

Completeness of registration of persons

This is the proportion of persons in the target population which is correctly classified in the registry. Methods for evaluation of completeness can be divided into two main groups.

An estimate of the degree of completeness can be obtained by **comparing the data source with one or more independent reference sources**, in which the whole (total) or part (partial) of the target population is registered (Goldberg *et al.*, 1980). The comparison is made on a case by case basis. Cases escape even the best registration systems. Some researchers have therefore compared different independent data sources, and the missing cases have been estimated in a capture–recapture model (Sørensen *et al.*, 1996). A mathematical capture–recapture analysis offers the opportunity to estimate the number of cases not registered in the registry and, if the background population is known as well, an estimate of the specificity can be obtained (Sørensen *et al.*, 1996).

Students are often confused by the many different terms that are used in registry validation research. I suggest using the standard terminology for epidemiologic measurement in this context. Validity is the extent to which the study measures what it is intended to measure. Lack of validity is referred to as bias. If this terminology is used, the two most often used validity measures are sensitivity and a predictive value of a positive registration.

The concept of completeness is closely linked to the concept of sensitivity. The validity concept of the registration of cases as used in the literature in the field of validation of registers, the ratio between the number of correctly registered persons (e.g. meningococcal disease) and all registered persons (e.g. all registered persons with meningococcal disease), is, however, closely linked to the concept of the predictive value of a positive registration. A comparison between two data sources alone does not provide the opportunity to estimate specificity. It can be assumed, though, that specificity will be close to one if the background population is large and the disease rather rare.

In the **aggregated methods** the total number of cases in the data source is compared with the total number in other sources, or the expected number of cases is calculated by applying epidemiologic rates from demographically similar populations or by the simulation method, which uses the information system to simulate patterns of incomplete reporting to examine the possible effect on a specific dependent variable (Goldberg *et al.*, 1980).

Record review methods are often used in the validation of diagnosis in hospital discharge registries by review of hospital records of registered cases. However, only one dimension of the validity is examined in this manner, namely the predictive value of the registrations and not the completeness.

Several types of problems limit the usefulness of discharge diagnoses in registry research (Steinberg *et al.*, 1990):

- variations in coding
- errors in coding
- incompleteness in coding, especially of comorbidities
- limits in the specificity of available codes
- errors and variation in clinical diagnosis.

The students must be aware that the demands for completeness and representativeness depend on the research question and design. For several analytical studies the degree of completeness may be less important than whether the misclassification is random or differential. Since valid measures of effect size only depend on the odds of exposed to non-exposed among cases and controls, not the completeness of the case ascertainment, incomplete case ascertainment may be critical in a follow-up study, but less troublesome in a case control design. As long as the case identification is unrelated to the exposure of interest, a case registry may be used as a valid source of candidates for a case control study (Sørensen *et al.*, 1996).

The validity of the registered data

The individual record in a registry will often contain several variables apart from the one by which the person is identified (exposure or outcome); for example, the results of certain diagnostic tests, diagnoses, age, gender, and other demographic data.

The validity of such registered data will often have to be evaluated by comparison with independent external criteria (Goldberg *et al.*, 1980) or by comparison with operational criteria by studying records (Tennis *et al.*, 1993). The validity of this sort of review is close to the concept of the predictive value of a positive registration.

Furthermore, the evaluation also includes the extent of missing data, since a significant degree of missing and incomplete data negates the value of the source (Connel *et al.*, 1987). For each single variable it should be considered whether missing information means that exposure or outcome has not taken place or whether the variable represents a missing value. Inaccurate or missing data tend to bias associations toward the null hypothesis rather than to cause spurious associations, as long as they occur in equal proportion in the groups to be compared (Sørensen *et al.*, 1996).

Another recurring problem with registry studies concerns missing information about potential confounders (Sørensen *et al.*, 1996; Brownson *et al.*, 1989). Potential confounders often lacking in registry data are smoking habits and other life style factors.

In summary, data quality problems can be categorized as follows: first, errors in the data set may reflect incorrect data entry or lack of entry of available information; and, second, the original source of information may be correctly entered into the data source but may not reflect the true condition or characteristic of the subject. There is an increasing tendency to combine primary data and registry data to reduce some of the problems with confounding; for example, to collect primary data about exposure and confounders and follow the individuals through registries to an outcome (Grønbæk *et al.*, 1998).

The size of the data source

Before designing the study, it is essential for the student to know how many persons and how many variables are registered in the data source. Furthermore, it may be relevant to know the distribution of the various variables and especially the number of outcomes since this may be of importance in designing the study to provide it with proper dimension (random error). Use of restriction and matching in the control of confounding factors and sources of selection often requires progressively more subjects as the number of matching variables increases, and some registries may even be too small to use these techniques. To reduce the magnitude of programming problems and computer capacity, a case control study can be an advantage compared to cohort studies (Mortensen *et al.*, 2000). A case control study often gives more familiarity with data, a better option to adjust for confounding, if for example the study population is very large.

The registration period

With respect to longitudinal studies, information concerning the registration period(s) is essential for the design to relate exposure and effect to possible **induction and** latent periods (Sørensen *et al.*, 1996). The induction period is the period required for a specific cause to produce disease, the latent period is the delay between the exposure and the period of manifestation of the disease. Data sources with observation periods of a few years will seldom be suitable for etiologic cancer research. The length of registration may also be of importance in ascertaining cases where the diagnosis is delayed, e.g. congenital heart diseases are often not diagnosed until after the neonatal period.

Furthermore, codes, and even the layout of records, are changed periodically. Changes in diagnostic criteria, classifications, and methods (e.g. the recent change from ICD-9-CM to ICD-10 disease classification system) frequently cause problems when comparing data over longer periods (Sørensen *et al.*, 1996).

Data accessibility, availability, and cost

It is often unclear who owns the registry data and who has the right to use them (accessibility). Some registry data are public, while others are owned by companies, e.g. some prescription databases. It is thus important to find out which authorities should approve the use of the data for research purposes. It must be emphasized to the students that general practitioners and hospitals do not always respond or accept the use of their records for research. This is mainly a problem for validation studies where registry data are compared with primary record data. Records may even have been destroyed.

It is additionally important to know the financial costs of using the data and for having them made available. Information on data confidentiality is also essential to ensure protection of confidentiality of data on individuals which are reported to the data sources, so that information on registered persons cannot reach unauthorized third parties (Coleman *et al.*, 1992).

Data format

Registry data will often be in the form of paper records from hospitals or may be computerized, e.g. many health insurance data (Connel *et al.*, 1987; Lauderdale *et al.*, 1993; Bright *et al.*, 1989; Ray and Griffin, 1989; Fisher *et al.*, 1990). Even computerized records can be formatted or structured in such a way that their use is made difficult for research, e.g. inappropriate format of variables (perhaps diagnostic categories, age bands). The student must critically review existing documentation to assess the appropriateness of the data for their intended use. If such documentation does not exist, the student must evaluate the data source. This involves the protocols, record layout and codes, data entry instructions, published material, analyses, technical reports, and the carrying out of appropriate studies of completeness and validity, all with respect to the specific context of the study (Connel *et al.*, 1987).

Possibilities of linkage with other data sources (record linkage)

The students must be given examples of important research results that have been obtained by linkage of different data sources (Roos and Wajda, 1991; Mortensen, 1995; Sørensen, 1997). Record linkage techniques can help to identify the same person in different files. The several computerized healthcare databases in North America can be used in teaching (Lauderdale *et al.*, 1993; Bright *et al.*, 1989; Ray and Griffin, 1989; Fisher *et al.*, 1990). By using computerized billing records, drug exposure is linked to files which include diagnoses (internal record linkage). Linkage is done via a personal identification number. Consequently, these databases constitute powerful tools for drug evaluation. However, a complete high quality record linkage may not always be possible. The best population-based data sources are probably the extensive data linkage networks in Scandinavia, where each person is assigned a unique personal registration number at birth (CPR number), allowing record linkage between several independent data systems and vital statistical registers (external record linkage) (Sørensen *et al.*, 1996; 1998).

Teaching method and format

Starting the new student off is not easy in registry research. The optimum introductory course consists of lectures, simple exercises, and reading of papers. The epidemiologic terminology should be in focus all the time. Use of registers is just one method of gathering data. Group exercises may include examining articles dealing with the same research question in which primary data collections or registers have been used, typically a case control study *versus* a cohort study. This gives the students a sense of strengths and weaknesses. Other examples should include the problems with inconsistent terminology. I avoid the use of computers when teaching introductory courses, except basic calculations on a pocket calculator. This is partly because these types of courses deal with the understanding of basic principles, and partly because the students often do not have the necessary qualifications for it to become meaningful. However, even simple examples of estimation on a pocket calculator can often be of value.

On more advanced courses it is relevant to use simple computer exercises, but analyses of, for example, dynamic cohorts demand an extensive programming insight. There is hardly any room for this during class, except when one is teaching experienced epidemiologists, as the programming problems will overshadow the aim of the teaching. However, exercises of simple case control studies are often very valuable.

Assessing students' achievements

I often evaluate the students by asking them to evaluate papers. Critique of articles dealing with registry-based research and the concepts provides valuable insight in the students' degree of learning. I often give them papers on the same topic based on primary and secondary data collection and ask them to identify strengths, limitations, and bias problems. I have sometimes used papers regarding oral contraceptives and venous thromboembolism, a topic that is covered by both primary and registry data (Spitzer *et al.*, 1996; Jick *et al.*, 1995). It can be an advantage for this evaluation exercise to delete the discussion sections of the papers and ask the students to write the discussion.

References

Bright, R. A., Avorn, J., Everitt, D. E. (1989). MEDICAID data as a resource for epidemiologic studies: strengths and limitations. *Journal of Clinical Epidemiology* **42**, 937–45.

Brownson, R. C., Davis, J. R., Chang, J. C., DiLorenzo, T. M., Keefe, T. J., Bagby, J. J. Jr. (1989). A study of the accuracy of cancer risk factor information reported to a central registry compared to that obtained by interview. *American Journal of Epidemiology* **129**, 616–24.

Coleman, M. P., Muir, L. S., Ménégoz, F. (1992). Confidentiality in the cancer registry. *British Journal of Cancer* **62**, 1138–49.

Connel, F. A., Diehr, P., Hart, L. G. (1987). The use of large data bases in health care studies. *Annual Review of Public Health* **8**, 51–74.

Fisher, E. S., Baron, J. A., Malenka, D. J., Barrett, J., Bubolz, T. A. (1990). Overcoming potential pitfalls in the use of Medicare data for epidemiologic research. *American Journal of Public Health* **86**, 1487–90.

Goldberg, J., Gelfand, H. M., Levy, P. S. (1980). Registry evaluation methods: a review and case study. *Epidemiological Review* 1980; **2**, 210–20.

Grønbæk, M., Becker, V., Johansen, D., Tønnesen, H. Sørensen, T. I. (1998). Population-based cohort study of the association between alcohol intake and cancer of the upper digestive tract. *British Medical Journal* **317**, 844–7.

Hansen, A. G. and Looft C. (1973). *Leprosy: in its clinical & pathological aspects.* John Wright & Co, Bristol.

Jick H., Jick, S. S., Gurewich, V., Myers M. W., Vasilakis C. (1995). *Risk of idiopathic cardiovascular death and nonfatal venous thromboembolism in women using oral contraceptives with differing progestagen components. Lancet* **346**, 1589–93.

Last, J. M. (1995). *A dictionary of epidemiology.* Oxford University Press, New York, Oxford, Toronto.

Lauderdale, D. S., Furner, S. E., Miles, T. P., Goldberg, J. (1993). Epidemiologic uses of Medicare data. *Epidemiologic Reviews* **15**, 319–27.

Mortensen, P. B. (1995). The untapped potential of case registers and record-linkage studies in psychiatric epidemiology. *Epidemiologic Reviews* **17**, 205–9.

Mortensen, P. B., Agerbo, E., Erikson, T., Qin, P., Westergaard-Nielsen, N. (2000). Psychiatric illness and risk factors for suicide in Denmark. *Lancet* **355**, 9–12.

Ray, W. A., Griffin, M. R. (1989). Use of MEDICAID data for pharmacoepidemiology. *American Journal of Epidemiololgy* **129**, 837–49.

Roos, L. L., Wajda, A. (1991). Record linkages strategies. *Methods of Information in Medicine* **30**, 117–23.

Spitzer W. O., Lewis M. A., Heinemann L. A, Thorogood M., MacRae K. D. (1996). Third generation oral contraceptives and risk of venous thromboembolic disorders: an international case-control study. *Transnational Research Group on Oral Contraceptives and the Health of Young Women BMJ* **312**, 83–8.

Sørensen, H. T. (1997). Regional administrative health registers as a resource in clinical epidemiology. A study of options, strengths, limitations and data quality provided with examples of use. *International Journal of Risk and Safety in Medicine* **10**, 1–22.

Sørensen H. T., Sabroe, S., Olsen, J. (1996). A framework for evaluation of secondary data sources for epidemiological research. *International Journal of Epidemiology* **25**, 435–42.

Sørensen, H. T., Mellemkjær, L., Steffensen, F. H., Olsen, J. H., Nielsen, G. L. (1998). The risk of a diagnosis of cancer after primary deep venous thrombosis and pulmonary embolism. *New England Journal of Medicine* **338**, 1169–73.

Steinberg, E. P., Whittle, J., Anderson, G. F. (1990). Impact of claims data research on clinical practice. *International Journal of Technological Assessment of Health Care* **6**, 282–7.

Tennis, P., Bombardier, C., Malcolm, E., Downey, W. (1993). Validity of rheumatoid arthritis diagnoses listed in the Saskatchewan hospital separations database. *Journal of Clinical Epidemiology* **46**, 675–83.

Chapter 10

Environment

Anders Ahlbom

Introduction

Interest in environmental epidemiology is on the increase and for good reasons. We currently face many environmental health issues which will depend on epidemiology for their resolution. These issues include:

+ The question of whether the deposition in the environment of hormone-disrupting substances such as PCBs affects reproductive outcomes or increases the risk of some other hormone-dependent health effect.

+ The identification of environmental causes of the increase in the incidence of allergy.

+ The resolution of the controversy of chronic health effects caused by air pollution, such as cardiovascular disease.

+ The resolution of the controversy surrounding possible effects of exposure to magnetic fields on cancer risk.

+ Response to the public's demand for more knowledge about possible health effects from mobile telephony.

It is also easy to foresee that major global phenomena, such as the thinning of the ozone layer, global warming, and rapid world population growth may result in quite a number of fundamental issues for scientists, including environmental epidemiologists, to address (McMichael, 1995).

The rapid advancement of molecular biology also raises new issues in environmental epidemiology, in particular the possibility of studying interactions between genes or gene products and environmental factors, thereby identifying sensitive subpopulations on which environmental factors may have a considerably strong effect.

The purpose of this chapter is to discuss, from the teacher's perspective, some methodologic aspects that are of particular importance in the application of epidemiology to environmental health problems. Many of those who become interested in environmental epidemiology do not have a background in epidemiology, but rather in other areas within environmental science or environmental health such as toxicology, chemistry, physics, or engineering. With a background in such a discipline the starting point is different from those in other branches of epidemiology. As a consequence, the observational, rather than the experimental, nature of most epidemiologic research tends to create a tension among environmental scientists, as does the epidemiologist's approach to exposure assessment. This may appear to lack precision for someone used to administering internal doses of radiation or a chemical substance to experimental animals in cages or cell cultures in Petri dishes. There are indeed both similarities and differences between epidemiology and experimental sciences, which should be kept in mind if teaching is to be successful.

Teaching objectives

After the course the students should be able to:

1. Appreciate the role of epidemiology in environmental health sciences.
2. Assess the relative importance of various sources of error and understand the principles to evaluate these errors and to control them in study design.

Teaching contents

Role of epidemiology

In virtually all areas within environmental health, epidemiology is only one of the scientific disciplines providing data. The final assessment of the evidence will be based on a synthesis across scientific disciplines. This has already been pointed out by Bradford Hill, who included biological plausibility in his classic list of criteria for causality (Hill, 1965). It may be important in teaching to emphasize the multidisciplinary nature of environmental medicine and also the role of epidemiology. It may seem obvious, but it is still worth stressing that in research aimed at clarifying the association between an environmental factor and a disease risk in humans, epidemiologic data are those that address this directly and are therefore of highest relevance and priority. Examples may be found in the preamble of any of the *IARC Monographs* on the evaluation of carcinogenic risks to humans such as IARC (1992). From *in vivo* and *in vitro* studies a generalization will always have to be made to the human situation and so external validity is always an issue. On the other hand, it is usually easier to achieve a higher internal validity in the experimental setting than in an observational epidemiologic study.

One should also emphasize, however, that all the involved scientific disciplines have weak and strong sides. Some of these weaknesses and strengths are, indeed, shared by all the disciplines, whereas others may be more accentuated in one type of data than in another. Among those that are shared is the need for replication of results because of the possibility of a systematic or random error. Moreover, randomized experimental studies may suffer from confounding and also controlled experiments may run into difficulties because of poor exposure characterization. Likewise, associations simply caused by random variability may occur in almost any given study regardless of its nature. A critical attitude towards all type of data, epidemiologic as well as other, is therefore of the essence.

Selection of study subjects

Selection of study subjects is presumably the most critical part for the validity of any epidemiologic study. The investigator has lots of flexibility when deciding which the study population is going to be and during which period it is going to be followed. This flexibility should be used to define a population with sufficient variation with respect to exposure levels and with sufficient size so that the expected number of cases is large enough. The population should also be chosen and defined in such a way that it can be observed and followed with respect to occurring cases and other relevant data. In particular, the investigator can choose the study population with a view to the possibility to assess exposure.

However, as soon as the study population has been defined, it is crucial to identify and follow the study subjects within that population in such a way that selection bias is avoided. Problems in this respect are the most common source of grossly invalid or erroneous results.

In a case control study, all cases that occur within the study population as it has been defined must be identified and included. It is unsatisfactory simply to take cases that come to the attention of the investigator, e.g. those treated in a particular hospital. The reason that this is so important is that the controls which are also required for the study must be representative of the population from which the cases come. If not all the cases in the defined population are used, there is no way of knowing which population the controls should represent and thus one does not know how to select the controls. As a consequence, bias may occur. Even with the cases successfully identified, the investigator is left with the task of finding representative controls. Again, the controls should be a representative sample from the population generating the cases. Without any doubt, the safest way of doing this is through a simple random sample procedure from a roster of the population, possibly after stratification for age and sex. In situations where such registries are unavailable, problems arise that have to be resolved as best as possible with the basic principle described here in mind. For an extensive discussion of selection of study subjects see current textbooks: particularly good discussions of this topic are found in Norell (1991) or Rothman (1986).

To understand this issue one can consider the example of cases recruited from a hospital and controls taken as patients with other diagnoses from the same hospital. The investigator would have to prove that the exposure distribution in this control group was representative of the exposure distribution in the population from which the cases came. This may be the case in some instances, but it is virtually impossible to know or to prove. One can hardly argue that a group of patients constitutes a random sample of the general population. Even if this control group could be exchanged for a sample from the population of the area in which the hospital is located, the problem would still remain unless one knows that all patients in this population are actually seen at this hospital and that no other patients are admitted to the hospital.

Often, when experts from experimental sciences discuss control selection in epidemiologic studies, a tight matching is assumed to be the safeguard against selection problems. Although this may be the case in randomized clinical trials and other randomized studies, the situation is completely different in case control studies. Matching in case-control studies is an entirely different matter that only has to do with how finely the population should be stratified before controls are randomly selected. Matching is best viewed as an extreme case of stratified sampling in which defined characteristics for each case serve as the definition of the strata. In no way does this take away the need for a specified and identified study population from which to draw controls. For an extended discussion of matching in case control studies, see again some current textbooks such as Rothman (1986).

In a cohort study, the investigator has, of course, the same flexibility as in the case control study to select the study population and observation period. Valid identification and selection of the subjects within the study population is equally essential, as in case control studies. The main concern here is that case identification must not be associated with exposure status. A situation one may encounter in environmental epidemiology is that the population in a particular neighborhood is studied to compare disease or mortality rates to those of some reference population. Various types of selection bias may occur in this situation.

One example that tends to result in underestimation of relative risks is the following. Consider a retrospective cohort study in which mortality rates are used. This study type requires a register of the population at the beginning of the follow-up, which in a retrospective setting refers to a point back in time. This register is then matched against a mortality register to identify cases of deaths. Suppose that such a registry indeed existed at the beginning but that it has been updated and that deceased subjects have been deleted. Then, of course, mortality rates would be underestimated. The magnitude of this underestimation depends on what proportion of the deaths were removed. That a registry may be updated in this way is a real possibility, and may occur, for example, if it serves as a mailing list. We experienced exactly this when planning a retrospective cohort study on air pollution based on the residents in a particular neighborhood. The first results indicated considerably low mortality rates. The reason was that deaths that had come to the attention of the administrators had been removed from the register to which we had access. This updating of the registry was performed because its main use was for sending out information to the residents.

Consider now a second example which tends to bias the results in the other direction. Suppose one wants to study the disease rate in a particular neighborhood and that the population at the beginning of the follow-up is known and that the cases that occur in this population are identified through various sources. If one does not make certain that the identified cases really correspond to the population at the beginning of the follow-up, bias might occur. This may happen if information about the population size and the morbidity rates come from different sources. For example, the population size information may come from a census, while the cases may all be identified cases with connection to the studied neighborhood. Such connections may not necessarily qualify for inclusion in the census. This type of mismatch between numerator and denominator certainly explains some of the disease clusters that have been reported.

Exposure assessment

Exposure assessment is often considered both crucial and difficult in environmental epidemiology, and rightly so. This is a critical issue both in studies where the purpose is to decide whether or not causality exists, and in the next level studies, where the aim is to establish the shape of a risk function for the purpose of risk assessment or evaluation. This is an area where a close collaboration with experts in the various areas of application is absolutely essential. It is, however, equally essential in this collaboration that the purpose of the exposure assessments are clear. Exposure assessments must be viewed in relation to their purpose, and measurements in a chemical or physical setting may have different aims than those in an epidemiologic study.

In studies with the aim of estimating a relative risk that measures the association between the exposure and the disease, the exposure assessment must be viewed in the context of that particular purpose. The validity of an exposure assessment depends on its ability to provide a valid relative risk estimate. The solution to this is not always to use the most sophisticated and extensive measurements that are available. One reason is that timing of the exposure is also important, and in many cases the epidemiologist requires an estimate of historic exposure, while sophisticated technical measurement may only be performed prospectively. In such situations it is indeed possible that questionnaire or interview information is to be preferred. One example arises from the study of magnetic fields and childhood leukemia. One case control study collected exposure information after the cases were diagnosed and simultaneously for the controls by means of personal monitors that were worn for an extended period of time. These monitors were able to collect detailed magnetic field data over extended periods. Despite the detailed information this may not necessarily be a good idea. Not only do these monitors capture the wrong time periods, but the method may also introduce a differential exposure misclassification if the case children have changed their habits and life style after diagnosis. One could make the case that estimating the exposure from power lines and other installations in the vicinity of the home, although crude, would still yield more valid relative risk estimates. In preparation for studies on potential health risks from mobile telephony, biophysicists are developing models that describe power density and temperature rise in various parts of the head for different types of phones and usage. This may prove immensely useful for mechanistic research and for the development of mitigation techniques. Epidemiology may also benefit from this work, but the results should be considered with a view to the uncertainties in the historic data on frequency of phone use, type of phone system, etc. So, for various reasons it may not prove feasible to take advantage directly of some measurement techniques which are available in principle. What one should try hard to accomplish instead is to use these measurement techniques for validation of a cruder method that may be used. For example, in a study on magnetic fields and cancer we used a method to estimate historic fields generated by high voltage power lines. This method was first applied to current fields and could thus be validated by the use of simultaneous measurements (Feychting and Ahlbom, 1993).

When criticized for using too crude exposure assessment methods, epidemiologists often defend themselves by referring to the principle of dilution because of non-differential exposure misclassification. This is of course a valid response, although it may be useful to keep in mind that there are also effects on the dose–response curve that are somewhat more complex (Dosemeci *et al.*, 1990). The essence of this is that crude exposure assessments do not give rise to spurious associations but to an under-estimation of effects, if there are any. However, if an effect occurs in a study with a particularly crude exposure methodology, the association may simply become implausible, in which case other candidates for explanation such as selection bias may become stronger. In environmental epidemiology one sometimes sees studies that simply use distance to a source of exposure, or residence in a region with a presumed exposure as markers for exposure. To be convincing such a marker may have to be backed up by measurements or some other validation. We have recently seen several such studies looking at populations living near radio transmission towers. Although the explanation for some of these clusters is not yet clear, chance or selection bias should be considered candidates.

The effects of crude exposure assessments should be considered in the planning phase of a study. The impact of the misclassification is determined by the specificity and sensitivity of the exposure assessment (Norell, 1991; Feychting and Ahlbom, 2000). The specificity is the probability of an unexposed subject being classified as unexposed, and the sensitivity is the probability of an exposed subject being classified as exposed. If both are 100% there will be no misclassification. However, that is hardly ever the case. Typically, if one increases the sensitivity, there is a trade-off in terms of decreased specificity and vice versa. Prevalence of exposure is a further factor that plays a role in determining the level of misclassification. Often in environmental epidemiol-ogy, the exposure prevalence is low, at least in the general population. In such situa-tions, sensitivity operates on a small exposed proportion of the population, while specificity operates on a large unexposed part of the population. The effect of this is that a reduction in sensitivity plays a minor role, while a reduction in specificity may be devastating. For example, with a true relative risk of 2.0 and an exposure prevalence of 10% the observed relative risk would be 1.96 if the specificity was 100% and the sen-sitivity 80%. That is, a 20% reduction in sensitivity makes little difference. However, consider the same population but with a different means for exposure assessment. With 80% specificity and 100% sensitivity the observed relative risk would come down to 1.36. That is, with a compromised specificity of this magnitude, 64% of the excess risk would disappear. This effect would be considerably more marked with a lower exposure prevalence. The conclusion of this discussion is that, with low exposure prevalence a high specificity is the priority while a high sensitivity is of less impor-tance. In other words, it is essential to use an exposure assessment technique that guar-antees that unexposed subjects are not included in the exposed group. At the same time it is not essential to identify and include all exposed subjects in the exposed group. For example, assume that one were interested in studying health effects from air pollution around an industry, and planned to do this by looking at people living with-in a circle surrounding the industry. Unless this circle is made very small, the exposure specificity will be compromised in that quite a number of those living within the circle will be unexposed. As a consequence, a severe underestimation of the effect, if there is one, is likely to occur. With this in mind the circle should be made small for validity reasons, unless some other study design can be developed. At the same time it is presumably tempting to make the circle wide because that would increase the size of the study population. However, this temptation should be resisted.

Confounding

Confounding may be defined as the presence of a baseline difference in incidence between exposed and unexposed subjects. That is, an incidence difference would exist even if the exposure had no effect. For example, if the age distribution differed between an exposed and an unexposed group, one would expect a difference in baseline incidence simply because most diseases are age-dependent. One would say that a relative risk comparing the exposed and the unexposed would be confounded by age. A classical example is the comparison of subjects with and without yellow fingers, the stain caused by nicotine. Such a comparison would most likely reveal an association between yellowness and lung cancer incidence. This comparison, however, would be confounded by smoking.

Both of these examples illustrate that, for confounding to occur, two associations must be in place simultaneously, namely between the confounder and the disease, and between the confounder and the exposure. Age distribution must be different between exposed and unexposed (association between confounder and exposure) and the disease must be age-dependent (association between confounder and disease). The situation is similar in the second example with smoking and yellowness being associated as well as smoking and lung cancer. In discussions of whether or not an observed association is caused by confounding it is often forgotten that both these associations are required for confounding to occur. For example, several studies have indicated that children living near power lines are at increased risk of leukemia. In discussions about the interpretation of this, it has been suggested that there may be a socioeconomic gradient such that people of lower socioeconomic status tend to live close to power lines. However, for this to result in socioeconomic confounding it would also be required that children of lower socioeconomic status were at increased risk of leukemia, for which there is little evidence.

In discussions of the possibility that an observed association is due to confounding rather than causation, one must also keep magnitude in mind. The magnitude of a confounding effect depends on the strength of the two involved associations. It has been shown that, for a confounder to have a sizeable effect, both the involved associations must be strong. Generally, one can not expect confounding to give rise to a spurious association with a relative risk exceeding, say, 1.5 or 2.0 and, even so, both associations would have to be quite strong. The association between smoking and lung cancer is one of the stronger in the epidemiologic literature. Yet it is not expected that smoking is likely to create a stronger confounding than 1.5–2.0 in occupational studies on lung cancer (Axelson, 1978). In a recent interesting approach, Langholz (2000) has shown that there is a maximal limit for a potential confounding effect that can be assessed given that the exposure distribution is known.

For people used to and trained in experimental and randomized sciences, confounding seems to appear as the major alternative to causality. Generally speaking, however, this is not in agreement with the literature, which points towards selection bias and also chance as being more important alternatives for consideration. Nevertheless, it is not uncommon, in a situation with an unexpected outcome of a study, that the findings are questioned with reference to the possibility that the explanation may indeed be confounded by some unknown factor X. This is, of course, correct. There is never a way of excluding confounding by some hitherto unknown risk factor as the explanation. This actually also holds both for studies with results as expected and even for randomized experiments. However, the crucial comment is that, for a critique of a study result to be useful, it should also be testable. For a critique invoking confounding as a possible explanation to be testable, it must identify the putative confounder. If this is done, one can, at least in principle, test this possibility by adjusting for the potential confounder either in presently existing data or in future studies.

Comments

The basic principles of environmental epidemiology are of course no different than those in other branches of epidemiology. This chapter underscores some of the principles that may be of particular interest when teaching epidemiology to an audience with a background in disciplines of other relevance to environmental medicine than epidemiology. In particular, the discussion has focused on some of the consequences that arise from the observational rather than experimental nature of most epidemiology. Other important aspects are the sometimes weak effects of environmental risk factors that create particular difficulties to the environmental epidemiologists. The prevalence of environmental exposures may sometimes be low but there are also instances with ubiquitous exposure. Both situations create challenges to the epidemiologist The rapidly evolving molecular biology will without any doubt provide new tools such as biomarkers and markers for individual susceptibility, and it will be essential to be able to incorporate these into study designs. The most important characteristic for environmental epidemiology is perhaps the need for a good collaboration with experts in related areas and, in particular, in areas of relevance for current chapter.

Teaching method and format

There is usually no guarantee that students in a course like this are familiar with the basics of epidemiology. I would therefore suggest that a course in environmental epidemiology has the overall structure of a general epidemiology course, but with emphasis on the areas discussed in the previous section.

1. Introduction to epidemiology
2. Measures on disease occurrence and effect
3. Causation
4. Cohort studies, including systematic and random errors
5. Case control studies, including systematic and random errors
6. Data analysis in epidemiology
7. Interpretation of epidemiologic studies

The teaching format I prefer is a combination of lectures, exercises, and case studies. Each topic would first be presented in a lecture. It would then be followed up with simple exercises. These are performed individually and reviewed in class at the next lecture. Each topic is also followed up with a case study, preferably in the form of a published article that is used to illustrate a particular topic. The students read the paper for themselves, together with specific questions related to the paper. They then discuss the questions in small groups and, finally, this is followed by a plenary discussion.

Assessing students' achievements

The method for evaluation of students depends on whether the course is taken for credits or not. It also depends on the length of the course, because one does not want to use too large a proportion of the time for the test. One should try to integrate the evaluation in the teaching and my preference is a series of quizzes. They may take only 15 minutes to do in class. If they are discussed afterwards, it may be an instructive way of reviewing certain topics.

References

Axelson, O. (1978). Aspects on confounding in occupational health epidemiology. *Scand J Work Environ Health* **4**, 85–9.

Dosemeci, M., Wacholder, S., Lubin, J. H. (1990). Does nondifferential misclassification of exposure always bias a true effect toward the null value? *Am J Epidemiol* **132**, 746–8.

Feychting, M., and Ahlbom, A. (1993). Magnetic fields and cancer in children residing near Swedish high voltage power lines. *Am J Epidemiol* **138**, 467–81.

Feychting, M., and Ahlbom, A. Exposure assessment in epidemiological studies – sensitivity, specificity and the impact of nondifferential exposure misclassification. In press.

Hill, B. A. (1965). The environment and disease, association or causation? *Proc R Soc Med* **58**, 295–300.

IARC Monographs of the Evaluation of Carcinogenic Risks to Humans (1992), vol. 55. *Solar and ultraviolet radiation*. Lyon: IARC.

Langholz, B. (2001). Factors that explain the power line configuration wiring code-leukemia association: what would they look like? *Bioelectromagnetics* Suppl 5: 519–31.

McMichael, A. J. (1995) *Planetary overload: global environmental change and the health of the human species*. Cambridge: Cambridge University Press.

Norell, S. E. (1989). The magnitude of the effect of misclassification on relative risk estimation. In: *Epidemiology, nutrition and health*. (eds Kohlmeier L, Helsing E).

Norell, S. E. (1991). *A short course in epidemiology*. New York: Raven Press.

Rothman, K. J. (1986). *Modern epidemiology*. Boston/Toronto: Little, Brown and company.

Chapter 11

Occupation

Neil Pearce

Introduction

Occupational epidemiology is the study of the distribution and causes of illness and injury that result from hazardous work place exposures (Checkoway *et al.*, 1989). Concerns about adverse health consequences of occupational exposures date back to Hippocrates' warnings to physicians to explore patients' environmental life style and vocational backgrounds. In 1700 the Italian physician Ramazzini described numerous diseases such as silicosis among stonemasons, ocular disorders among glass blowers, and neurologic toxicity among tradesman exposed to mercury. More recent descriptions of occupational diseases have included pneumoconiosis among miners of gold and silver in Germany and the former Czechoslovakia, the identification of soot as the cause of scrotal cancer in London chimney sweeps by Percival Pott in 1775, and the recognition of asbestos-associated disease including asbestosis, lung cancer, and mesothelioma (Checkoway *et al.*, 1989). More recent examples include evidence supporting associations of industrial solvents with Alzheimer's disease (Kukull *et al.*, 1995) and various metals (Gorrell *et al.*, 1997), and pesticides with Parkinson's disease (Seider *et al.*, 1996; Lion *et al.*, 1997). Until recently, most occupational epidemiology studies have been conducted in western countries. However, the number of workers in industries involving a risk of cancer and other occupational disease is increasing in developing countries, partly as a result of the transfer of hazardous industry from industrialized countries (Pearce *et al.*, 1994). Thus, it is increasingly important to take a global view of occupational disease.

Teaching objectives

Students on occupational epidemiology courses may include trained epidemiologists who are learning about occupational epidemiology for the first time, as well as occupational hygienists, and healthcare professionals (e.g. occupational physicians, occupational health nurses, and students of medicine and nursing) also learning about these methods for the first time. It is important to distinguish between teaching occupational epidemiology to researchers and to public health officers and occupational physicians, since researchers often have a stronger interest in theoretical issues, whereas the latter groups may have a stronger interest in specific occupational health problems (Merletti and Comba, 1992). In this chapter it is assumed that students have previously undertaken an introductory epidemiology course, and the focus is on issues which are relatively unique, or which receive greater emphasis in occupational epidemiology. A problem-based approach is emphasized which involves learning occupational epidemiology in the context of active experience in developing, conducting, and reporting on a (hypothetical) occupational epidemiology study. By the end of the course, participants should be able to:

+ Describe the strengths and limitations of occupational epidemiology, and particularly its potential for use in solving real work place health problems and developing preventive interventions.

+ Discuss the key features of occupational epidemiology that distinguish it from other fields of epidemiology.

+ Consult with managers, unions, workers, researchers, government agencies, and other interested parties in developing a research question.

+ Design an occupational epidemiology study that addresses this research question.

+ Write a research proposal suitable for submission for funding.

+ Communicate the findings of research both in academic form and in the form of a press statement for the general media.

Of course, these objectives will be met to a greater or lesser extent depending on the background, experience, and ability of the course participants, but the specific course content and the level of detail and methodologic rigour expected of the research proposal, can be modified accordingly.

Teaching contents

In this section, the key topics that should be covered as a complement to a more general introductory epidemiology course are discussed.

Reasons for conducting occupational epidemiology studies

The primary objective of occupational epidemiology is to identify hazardous work place exposures to prevent occupational disease (Checkoway *et al.*, 1989). The potential for prevention is often much greater than in other fields of epidemiology since work place exposures can often be readily identified and removed. This can be illustrated using examples of successful prevention (Merletti and Comba, 1992), including non-introduction of hazards into the work place, removal of hazards, reduction in exposure levels, reduction in hazardous activities, and increased protection (Swerdlow, 1990). It is therefore valuable to discuss current work place health and safety issues with management, unions, and workers, and to identify the potential health hazards that are currently of most concern and for which there is the greatest potential for prevention.

A second objective of occupational epidemiology is to provide information that can be used in risk assessment and in the prevention of hazards in the general population. For example, it is notoriously difficult to study the health effects of occasional low level pesticide exposure in the general population, and it is more valuable to conduct studies of heavily exposed pesticide production workers and sprayers, and to use the findings from these studies to estimate the risk from lower levels of exposure in the general population. Once again, a problem-based approach can be valuable. For example, students can be introduced to these issues by discussing a problem that is currently of community concern (e.g. the risks of environmental pesticide exposure, exposure to electromagnetic fields, asbestos exposure in the home), and by discussions with some of the interested parties in the community and in industry.

A further reason for conducting occupational epidemiology studies is to evaluate the effects of work place interventions, such as the removal of a hazardous exposure and its replacement with a substitute believed to be less hazardous. For example, asbestos has increasingly been replaced by various man-made mineral fibers which appear also to involve an increased risk of asbestos-related diseases such as lung cancer. It is therefore important to emphasize the importance of following up on previous epidemiologic studies, ascertaining what preventive measures have been adopted in response to their findings, and how effective these measures have been. For example, in a longitudinal study of occupational respiratory disease it is relatively straightforward to assess changes in health and safety practices, and provision of protective equipment over time (Slater *et al.*, 2000).

Political and ethical issues

A problem-based approach will inevitably lead to discussion of controversies in occupational epidemiology and risk assessment. Discussing such controversies can be valuable in demonstrating the strengths and weaknesses of occupational epidemiology, its wider role in causal assessment and risk assessment, and the political, economic, and social influences that often affect which hypotheses are chosen for study, which methods are used, and how the findings are interpreted. These issues are relevant to all epidemiologic studies, but are often particularly acute in occupational epidemiology, as well as in other fields of epidemiology that involve vested interests (e.g. environmental epidemiology and pharmacoepidemiology).

Unfortunately, such discussions can often involve an undue emphasis on criticism of published studies, and this is often encouraged in courses that overemphasize the role of criticism under a simplistic interpretation of the Popperian philosophy of science. Such a one-sided emphasis on criticism can lead to disillusionment amongst students as to the validity and value of occupational epidemiology. Thus, it is valuable to ask students to design a study of a specific issue and to write a research protocol for it, rather than asking them merely to write a critique on a published paper. This approach is not only invaluable in terms of practical experience with epidemiologic study design, but can also teach students the practical compromises that are often involved in conducting occupational epidemiology studies. They can therefore learn that no study can be perfect or definitive, and that the aim of a single study should be to contribute to the pool of information available for scientific and public health decision-making. In the latter context, decisions are often made on the basis of the 'balance of evidence' rather than requiring hazard or safety to be proven with certainty or even 'beyond reasonable doubt'.

The potential for preventive action, and the considerable vested interests which may hasten or delay such action, means that ethical issues play a major role in occupational epidemiology (Merletti and Comba, 1992). In particular, the need to conduct further epidemiologic studies should not be a reason to delay preventive measures. Furthermore, it is important that reports of occupational epidemiology studies, and criticisms of these reports, should openly acknowledge sources of funding and any other potential conflicts of interest.

Methodological issues

Healthy worker effect

A major issue in occupational studies is the healthy worker effect (Checkoway *et al.*, 1989). The typically lower relative risk of death or chronic disease in an occupational cohort occurs because relatively healthy individuals are likely to gain employment, and to remain employed. Thus, the initial selection occurs at the time of hire in that relatively healthy persons are more likely to seek and to be offered employment; the most direct way to control for this phenomenon partially is to stratify on initial employment status, i.e. to compare the asthma morbidity rate of a particular work force with that of other employed persons rather than with a general population sample (which includes invalids and the unemployed). The second key aspect of the healthy worker effect is the selection of unhealthy persons out of the work force. In some instances, this problem can be partially addressed by considering each worker's employment status (i.e. active or non-active worker) at a particular time and controlling for it as a confounder (Pearce, 1992a; Steenland and Stayner, 1991). Furthermore, for many occupations the strength of the healthy worker effect tends to diminish with increasing time since first employment; this problem can be addressed by controlling for length of follow-up.

The healthy worker effect means that considerable attention should be given to the selection of appropriate comparison populations. Despite the limitations of standardized mortality ratio (SMR) analyses using the general population as a comparison, this is usually the most practical option for initial analyses. However, alternative comparison populations (e.g. regional mortality rates, other employed workers) should also be considered. The value of internal comparisons and the importance of defining a cohort so that such comparisons are feasible and meaningful should also be emphasized.

However, although the use of an internal reference group may control for initial employment status and therefore for the initial selection into employment (aspect 1 of the healthy worker effect), it will not necessarily eliminate other forms of bias. In particular, exposure (or the termination of exposure through leaving employment) can be a cause and/or a consequence of occupational disease, and can affect the subsequent risk of mortality. Such 'intermediate variables' should not be routinely controlled using standard techniques, and special techniques are required to avoid adding bias (Robins, 1989; Pearce, 1992b).

Exposure data

A feature of occupational epidemiology studies is the frequent use of job exposure matrices to estimate historic exposures. The sources of data for a job exposure matrix include industrial hygiene sampling data, process descriptions and flow charts, plant production records, inspection and accident reports, engineering documentation, and biologic monitoring data (Checkoway *et al.*, 1989). However, the starting point for development of job exposure matrices and the estimation of individual historic exposures is the personnel records. It is therefore important to use real examples of personnel records in teaching, and to discuss the practical aspects of classifying and grouping departments and job titles.

Recently, there has been increasing emphasis on the use of molecular markers of internal dose (Schulte and Perera, 1993). In fact, there are a number of major limitations of currently available biomarkers of exposure (Armstrong *et al.*, 1992), particularly with regard to historic exposures (Pearce *et al.*, 1995). Some biomarkers are better than others in this respect (particularly markers of exposure to biologic agents), but even the best markers of chemical exposures usually reflect only the last few weeks or months of exposure. Thus, the use of work history records in combination with a job exposure matrix (based on historic exposure measurements of work areas rather than individuals) is often more valid than current exposure measurements (whether based on environmental measurements or biomarkers) if the aim is to estimate historic exposure levels (Checkoway *et al.*, 1989). The emphasis should be on using 'appropriate technology', and that the most appropriate approach (questionnaires, environmental measurements, or biological measurements) will vary from study to study, and from exposure to exposure within the same study (or within the same complex chemical mixture, e.g. in welding fumes). This can be illustrated by a problem-based approach in which different exposure estimation methods are shown to be appropriate for different studies (Steenland, 1993).

Confounding

Confounding is of concern in occupational epidemiology, as in other fields of epidemiology. However, to be a significant confounder, a factor must be strongly predictive of disease and strongly associated with exposure. Thus, confounding is often relatively weak in occupational studies, particularly when comparing 'exposed' and 'non-exposed' manual ('blue collar') workers since there are usually few important differences in life style between different groups of workers. For example, Siemiatycki *et al.* (1988) found that confounding by smoking is generally very weak for internal comparisons in which exposed workers are compared with non-exposed workers in the same factory or industry. If it is not possible to obtain confounder information for any study subjects, it may still be possible to estimate how strong the confounding is likely to be from particular risk factors. This is often done in studies of occupational causes of lung cancer, where smoking is a potential confounder, but smoking information is rarely available. For example, Axelson (1978) found that, for plausible estimates of the smoking prevalence in occupational populations, confounding by smoking can rarely account for a relative risk of lung cancer of greater than 1.5. Course participants can repeat this exercise for other situations, e.g. by estimating the potential for confounding in their proposed study.

However, it should also be emphasized that occupational exposures often involve complex mixtures such as welding fumes. In this situation, confounding by 'external' exposures such as smoking is likely to be weak, but there may be a significant 'identification problem' with regard to the etiologically relevant constituent(s) of the complex occupational exposures.

Study designs

The study design options in occupational epidemiology are the same as for other fields of epidemiology (Checkoway *et al.*, 1989), but the methodologic issues involved may differ (see above), as may the emphasis given to specific study designs. In particular, cohort studies are relatively common in occupational epidemiology since most occupational exposures are 'rare' in the general population. Thus, it is valuable to review the standard study design options, but to give particular attention to the specific issues and methodologic characteristics of occupational studies.

Routine mortality and morbidity data

In many countries, death certificates include the deceased person's current or most recent occupation, and it is therefore possible to estimate national or regional death rates for specific occupations. Occupational information may also be available for hospital admissions and for registers of diseases such as cancer. Thus, analyses of existing data sources play an important role in occupational epidemiology (Melius *et al.*, 1989; Merletti and Comba, 1992). Direct age standardization and other methods for 'descriptive' analyses are therefore particularly relevant and may not have been covered in general introductory courses. In the past, analyses of routine data sources have often included proportional mortality ratio (PMR) analyses. However, this is just an outdated variant of the case control approach in which non-case deaths are used as controls (Miettinen and Wang, 1981). Thus, PMR analyses should ideally be discussed in the context of case control studies (see below) rather than as a variant of SMR analyses.

Clusters

Many occupational epidemiology studies are motivated by reports of work place clusters of disease. A cluster investigation initially involves defining the population in the time period under study (the study base), and ascertaining whether the disease occurrence in this study base is greater than expected. However, the occurrence of a statistically significant cluster of occupational disease can merely establish a hypothesis that requires further scrutiny in another study base. For this reason, it is often argued that the investigation of disease clusters is a public health 'social service', but has little scientific value. However, most causes of chronic occupational disease were discovered through cluster investigations, and such investigations will continue to be an important method for identifying new causes of chronic occupational disease (Pearce, 1994). Cluster investigations are also of particular interest for occupational physicians and public health officers since they regularly encounter cluster reports in the course of their work. In particular, occupational health professionals, as well as general practitioners, can play a major role in identifying and investigating such clusters (Merletti and Comba, 1992). This can be illustrated by an exercise in which a cluster report is presented and a group of course participants is asked to define the cluster (in terms of the population at risk and the outcomes which will be considered), and to design an appropriate study (in the defined population and/or another population), as well as an interim press statement describing the cluster and what further action is being taken.

Incidence (cohort) studies

Occupational epidemiology frequently involves rare exposures, and the availability of personnel records and historical industrial hygiene information makes historical cohort studies much more feasible than in many other branches of epidemiology.

Cohort studies are usually based on personnel records, and the importance of storing such records in perpetuity should be emphasized. However, they can also be based on registries for exposures such as asbestos and vinyl chloride (Merletti and Comba, 1992). Such registries can also play a valuable role in raising awareness of work place hazards and stimulating preventive measures (Ahlo *et al.*, 1988).

In occupational cohort studies, methods of cohort enumeration (using personnel records), exposure ascertainment (using job exposure matrices), and follow-up (using national or regional mortality and/or disease registration records) are frequently different from community-based cohort studies. Other issues include verification of the completeness of cohorts using alternative data sources, and verification of vital status using a variety of data sources (e.g. death registrations, superannuation records, electoral rolls, driver's license records). It is important to discuss cohort studies in considerable practical detail, including practical examples of individual exposure assessment, exercises involving the actual calculation of individual person–time data, and its use in calculating expected mortality and/or incidence rates, since the use of such data is often difficult to understand without practical experience.

Incidence case control studies

Case control studies can then be introduced in the context of studies nested within a defined occupational cohort. It can be readily demonstrated that a nested case control study can be considerably more efficient than a full cohort analysis, with no loss of validity and only a minimal loss in precision (Checkoway *et al.*, 1989). The cohort (study base) must still be defined and enumerated, and incident cases must be identified. However, it is only necessary to collect exposure history information on the cases and on a sample of controls selected from the cohort, rather than on the entire cohort. Nested case control studies thereby combine the advantages of cohort studies for investigating rare exposures, and of case control studies for investigating rare outcomes.

The effect measure which the odds ratio obtained from nested case control studies will estimate depends on the manner in which controls are selected. The three main methods of control sampling (cumulative sampling, case–base sampling, and density sampling) can be illustrated using a single dataset (Pearce, 1993).

Although occupational case control studies can best be introduced and discussed in the context of nested studies, there are also some occupational exposures (e.g. farming) which are relatively common, but for which it is difficult to identify and enumerate a historical cohort. In this situation, population-based case control studies can be conducted based on a geographically defined population. Although such studies have traditionally been presented in terms of cumulative sampling, in fact most case control studies actually involve density sampling (often with matching on a time variable such as calendar time or age), and therefore estimate the rate ratio without the need for any rare disease assumption (Miettinen, 1976).

Prevalence studies

Another feature of occupational epidemiology is the relatively frequent use of cross-sectional studies of non-fatal occupational diseases, such as occupational asthma (Pearce *et al.*, 1998). For example, a prevalence study, or a prevalence case control study, may estimate the prevalence odds ratio for asthma associated with a specific occupational exposure such as welding fumes. This approach is often appropriate and convenient, but the healthy worker effect may be of particular concern since workers with work-related symptoms may have left employment (Checkoway *et al.*, 1989). This problem may be particularly strong for non-fatal chronic diseases such as occupational asthma (Eisen *et al.*, 1995). Furthermore, Krzyanowski and Kauffmann (1988) have noted that most such studies have focused on industrial groups with high levels of exposure, and that these groups may be particularly affected by selection effects (Graham and Graham-Tomasi, 1985).

Teaching method and format

As indicated above, the study design options in occupational epidemiology are the same as for other fields of epidemiology, but the emphases given to specific study designs and the methodologic issues involved, may differ. Therefore, much of the formal content of an occupational epidemiology course may cover the same general topics as for a general epidemiology course, including the various study design options, study design issues, and detailed consideration of the different possible study designs (see above). However, the detailed content will usually differ considerably.

As noted above, it is useful to teach these methods in the context of developing a research protocol, and reporting on research findings. This can be done as an individual activity, but is often more valuable as a group activity. Thus, the course participants can be divided into groups early on, and these groups can hold regular meetings to develop a research question and design an appropriate study.

This approach can be applied to almost any course at any level, with appropriate variations in the amount of detail and methodologic rigor required. Even with an introductory course of five or six sessions, it is usually possible for the participants to divide into groups, develop a hypothesis, design a basic protocol, and present it at the final session. With a longer and more advanced course, it is often possible to develop a fully fledged protocol. This process can be assisted by:

+ Regular presentations (interspersed with the methodologic teaching) from managers, unions, and government agencies regarding their priorities for occupational health research

- 'Consultation' meetings with the course coordinator to discuss the preliminary research question and the provisional study design
- Presentation, by each group or individual, of the research question and preliminary protocol to the other course participants
- Presentation of the proposal to an appropriate 'client' (e.g. the Occupational Safety and Health agency, or a particular company or union) if one is available, and if there is a prospect that the proposal may lead to a real research project.

The more generic methods (see above) can then be covered in conventional teaching sessions using the standard topics outlined above, but with a particular emphasis on methodologic issues relevant to the protocols under development. Relatively brief exercises on specific methods (e.g. calculation of SMRs) can be completed on an individual basis, but the bulk of practical time can be devoted to protocol development. Thus, one possible course timetable could involve sessions on:

- Reasons for conducting occupational epidemiology studies
- Introduction to developing a research protocol
- Sessions with managers, unions, and interested government agencies
- Overview of study designs
- Overview of issues of bias
- Measuring occupational exposures
- Preliminary discussion of research protocols with the course coordinator and the course participants
- Routine mortality and morbidity rate analyses
- Clusters
- Cohort studies
- Case control studies
- Cross-sectional studies
- Current topics in occupational epidemiology
- Political and ethical issues
- Presentation of research protocols

Assessing students' achievements

Under this approach, the methodologic course exercises (e.g. calculation of SMRs) form a small part of the coursework and can usually be completed on an individual basis in the evening or day after the discussion of the relevant topic. The course assessment is then primarily or solely based on the research proposal. This can be developed as an individual or a group activity (the latter is often preferable), and can be presented in oral or written form, depending on the resources and the time available. The protocol can then be assessed with an oral or written review, as would be provided for a grant application. The review should ideally follow as closely as possible the actual format used for reviews of grant applications from the principal occupational health research funding body (e.g. National Institutes for Health).

In addition, it is often useful for course participants to draw up a few simple tables of hypothetical results for the proposed study, which follow the same format as would be used in a journal publication, and to write a brief press statement summarizing the results. These 'findings' can also be presented and discussed (in oral and/or written form) when the final protocol is presented.

Acknowledgements

The Centre for Public Health Research is funded by a Programme Grant from the Health Research Council of New Zealand.

References

Ahlo, J., Kauppinen, T., Sundquist, E. (1988). Use of exposure registration in the prevention of occupational cancer in Finland. *Am J Ind Med* **13**, 581–92.

Armstrong, B. K., White, E., Saracci, R. *Principles of exposure measurement in epidemiology.* New York: Oxford University Press, 1992.

Axelson, O. (1978). Aspects on confounding in occupational health epidemiology. *Scand J Work Environ Health* **4**, 85–9.

Checkoway, H., Pearce, N. E., Crawford-Brown, D. J. (1989). *Research methods in occupational epidemiology.* New York: Oxford University Press.

Eisen, E. A., Wegman, D. H., Louis, T. A. *et al.* (1995). Healthy worker effect in a longitudinal study of one-second forced expiratory volume (FEV_1) and chronic exposure to granite dust. *Int J Epidemiol* **24**, 1154–62.

Gorrell, J. M., Johnson, C. C., Rybicki, B. A. *et al.* (1997). Occupational exposures to metals as risk factors for Parkinson's disease. *Neurology* **48**, 650–8.

Graham, S., Graham-Tomasi, R. (1985). Achieved status as a risk factor in epidemiology. *Am J Epidemiol* **122**, 553–8.

Krzyanowski, M., Kauffmann, F. (1988). The relation of respiratory symptoms and ventilatory function to moderate occupational exposure in a general population. *Int J Epidemiol* **17**, 397–406.

Kukull, W. A., Larson, E. B., Bowen, J. D. *et al.* (1995). Solvent exposure as a risk factor for Alzheimer's disease: a case-control study. *Am J Epidemiol* **141**, 1059–71.

Liou, H. H., Tsai, M. C., Chen, C. J. *et al.* (1997). Environmental risk factors for Parkinson's disease: a case-control study in Taiwan. *Neurology* **48**, 1583–8.

Melius, J. M., Sestito, J. P., Seligman, P. J. (1989). Occupational disease surveillance with existing data sources. *Am J Publ Health* **79** (Suppl.): 46–52.

Merletti, F., Comba, P. (1992). Occupational epidemiology. In: Olsen, J., Trichopolous, D., Saracci, R. (eds). *Teaching epidemiology.* Oxford: Oxford University Press.

Miettinen, O. S. (1976). Estimability and estimation in case-referent studies. *Am J Epidemiol* **103**, 226–35.

Miettinen, O. S. and Wang, J.-D. (1981). An alternative to the proportionate mortality ratio. *Am J Epidemiol* **114**, 144–8.

Pearce, N. E. (1992a). Methodological problems of time-related variables in occupational cohort studies. *Rev Epidem et Santé Publ* **40**, S43-S54.

Pearce, N. E. (1992b). Time-related confounders and intermediate variables in epidemiologic studies. *Epidemiology* **3**, 279–81.

Pearce, N. E. (1993). What does the odds ratio estimate in a case-control study? *Int J Epidemiol* **22**, 1189–92.

Pearce, N. (1994). Disease clusters and high-risk occupations. People and Work. Research Reports 1. *Proceedings of the International Symposium on New Epidemics in Occupational Health.* Helsinki, Finnish Institute of Occupational Health, pp. 214–20.

Pearce, N. E., Matos, E., Vainio, H. *et al.* (eds) (1994). *Occupational cancer in developing countries.* Lyon: IARC.

Pearce, N., Sanjose, S., Boffetta, P. *et al.* (1995). Limitations of biomarkers of exposure in cancer epidemiology. *Epidemiology* **6**, 190–4.

Pearce, N., Beasley, R., Burgess, C., Crane, J. (1998). *Asthma epidemiology: principles and methods.* New York: Oxford University Press.

Robins, J. (1989). The control of confounding by intermediate variables. *Stat Med* **8**, 679–701.

Schulte, P., Perera, F. P. *Molecular epidemiology: principles and practices.* New York: Academic Press, 1993, pp. 3–44.

Seider, A., Hellenbrand, W., Robra, B.-P. *et al.* (1996). Possible environmental, occupational, and other etiologic factors for Parkinson's disease: a case-control study in Germany. *Neurology* **46**, 1275–84.

Siemiatycki, J., Wacholder, S., Dewar, R. *et al.* (1988). Smoking and degree of occupational exposure: are internal analyses in cohort studies likely to be confounded by smoking status? *Am J Ind Med* **13**, 59–69.

Slater, T., Erkinjuntti-Pekkanen, R., Fishwick, D. *et al.* (2000). Changes in work practice after a respiratory health survey among welders in New Zealand. *NZ Med J*, **113**, 305–8.

Steenland, K. (ed.) (1993). *Case studies in occupational epidemiology.* New York: Oxford University Press.

Steenland, K., Stayner, L. (1991). The importance of employment status in occupational cohort mortality studies. *Epidemiology* **2**, 418–23.

Swerdlow, A. J. (1990). Effectiveness of primary prevention of occupational exposures on cancer risk. In: Hakama, M., Beral, V., Cullen. J. W., Parkin, D. M. (eds). *Evaluating effectiveness of primary prevention of cancer.* Lyon: IARC, pp. 23–56.

Chapter 12

Life style and life course

A. J. McMichael and A. R. Britton

Introduction

This chapter addresses the aspects of exposure-orientated epidemiology which are broadly referred to as 'life style' exposures and which occur over an individual's 'life course'. Whilst certain elements are covered in other chapters in this book, teachers may find it helpful to timetable a separate session on life style exposure to ensure their students are fully aware of the implications.

This chapter will cover the major components of a life style and life course perspective, the research designs and levels of analysis most amenable to their measurement, the advantages of such an approach, and finally suggested teaching techniques. It is envisaged that the material covered here will be suitable for both novice epidemiologists and those undertaking postgraduate courses.

Teaching objectives

The material covered in this chapter will enable students to:

♦ demonstrate an understanding of the importance of a life style and life course perspective

♦ demonstrate an understanding of confounding and interaction between life style variables

♦ evaluate research designs for measuring life style and life course exposures

♦ describe the different levels of assessment

♦ discuss the use of attributable risks for life style exposures

Teaching contents

The following section outlines the key concepts and items which should be covered. The first six sections are essential for students at all levels, whilst the last two will be more appropriate to those studying epidemiology at a more advanced level.

Defining 'life style'

At the outset of the teaching session it is vital that the students have a clear definition of what is meant by 'life style' in the context of exposure assessment. 'Life style' is usually viewed as a set of discretionary, or voluntary, behaviors that represent an individual's choices, exercised within a particular context of choice of commodities and behavioral opportunity. The implication is that life style is essentially a voluntary component of one's life situation. This idea is applied particularly to liberal consumer populations such as typify westernized urban industrialized societies.

The life style idea became prominent in epidemiologic research in the 1970s and 1980s, as it became evident that many chronic non-communicable diseases of later adulthood were strongly influenced by factors such as personal diet, smoking behavior, alcohol consumption, physical activity, and oral contraceptive usage. This life style model of disease etiology evolved in contrasting counterpoint to the continuing study of the health impacts of essentially involuntary occupational and environmental exposures.

During the 1990s, there was a growth of epidemiologic research interest in the broader influences of socioeconomic status, of psychosocial experiences, and of national socioeconomic transition (Krieger, 1994). This has necessarily led to some reconsideration of the extent to which life style is a manifestation of socioeconomic circumstances and of subculture (Kaufman and Cooper, 1998). To what extent are personal behaviors the result of free choice? A fuller 'social causation' model recognizes the 'upstream' factors that determine patterns of groups and individual behavior and, hence, the distribution of risk behaviors within a population, and also of the 'downstream' disease-specific impacts of these risk behaviors (McMichael, 1999).

Some particular sharpening of this debate occurred in response to the advent of HIV/AIDS within western societies in the 1980s (Krieger and Zierler, 1996). Was the infection the result of the individual's sexual or drug-use 'life style'? Was it therefore attributable to that individual's freely chosen behaviors? Or did certain characteristics of societies predispose to particular patterns of high risk behavior? Would we regard HIV/AIDS as a 'life style disease' among poor rural women in Africa or India?

It is important in teaching about 'life style' factors to encourage a critical discussion of their defining characteristics. Students should be asked to reflect on the extent to which their own social milieu, their own subculture, influences their perception of 'life style' factors in relation to epidemiology.

Life style *versus* way-of-life

The notion of life style may seem to imply a variable composite of specific behaviors, each constituting an independent 'risk factor'. Many social scientists contend, however, that behaviors tend to cluster in ways that reflect not so much a discretionary life style but a subcultural way-of-life. For example, there is the 'Mediterranean life style' – a particular dietary profile (pasta, fresh vegetables, olive oil, etc.), consumption of wine with meals, communal eating habits, and midday siestas. This way-of-life is associated with a relatively low risk of various diseases, especially coronary heart disease, stroke, and cancers of the large bowel and breast. The phrase 'way-of-life' acknowledges a shared *pattern* of behaviors, grounded in local culture, custom, and socioeconomic circumstance.

'Life style' is an open-ended category of behaviors, ranging from obvious interindividual differences in such things as dietary behaviors, smoking, alcohol consumption – all with major known influences on disease etiology – to relaxation patterns, sleep habits, vitamin supplementation, beverage preferences, clothing, and work patterns. The behaviors most relevant to epidemiology are those with metabolic, hormonal, pharmacologic or toxicologic consequences.

Eight important individual behavioral risk factors, each with a range of health consequences, are shown in Table 12.1. Alcohol consumption, for example, affects blood pressure, blood clotting tendency, blood lipid profile (beneficial), cancers of the upper aerodigestive tract, cancer of the female breast, gallstone disease (protective), liver cirrhosis, fetal development, organic brain disease and dementia, antisocial behaviors, and road trauma. The relative importance of the main biological pathways of action, for each of these behaviors, is indicated.

Level of analysis: individual, community, or population

Epidemiologists usually assume that life style-orientated research should, wherever possible, be conducted at the individual level (as in cohort or case control studies). However, for some of these variables (such as dietary fat consumption) the interindividual range of exposure within a particular population may be rather small, and stronger comparisons may well be possible at the group or population level. Likewise, there may be striking variations in exposure over time in a population.

Therefore, some of the most persuasive evidence linking life style factors with disease risk has come from comparisons of countries or regions, from studies of subpopulations such as vegetarians, or from observations on migrant populations undergoing 'east-to-west' shifts in their dietary habits (McMichael et al., 1980; McMichael and Giles, 1988). The role of 'ecological' (population level) studies in relation to life style variables should therefore be discussed critically.

Likewise, students should examine critically the ideas developed by the British epidemiologist Geoffrey Rose, who contrasted 'sick individuals' with 'sick populations' (Rose, 1985). Rose noted that the emphasis on individual life style as a cause of disease implies that the appropriate intervention is to identify the high risk individuals within the population, and to modify their behaviors. The real public health problem, he argued, is typically that the whole population has moved 'to the right' (i.e. higher) on the risk factor axis. It is therefore the population's way-of-life rather than the 'high-risk' individual's life style that accounts for most of the increased incidence of disease. Whereas high-risk individuals are, usually, at markedly above average risk of developing a particular disease, most cases of disease arise from the much larger number of medium risk persons.

Rose also noted that it is usually difficult to persuade high risk individuals to alter their behaviors, especially when the society at large has a tendency towards an elevated risk level. For example, urbanized societies with a high intake of processed foods typically have a rather high intake of salt. In such a setting, it is not easy to get those individuals with a particularly high salt intake to cut back substantially.

Table 12.1 Eight important individual behavioral risk factors. The relative importance of the main biologic pathways of action, for each of these eight behaviors is shown.

Behaviour	Mode of action							
	Metabolic	Physiologic	Pharmacologic	Toxicologic	Immunologic	Hormonal	Infectious	Physical
Diet	++++	+		+	++	++		
Physical activity	++	+++				+		
Alcohol consumption	++		+++	+++	+	+		
Smoking	+	+	++	++++	+			
Oral contraception (and HRT)					(+)	++++		
Sexual activity						+	++++	
Recreational drugs		+	++++	+	+	+	++ (intravenous)	
Solar exposure	+				++			++++

Confounding and effect modification between life style variables

Students must understand the conceptual difference between confounding (a consequence of the non-random distribution of two or more risk factors for the disease under investigation) and effect modification (a consequence of the biologic amplification of the effect of one variable caused by the enhancing effect of another variable). Confounding is a potential source of bias that the investigator hopes to prevent or to remove (by stratification or adjustment). However, effect modification is a real phenomenon, wherein the health impact of one variable is conditional on the coincident level of some other variable. Effect modification (which is sometimes called 'interaction', although many statisticians regard interaction as a mathematically defined entity) is therefore to be sought out and reported, rather than avoided.

Confounding

The frequent correlations between life style factors create a considerable potential for confounding in this topic area. For example, vegetarians tend disproportionately to be non-smokers and moderate consumers of alcohol. In many cultures, persons who smoke also tend to drink alcohol – and are often above average consumers of coffee. A good discussion of this general issue is contained in the paper by Johansson and colleagues (1999).

Effect modification

The frequent occurrence of coexistent risk behaviors creates many possibilities for biologic interaction, often referred to as effect modification. Two of the best known examples are the effect modifications of alcohol and smoking in the induction of cancers of the mouth, throat, oesophagus, and larynx, and of oral contraceptive usage and cigarette smoking in the risk of thrombotic stroke in young women. The former interaction is well illustrated by the case control study of Rothman and Keller (1972) and for a more general discussion students should be directed to Rothman and Greenland (1998).

Life style factors also interact with other categories of factors. Of increasing interest, given the rise of molecular genetics and knowledge of metabolic polymorphisms, it is becoming important to consider interaction between life style exposures and genetically based susceptibility. For example, the increasing risk of colon cancer in relation to increasing level of meat consumption appears to be largely confined to persons who are 'fast acetylators', one of the two metabolic phenotypes determined by the *NAT2* gene (Roberts-Thomson *et al.*, 1996). The results of this type of study, presented in stratified fashion, provide illuminating examples of the effect modification phenomenon.

The 'life course' perspective

Another perspective receiving increasing attention from epidemiologists is the recognition that life's experiences, extending from antenatal life, through childhood, adolescence, and adulthood, comprise a longitudinal and dynamic process within which the risks of various chronic diseases evolve (Kuh and Ben-Shlomo, 1997; Brunner *et al.*, 1999; Blane, 1999).

The 'life course' perspective thus recognizes the following:

1. That many disease processes of later life have their origins in early, even, antenatal experiences.
2. That many disease 'risks' evolve over the course of a lifetime, and the influence of a specific 'factor' is usually conditioned by the presence of other factors.
3. This interactive 'system' of influences encompasses genetic, environmental, social, and behavioral factors.

Coronary heart disease (CHD) provides a ready example. There is a range of genetic influences on this disease, predisposing to hyperlipidemia, hypertension, insulin resistance and so on. It is also evident that some aspects of fetal life associated with impaired development and low birth weight cause modulation of physiologic and metabolic functions that affect the risk of this disease process (Barker, 1994). During childhood and adolescence, aspects of 'social positioning' and the associated nutritional, social, and environmental experiences, affecting such things as bodily growth trajectory and patterns of cortisol secretion in response to stressful situations, contribute further to the evolution of CHD risk (Blane, 1999).

The relative importance of early life and adult life influences varies between categories of disease outcome. For example, a cohort study of Scottish men found that the risk of stroke and stomach cancer mortality depended primarily on childhood socioeconomic conditions, whereas heart disease mortality was influenced by conditions in both childhood and adulthood (Davey Smith *et al.*, 1998). Early life experiences may critically affect some heart disease risk factors such as triglyceride levels, while cholesterol level and blood pressure are affected by both early and adult life (Davey Smith *et al.*, 1997).

Note that these contributory influences are not necessarily merely sequential, and additive. Rather, the 'life course' model assumes that there will be interactions between these several domains of causal influence: genetic, environmental, nutritional, and psychosocial. Note also that, within this etiologic model, the role of 'life style' factors, that is, personally chosen, independent risk factors, is merely a part of the overall etiologic configuration. Life style is subsumed within life course. Indeed, there is a further conceptual shift. The conventional conception of life style variables has been of behaviors that emerged in adulthood, such as smoking and alcohol consumption. The notion of 'dose' was implicit, and, where appropriate, duration of the behavior was therefore usually estimated. Nevertheless, many cohort studies and case control studies used one-off estimates of the exposure which led to a rather modular statistical model based on static measures of exposure (McMichael, 1999).

This genre of research will require various new techniques of analysing data, such as repeated-measures techniques, multistate modeling, and adaptive genetic algorithms. The 'life course' model of disease etiology also, of course, has important implications for disease prevention. More advanced students should be directed to Cox and Wermuth, 1996 and Greenland *et al.*, 1999 for modeling techniques.

Choosing a research design

Population level analyses

There is, at first sight, a seeming incongruity in using population level analyses to examine the disease risks associated with a variable that is considered to be an individual level 'life style' variable. However, population level analyses are particularly useful in identifying or corroborating relationships. This is well illustrated by the Seven Countries Study from the 1970s, which showed how variations in blood cholesterol and blood pressure correlated with CHD rates (Keys *et al.*, 1986).

Population level analyses are also useful in identifying rapid changes in cause-specific mortality rates following an abrupt change in population exposure level. This occurred in France, when wartime constraints on alcohol consumption were followed by a rapid downturn in liver cirrhosis mortality, in Norway when heart disease mortality rates dropped immediately after the occupying German army commandeered the meat, eggs, and dairy products, and in Poland during the 1990s after the transformation of the nation's food supply that led to a substantial switching from polyunsaturated fats to saturated fats (Zatonski *et al.*, 1998).

One interesting sidelight on these studies is that many of them indicate, in ways not easily studied in individual level studies, the role of the life style exposure in the late-stage processes of the disease: i.e. in the transition from advanced disease to fatal disease. This apparently accounts for the surprisingly rapid downturn in cause-specific death rates following cessation of exposure.

Students should be challenged to think critically about the circumstances in which population level analyses are informative, and indeed may be the preferred or the only source of useful information. Considerations include differences in exposure ranges within and between populations, the opportunity to test for the effect of different time lags, and the opportunity afforded by migrant populations to assess critical ages of first exposure.

Cohort studies

Whereas cohort studies of environmental and occupational exposures must often settle for comparing groups of individuals defined by job, residential location or some other index of presumed shared 'exposure', life style factors can often be readily and well studied at the individual level. Indeed, many of the modern methods in cohort study design and analysis have evolved via studies of life style and disease risk.

Teachers should ensure that they are familiar with the well known examples of cohort studies such as the Framingham Study of individual behaviors and biomedical factors in relation to coronary heart disease (Kannel *et al.*, 1961), the British Doctors study of cigarette smoking, lung cancer, and other diseases (Doll *et al.*, 1994), and the American Cancer Society's large cohort study (Boffetta and Garfinkel, 1990).

Case control studies

As with cohort studies, the modern case control study has been strongly shaped by the experience of relating disease outcome to a detailed history of prior life style behaviors. Much of the early information about the relationships of specific cancers to diet, alcohol, smoking, coffee consumption, oral contraception, and sexual behaviors came from case control studies. This retrospective focus on previous exposures provided a strong stimulus to the development of semiquantitative questionnaires for the assessment of long-term (perhaps whole-of-life) exposures to diet, alcohol, sunlight, and so on.

These case control studies have also afforded many examples of various types of bias, both classification and selection biases. Classification biases, particularly with respect to self-reported exposure history, are discussed below under 'measuring exposure to life style factors'. The following are two interesting examples of selection biases occurring in case control studies. First, an initial report that pancreatic cancer was associated with coffee consumption was later attributed to the fact that the control group, comprising cancer-free hospital patients from a gastrointestinal clinic, had below average consumption of coffee. Second, several studies have reported an inverse relationship between Alzheimer's disease and cigarette smoking. However, it appears that hypercholesterolemia, which is a true risk factor for the disease, combines with cigarette smoking to cause premature death (via cardiovascular disease) in smokers, which leaves the surviving non-smoking hypercholesterolemics prone to subsequent Alzheimer's disease.

Intervention studies

Experimental studies are possible at several spatial levels. Well known examples of whole-community studies include the North Karelia study, in which a life style modification public education program was mounted in this region of Finland in an attempt to reduce the unusually high rate of coronary heart disease mortality (Puska et al., 1985). Comparison over time was made with the adjoining, non-intervention region. Surprisingly, there was little difference in the subsequent time trends in CHD mortality rates in the two populations, an observation that was attributed to the uncontrollable spread of health-promoting information and ideas into the control community.

Many experimental studies have been conducted at the individual level, particularly studies in high risk individuals. Students should become acquainted with the well known examples such as the Oslo Study of smoking intervention (Hjermann et al., 1981) and the Multiple Risk Factor Intervention Trial (MRFIT) in middle-aged US males at high risk of coronary heart disease (Mr Fit Research Group, 1982).

Measuring exposure to life style factors

The general issues in exposure assessment have been well reviewed elsewhere (Armstrong et al., 1992). However, epidemiology students should be reminded that many 'exposures' change over time. For example, the formulation of the oral contraceptive pill keeps changing. Likewise, cigarettes today in countries with a high income tend to have markedly less nicotine than those of earlier decades. Hence, we may sometimes be estimating risks of today's chronic disease outcomes in relation to a superseded exposure.

Individual level assessment

There are three main strategies for estimating an individual's life style. They are:

+ interview, questionnaire or short-term diary
+ biologic markers
+ surrogate data (e.g. membership of a vegetarian society, or of an abstaining religious sect).

Because of the strong normative values attached to many of these behaviors – such as smoking habits, number of sexual partners, and drinking behaviors – there is a recurring problem of respondent bias (so-called classification bias). Very often, respondents give socially acceptable answers. Students should consider how this type of bias could be minimized.

Group or population level assessment

At the group level, the four main options for exposure assessment are:

+ centrally held records (e.g. sales of alcohol, imports and exports, household surveys, etc.)
+ interviews, questionnaires or short-term diaries for cross-sectional assessment of the mean and variance of group level behavior
+ surrogate variables (e.g. cirrhosis rates for levels of heavy alcohol consumption)
+ biologic markers

Biologic indices of exposure

Students should be asked to consider the role of independent biologic markers of 'exposure', both as definitive exposure indices and as validation indices. A key concept here is that interindividual variation in biologic index usually reflects much more than the original variation in external exposure. It also incorporates 'host' differences in the way the individual absorbs, transports, metabolizes, and excretes the exposure factor.

Wherever possible, and affordable, epidemiologists prefer to obtain biologic indicators of dietary 'exposure'. However, there are few ways of obtaining an integrated measure of dietary intake over a long period of time. Hair and nails provide measures of intake of certain elements over a succession of months. In relation to large bowel cancer and other bowel disorders, fecal samples have been used to assess the integrated impact of diet, conditioned by endogenous host characteristics, upon acidity, metabolism of bile acids, transit speed, and bacterial profile. Used judiciously, these biomarkers can provide useful 'ecologic' comparison of samples of populations known to be at differing risk of some specified disease.

Differentiating 'upstream' from 'downstream' variables: choosing an appropriate analytic strategy

More advanced epidemiology students should be able to make informed and knowledgeable judgements on appropriate analytic strategies. It is important to remind them that 'life style' variables are 'downstream' variables. As individual behaviors, these variables have their origins in culture, socioeconomic status, patterns of peer group behavior, local conditions and opportunities. It is common for epidemiologists to construct multivariate models that entail cross-level mixing of variables, e.g. socioeconomic status, smoking behavior, and blood cholesterol. The assigning of partial risk coefficients to each of these on the basis of standard multiple (logistic) regression analysis, assumes that they act in parallel. In fact, each of these three variables represents different segments of a generic causal change: the sociocultural milieu, individual behaviors, and biologic indicators. That is, they are differing 'distances' from the health outcome variable. Hence, it is important to use an appropriate modeling approach to the phenomenon of hierarchical, sequential, causation. Hierarchical models and pathway analysis are two options that will often give less biased and more informative results when the dataset transcends several 'levels' of causation.

Estimating attributable risks

Students at a more advanced level need to give critical consideration to several issues in the estimation of the 'attributable' risks for life style factors.

Compared to what?

A primary decision is the choice of reference category. For occupational or ambient environmental exposures the reference category is often zero dose. Likewise, in the life style domain, it is intuitively appealing to use the zero dose category for assessing the attributable risk of disease to smoking, alcohol, or oral contraceptive use.

However, two caveats apply here. First, for a number of life style variables, such as physical activity and dietary (macronutrient and micronutrient) intakes, the comparison must often be to some *non*-zero category (e.g. there are no no-fat consumers!). Second, there is a hierarchy of 'reasonableness' that applies in seeking to estimate how much disease is actually preventable within a specified population. Murray and Lopez (1999) propose four levels of estimated disease 'preventability' as a function of the proportion of exposure within the population that is eliminated: namely, what is:

- theoretically possible (all exposure is eliminated)
- plausible (how much could be eliminated in ideal circumstances)
- feasible (how much could be eliminated realistically)
- affordable (what intervention is actually cost-effective).

We read that in today's world there are approximately three million deaths annually attributable to cigarette smoking, and that by 2020 this figure will have grown to ten million deaths annually. In advising policy makers, can we say more realistically what proportion of these deaths could be avoided by available interventions such as banning advertising or doubling the retail price?

Single or multiple health outcomes (i.e. full cost accounting)

An important consideration is taking account of the full balance sheet of health gains and losses associated with a specified change in life style. Two ready examples are alcohol consumption and oral contraceptive use. For each it is likely to be misleading to base public health policy advice on just one health outcome. Students should be asked to review the literature and identify the panoply of health risk shifts associated with these and other life style exposures.

Alcohol consumption, for example, increases the risk of breast cancer, various other cancers, cirrhosis of the liver, dementia, risk of physical injury (especially on the roads), and antisocial violent behaviors. On the other hand, it reduces the risk of coronary heart disease mortality, gallstone disease and, in moderation, it can assist in reducing stress levels.

Likewise, the use of oral contraceptives, depending on type, age of use, duration of use, and association with cigarette smoking, can increase the risks of breast cancer (but only marginally), venous thrombosis, and subarachnoid hemorrhage. On the other hand it reduces the risks associated with unwanted pregnancy (e.g. abortion, especially if illegal, and childbirth), and the risk of occurrence of ovarian cancer and, perhaps, colon cancer.

This issue challenges the student to consider how to do the balance sheet 'arithmetic'. This array of health outcomes is heterogeneous. How can the estimated gains and losses be compared? Is there some common metric that can be applied to enable direct quantitative comparison? Pursuit of this question should open up the interesting discussion about the merits and demerits of using measures such as DALYs, disability-adjusted life years (Murray and Lopez, 1996).

Teaching method and format

The teaching of a life style and life course perspective can be integrated into a single module of a basic epidemiology course or, when covered more extensively, it can warrant a whole separate study unit, perhaps consisting of several sequential sessions over a term. There are ample opportunities for varied and innovative teaching techniques, with the aim of engaging the students and encouraging active learning.

Suggested teaching formats and exercises are now given for the components discussed above.

Introducing life style and life course perspective

This could consist of a preliminary lecture in which the basic concepts are introduced and the course content outlined. The students could be directed towards resources for self-learning, such as key textbooks in this field (*A life course approach to chronic disease epidemiology* edited by Kuh and Ben-Shlomo, 1997 and *The LS factor* by Hetzel and McMichael, 1987).

Research designs and measuring life style exposures

This topic lends itself well to a small groupwork exercise. Students could be introduced to the concepts in a lecture, followed by a practical session in which the students are asked to design a suitable study. Working in groups of about four or five, the students could be given research questions, such as 'What is the breast cancer risk associated with use of the oral contraception pill?' They will need to describe an appropriate study design, giving particular consideration to how they would measure exposure (acknowledging the changes in pill formulation over time), confounding variables, and so on. The students then present their design to the rest of the group for comment and further discussion.

Confounding and effect modification

A problem-based exercise, either working alone or in small groups, could be devised to introduce students to the problems arising from confounding and effect modification, and the difference between the two concepts. Some of the best known cohort studies (see above) could be used as the basis of material to illustrate the type of confounding and effect modification issues which arise when assessing life style exposures and the possible techniques for addressing them (both in the study design and analysis stages).

Estimating attributable risks

Students could be provided with several recent research papers and asked to review the literature critically and see whether a distinction is made between 'attributability' and 'preventability' of disease risks in association with proposed alterations to life style. A group discussion could then follow about the feasibility of health promotion policy proposals. The importance of assessing all heath outcomes associated with changing life style exposure (both positive and negative, to individuals and society, and immediate or delayed) needs to be stressed.

Assessing students' achievements

The methods of evaluating students' understanding can range from a more formal written examination to informal class presentations. A quick and easy way to assess students' basic understanding is through the use of a multiple choice question paper. This could cover the key concepts and be used early in a course to monitor students' progress and pick up on any weaknesses in their understanding. At the end of a course, it may be more appropriate to evaluate their application of principles by setting a small project to be worked on individually or in small groups. This might, for instance, involve setting a research question for which the students are asked to outline an appropriate study design and analysis strategy.

A more integrated question could be set which incorporates the other aspects of exposure-orientated epidemiology (environment, occupation, social factors, etc.). This would challenge students to consider a wider perspective and the degree to which some exposures are more amenable to modification and their relative anticipated health gains.

References

Armstrong, B. K., White, E., Sarraci R. (1992). *Principles of exposure measurement in epidemiology*. Oxford University Press, Oxford.

Barker, D. J. P. (1994). *Mothers, Babies and Disease in Later Life*. BMJ Publishing, London.

Blane, D. (1999). The life course, the social gradient, and health. In: *Social Determinants of Health* (eds M. G. Marmot and R. Wilkinson), pp. 64–80. Oxford University Press, Oxford.

Boffetta, P. and Garfinkel, L. (1990) Alcohol drinking and mortality among men enrolled in an American Cancer Society prospective study. *Epidemiology* 1, 342–8.

Brunner, E., Shipley, M. J., Blane, D., Davey Smith, G., Marmot. M. G. (1999). When does cardiovascular risk start? Past and present socioeconomic circumstances and risk factors in adulthood. *Journal of Epidemiology and Community Health*, 53, 757–64.

Cox, D. R. and Wermuth, N. (1996). *Multivariate Dependencies. Models, analysis and interpretation.* Chapman and Hall, London.

Davey Smith, G., Hart, C., Blane, D., Gillis, C., Hawthorne, V. (1997). Lifetime socioeconomic position and mortality: prospective observational study. *British Medical Journal*, 314, 547–52.

Davey Smith, G., Hart, C., Blane, D., Hole, D. (1998). Adverse socioeconomic conditions in childhood and cause-specific adult mortality: prospective observational study. *British Medical Journal*, 316, 1631–5.

Doll, R., Peto, R., Wheatley, K., Gray, R., Sutherland, I. (1994). Mortality in relation to smoking: 40 years' observations on male British doctors. *British Medical Journal*, 309, 901–11.

Greenland, S., Pearl, J., Robins, J. M. (1999). Causal diagrams for epidemiological research. *Epidemiology*, 10, 37–48.

Hetzel, B. and McMichael, T. (1987). *The LS factor.* Penguin Books, Australia.

Hjermann, I., Vevke, J. B., Holme, I., Leren, P. (1981). Effect of diet and smoking intervention on the incidence of coronary heart disease. Report from the Oslo Study Group of a randomised trial in healthy men. *Lancet.* ii(8259), 1303–10

Johansson, L., Thelle, D. S., Solvoll, K., Bjorneboe, G. E., Drevon, C. A. (1999). Health dietary habits in relation to social determinants and life style factors. *British Journal of Nutrition*, 81, 211–20.

Kannel, W. B., Dawber, T. R., Kagan, A. *et al.* (1961). Factors of risk in the development of coronary heart disease – six year follow-up experience: the Framingham Study. *Annals of Internal Medicine*, 55, 33–50.

Kaufman, J. S., Cooper, R. S. (1998). Seeking causal explanations in social epidemiology. *American Journal of Epidemiology*, 150, 113–20.

Keys, A., Menotti, A., Karvonen, M. J., Aravanis, C., Blackburn, H., Buzina, R., *et al.* (1986). The diet and 15-year death rate in the Seven Countries Study. *American Journal of Epidemiology*, 124, 903–15.

Krieger, N. (1994). Epidemiology and the web of causation: has anyone seen the spider? *Social Science and Medicine*, 39, 887–903.

Krieger, N., Zierler, S. (1996). What explains the public's health? A call for epidemiologic theory. *Epidemiology*, 7, 107–9.

Kuh, D. and Ben-Shlomo, Y. eds (1997). *A Life Course Approach to Chronic Disease Epidemiology.* Oxford University Press, Oxford.

McMichael, A. J. (1999). Prisoners of the proximate: loosening the constraints on epidemiology in an age of change. *American Journal of Epidemiology*, 149, 887–97.

McMichael, A. J., McCall, M. G., Hartshorne, J. M., Woodings, T. L. (1980). Patterns of gastro-intestinal cancer in European migrants to Australia: the role of dietary change. *International Journal of Cancer*, 25, 431–7.

McMichael, A. J., Giles, G. G. (1988). Cancer in migrants to Australia: extending the descriptive epidemiological data. *Cancer Research*, 48, 751–6.

Mr Fit Research Group. (1982). Multiple-risk Factor Intervention Trial. *Journal of the American Medical Association*, **248**, 1465–77.

Murray, C. J. and Lopez, A. (1999). On the comparable quantification of health risks: lessons from the Global Burden of Disease Study. *Epidemiology*, **10**, 594–605.

Murray, C. J. L. and Lopez, A. D., eds. (1996). *The Global Burden of Disease: a comprehensive assessment of mortality and disability from diseases, injuries, and risk factors in 1990 and projected to 2020*. Harvard University Press, Cambridge.

Puska, P., Nissinen, A., Tuomilehto, J. (1985). The community-based strategy to prevent coronary heart disease. Conclusions from the ten years of the North Karelia project. *Annual Review of Public Health*, **6**, 147–93.

Roberts-Thomson, I., Ryan, P. R., Khoo, K., Hart, W. J., McMichael, A. J., Butler, R. N. (1996) Diet, acetylator phenotype and risk of colorectal neoplasia. *Lancet*, **347**, 1372–4.

Rose, G. (1985). Sick individuals and sick populations? *International Journal of Epidemiology* **14**, 32–8.

Rothman, K. J. and Keller, A. Z. (1972). The effect of joint exposure to alcohol and tobacco on risk of cancer of the mouth and pharynx. *American Journal of Public Health*, **25**, 711–16.

Rothman, K. J. and Greenland, S. (1998). *Modern Epidemiology*, 2nd edn, Lippincott-Raven, Philadelphia, USA: pp. 329–42.

Zatonski, W., McMichael, A. J., Powles, J. W. (1998). Ecological study of reasons for sharp decline in mortality from ischaemic heart disease in Poland since 1991. *British Medical Journal*, **316**, 1045–7.

Chapter 13

Pharmacoepidemiology

Susan S. Jick

Introduction

This chapter provides an approach to teaching drug epidemiology (often called pharmacoepidemiology) that focuses primarily on techniques for conducting drug safety studies. However, these techniques can also be applied to pharmacoeconomic and outcomes research studies since the important principles covered in the drug safety area also form the foundation for other types of drug studies. The teaching is targeted towards students of epidemiology since the principles involved are fairly advanced and would be difficult to cover in an undergraduate class.

Teaching objectives

Students completing this course should be able to review the literature in the drug safety area critically as well as to design simple drug safety studies.

Teaching contents (key concepts and items that need to be taught)

As with any discipline it is important first to set out the basic principles and methods of the field of study. Drug epidemiology is similar to other areas of epidemiology in that the basic methods of clear case and exposure definition are critical to the success of a study. However, in pharmacoepidemiology, providing clear definitions is more complex than in classic epidemiology because drug exposures are constantly varying and are thus difficult to define precisely, and because the outcomes are often associated in some way to the exposure, creating biases and confounding that are essential to understand and properly adjust for in the study design. This chapter attempts to provide the necessary material for teaching the methods essential to the conduct of a well designed drug safety study.

Teaching method and contents

I begin this course by discussing how formalized studies of drug safety were first precipitated and provide past examples of serious drug safety problems such as thalidomide and phocomelia, or isotretinoin and birth defects. It is also helpful to discuss the different areas of pharmacoepidemiology such as drug utilization, outcomes research, and regulatory issues, as well as drug safety. I stress the methods of drug safety research in this course but briefly discuss the role of these other areas. A challenge for every course is to interest the students in the material presented in class. The exercises provided at the end of the chapter have stimulated much excitement and interest in this area of epidemiology and have inspired some very creative and thoughtful responses from the students. I encourage class participation and discussion through-out the course and challenge the students to work through the implications of using the different methodologies presented.

Below are described the key elements of drug epidemiology that need to be taught to begin to grasp the scope of the field and to be able to review the literature critically as well as to think about study designs. With each element there is a brief summary of the main points to be made.

Considerations for all drug safety studies

Basis for defining drug/disease relation

To design a drug epidemiology study properly one must first determine the nature of the outcome and the drug to be studied. Students should be presented with the various ways of thinking about drugs and drug effects. There are several ways to think about the exposure and outcome in drug safety studies. Is the outcome rare or common, serious or mild? Is it a pharmacologic, idiosyncratic, or allergic disorder? Is it a functional, biochemical, or structural problem? Is it caused by short-term use, long-term use, or both? Is the effect acute, continuous, or delayed? Is the drug newly marketed, recently marketed, or has it been marketed for many years?

All of these determinations help to frame the question at hand which in turn leads to the use of the appropriate methodology and data resources. For example, if a drug is not widely used one will need a very large database to find enough exposed subjects. If the effect is delayed one will need to follow up study subjects for a long period to detect the outcomes of interest. These elements must be sorted out before starting a study. The teacher should go through several scenarios to help the students grasp the variety in drug and outcome types.

In teaching a class pharmacoepidemiology, I carefully review the association between drugs and diseases. Some safety studies evaluate the relation between a drug that has no clinical relation to the outcome of interest (antidepressant drugs and liver disease, for example), while other drug–disease relations are more complicated (such as antibiotics and seizures). It is important that the disease under study not be associated with the drug under investigation. Also, the outcome must be idiopathic, that is, not due to another proximate cause. For example, in a study of drug-induced liver disease one must exclude as possible cases all persons with viral hepatitis, as this is a sufficient cause of liver disease and is unlikely to be drug-induced. One is interested in discovering possible cases of drug-induced illness in the absence of other apparent causes. If non-drug-induced illnesses are included as cases it is likely that a true effect will be obscured. It is helpful to provide examples of studies that are performed incorrectly in which a null result is found and compare it to a study that excludes non-idiopathic cases and finds a positive association between the drug and the outcome. It is also important to stress the limitations of observational studies of drug effects. Such studies cannot meaningfully evaluate an effect of a pre-existing illness, so that in a study of drug-induced seizures one must exclude all people with a previous history of epilepsy. It is rarely possible in observational studies to determine confidently if a drug causes worsening of seizures or increases the rate of seizures in someone with pre-existing disease. It would be useful at this point to have a discussion of prescribing bias where the teacher should provide (and solicit from the students) examples. One example of this type of bias is found in the study of antibiotic-associated seizures. If a subject already has a seizure disorder, does the receipt of an antibiotic worsen the condition? It is not possible to know if the antibiotic or the illness being treated by the antibiotic is causing the seizure, or if neither of the two are related. To study worsening of disease one must conduct a clinical trial as observational studies are inherently biased in ways that would yield uninterpretable results (Jick *et al.*, 1998; Ray, 1998).

Similarly, it is difficult, if not impossible, to interpret results when study drugs are used to treat diseases that are risk factors for the outcome under study using observational data. For example, the results of a study of suicide in users of antidepressants would be difficult to interpret as people on antidepressants are depressed and would be expected to commit suicide more often than those not exposed. Further, it is likely that people taking different antidepressants have varying severity of depression so the suicide rate would be different among the users of the various antidepressants. It is again helpful to have the students think through the logic in this example and to come up with other examples of such situations.

Control of confounding

Confounding is a concern in all epidemiologic studies and is covered in basic methodology classes. However, when I teach this course several factors in drug epidemiology studies that must be controlled or, at the very least, evaluated as potential confounders are discussed. These are age, sex, geography, and calendar time. Each of these factors is frequently correlated with the incidence of disease and always with the exposure variable. Drug use changes from one part of the world to another, it varies between men and women, and between age groups. It also varies over time as new drugs become available. Rates of illness may also vary across these four factors and thus must be taken into account in study design and analysis. Providing examples of these types of variation is useful in demonstrating their potential effects on a study result.

Confounding by indication

Confounding by indication is a bias that occurs when the drug of interest is selectively used or not used by those who develop the outcome of interest. This occurs when the drug is used to treat a diagnosis that is in the causal pathway of the outcome of interest. For example, if one were studying non-steroidal anti-inflammatory drugs (NSAIDs) in relation to renal cancer then one should be concerned that the NSAIDs were used to treat the early pain symptoms of the cancer. This bias presents some of the larger challenges in pharmacoepidemiologic studies and should be discussed thoroughly in class. Here again, working through examples will help the student grasp the nature and importance of this form of bias. Another example is found in the study of cimetidine and gastric cancer, where people with early symptoms of gastric cancer are likely to receive cimetidine to treat the symptoms. In this instance, if confounding by indication is not adequately controlled, then the researchers might incorrectly conclude that there is a positive association between the drug and the disease (Schumacher *et al.*, 1990). It is not always possible to control for this type of confounding and some studies simply cannot be done or, if they are done, the results are not interpretable. Randomized clinical trials are often the only reliable means of evaluating drug–disease relations in these circumstances. When I teach this I always describe a study that is subject to confounding by indication and then describe the proper methodology to avoid the problem (Schumacher *et al.*, 1990). It is also helpful to work through the result that would be obtained if the proper methodology were not employed.

Exposure ascertainment

Another challenge in the area of pharmacoepidemiology is obtaining accurate and complete exposure information. The classic way to obtain the data is to ask people what drugs they have taken. It is very revealing to ask students in the class what drugs they have taken in the past 3 years, for how long they took the drugs and what the dosages were. Most people do not remember what they took last week, never mind what they took last year. The point of this exercise is to demonstrate how difficult it can be to find reliable exposure information. It is then helpful to work through examples that illustrate the effects of misinformation on a study result. I like to go one step further and describe the importance of procuring timely data on exposure. It is not helpful to have information on drugs collected 10 years before the outcome under study. For most studies, drug exposure data must be gathered over time and must reflect changes in drug use that occur up until the diagnosis of the outcome. It is helpful to provide examples of studies that do not have complete drug information and to discuss the implications for the study results.

Considerations for cohort studies

Defining the cohorts

Selecting an exposed cohort and an appropriate comparison group is key in the design of a study. It is important for students in the class to think through the possible ways of defining the study cohorts. It is not always best to compare users of a drug to non-users. There are times when another drug exposure provides a more appropriate comparison. Subjects in the comparison cohort should be as similar to the exposed group as possible except that they have not received the study drug. For example, in studying the effect of an antibiotic drug it would be useful to compare the outcome to that of another antibiotic used to treat the same conditions. In this way one controls for the presence of underlying disease (the indication for drug use) which could be associated with the outcome under study. Sometimes a non-exposed cohort is the only reasonable choice for a comparison group. At other times one might choose, for efficiency, to have a non-exposed cohort *and* a cohort exposed to another drug (Jick,

1998). When teaching this class I always discuss the problems related to exposure definition that stem from changing and discontinuing drug use. Students should think through the design implications of changing exposure status; this is one of the challenges of pharmacoepidemiology. Remember that people are constantly changing their drug prescriptions and are often exposed to more than one study drug at a time. Taking the students through a study and discussing the implications of these issues is very helpful in thinking through proper exposure definition.

It is important to remind students that people receive drugs to treat medical problems. This means that, by definition, exposed study subjects will all have some medical condition (except in rare circumstances such as women using oral contraceptives). Yet, to be eligible to enter any of the study cohorts a subject must not have had the study outcome before entry into the study. In drug safety studies one should always look at newly diagnosed disease. In so doing, one is by definition excluding anyone who had the disease before receiving the study drug. For the same reason the investigator must exclude people who have predisposing conditions that are present before entry into the study as these conditions are the more likely cause of any subsequent development of the outcome under study and may influence later exposure to the study drug. This is discussed further in the section on Considerations for case control studies.

Defining the exposure window

The appropriate window(s) of exposure must be determined for each new study separately as it is dependent on the outcome under study and the drug under investigation. In this class I like to go through different scenarios to be sure that the students understand how the exposure window relates to the outcomes. For acute outcomes such as liver disease, renal disease, serious skin diseases, etc., a short window such as 45 or 60 days following discontinuation of therapy is appropriate. However, if one is studying the association between a drug and a delayed outcome such as cancer or cataracts then one might need to look at all time after exposure, taking into account duration of use, recency of use, cumulative dose, etc.

Expressing exposure

Students should have some familiarity with the different ways of expressing exposure. Exposure can be described in terms of person–time of exposure, or as counts of people exposed *versus* non-exposed. Each method is based on different assumptions. It is helpful for the students to grasp these differences by giving examples. For person counts to be a valid approach there must be comparable follow-up for all study subjects. This would apply in the study of an acute effect of an antibiotic, for example, where each person is followed for only 45 days. However, in a study of a chronically used drug, use will stop, start, change over time, and vary from one person to another. In this situation the contribution of each individual can be accumulated using person–time. The use of person–time for detailed evaluation of drug–disease exposures has limitations, however. It is difficult to assess duration, dose, and timing of use for each individual in a large study, and an essential element in drug studies, controling for calendar time, is difficult in this circumstance. In this situation it is advisable to use a case control analysis within the cohort to control for details of drug use as well as for confounding (see section on Case control studies).

Considerations in case control studies

Selections of cases and controls

In any drug safety study it is important to select cases with a newly diagnosed illness that has no other apparent non-drug cause. Case selection should always be accomplished without knowledge of the subject's exposure status to avoid biased case selection. One is not interested in studying prevalent disease. Put another way, if a disease is present before receipt of the drug then there is no possibility that the drug caused the disease, and therefore that person should not be included as a case. Similarly, if a subject has another proximate cause present for the illness of interest that is the most likely cause of the outcome, then that person should not be included as a case (Jick and Vessey, 1978). For example, in the case of a person who has just had surgery and develops a venous thromboembolism, the illness is most likely a result of the surgery and the drug should not be considered as a possible cause. Here again it is helpful to the students to demonstrate the importance of this lesson by providing examples and showing how the results differ when 'all' cases are included instead of only idiopathic cases.

When selecting controls any exclusion criteria applied to the cases must also be applied to the controls. Put another way, the base population from which the controls are drawn should be properly selected so that the cases and controls are equally likely to be exposed to the study drug in the absence of a drug effect. If studying estrogens and endometrial cancer, all women in the study population from whence cases and controls are drawn should have an intact uterus. A woman without a uterus could not become a case, nor does she have the same likelihood of being exposed to estrogens.

It is often helpful to match controls to cases on age, sex, and location to facilitate control of these potential confounding factors. In addition, matching the index date of the case to a set of matched controls achieves control of calendar time in an efficient manner. It should be noted, however, that if one matches on a factor then the independent effects of that factor cannot be evaluated in the analysis and the analysis must take the matching into account.

Selection of controls in a drug safety study should be discussed in depth with the students. It is helpful to go through several examples to illustrate the principles involved here. If one is selecting controls from a hospital population it is important that the controls not be admitted to the hospital for a reason related to the outcome or the exposure under study. For example, in a study of oral contraceptives and breast cancer, it is important that controls not be selected from a cardiovascular ward as these women are less likely to be taking oral contraceptives since women with cardiovascular problems are selectively not prescribed the drug. Selecting controls from this population would bias the likelihood of exposure in a way that could create a spurious positive association between oral contraceptives and breast cancer. Similarly, it is important that the controls not be more likely to be exposed to the drug of interest. For example, if one were studying the association between antidepressants and convulsions one would not select controls from the psychiatric ward as they would be more likely to be taking antidepressant medications. It would be appropriate to select controls from among those who were admitted for a condition that was unrelated to any psychiatric or neurologic problem (Jick and Vessey, 1978).

Expressing exposure

In a case control study, exposure is assessed for each case and each control at the time of the index date going back in time to see what exposure had occurred before the index date. Subjects are categorized into a predefined set of exposure categories such as current user, past user, non-user, etc. Exposure can then be further divided into categories of duration or dose of use. It is also feasible to assign values to each of the potential confounders at the time of the index date (age, sex, geography, and calendar time as well as other factors such as smoking, body mass index, etc.), allowing for control of confounding. It is useful to discuss how to define the different exposure, dose and duration categories, and to illustrate how the definitions would change for different drug–disease relations.

Defining exposure windows

Exposure windows in case control studies have the same considerations as in cohort studies. One may be interested only in exposures that occurred in the 45 or 60 days before the index date, or one may be interested in knowing about all study drug exposure before that date.

Drugs in relation to congenital anomalies

The study of congenital anomalies in relation to drug exposures has special considerations. A congenital anomaly, strictly speaking, is a prevalent condition. However, it remains true that one is interested in studying exposure to drugs that occurs before the development of the anomaly *in utero*. If a woman takes a drug in the third trimester of pregnancy, after the fetus is developed, it could not be responsible for causing spina bifida, for example, as the neural tube is already formed at this time. In general, one would like to know of all exposures that occurred just before conception and during the first trimester of pregnancy when the development of the body organs and limbs occurs. The exposure that occurs at the time the anomaly becomes manifest (at birth) is not relevant to the etiology of the outcome. This can pose a problem for ascertaining accurate exposure information since the exposure occurred long before the outcome was known. The issues here are not unlike those present in studies of cancer and other chronic diseases where there is a delay between exposure and diagnosis of disease. A discussion of which data resources would best suited for these studies is helpful in thinking through these issues.

Data resources

I like to describe some of the resources that are available for conducting drug safety research. There are more and more resources available, but below are some that have been used repeatedly and have been shown to be of high quality for this kind of research.

In-hospital monitoring study

The first formal data collected to study adverse drug effects was the Boston Collaborative Drug Surveillance Program's (1974) in-hospital monitoring study. Thousands of people who were admitted to hospitals around the world were interviewed by trained nurse monitors to collect information on demographics, reason for admission, and medical history. All drugs received in the hospital were recorded on data sheets, along with all dosing, starting, and stopping information, including the reason for stopping the drug. Any new medical events that occurred in the hospital were also recorded. This database provided information for many of the earliest drug safety studies (Jick *et al.*, 1970).

Ad hoc studies

These are drug safety studies for which all data were collected in a prospective manner over a long period of time. The Oxford Family Planning Association Contraceptive study is one such study. In this study there was interest in studying the long-term effects of oral contraceptive pills. A group of women who took oral contraceptives was followed over a long period of time and compared to a group of women who used other contraceptive methods. The study required identifying and interviewing many women, and then following them and repeatedly interviewing them over time to maintain accurate records of exposure and outcome information (Vessey, 1998). Other similar studies exist but there are few that were designed specifically to study drug effects.

Automated data resources

In the past 2 decades the use of automated data for conducting drug safety studies has increased greatly as more resources have become available. In the late 1970s, data from Group Health Cooperative of Puget Sound in Seattle Washington was first used to study drug–disease associations. Other automated databases have since been used regularly for the study of drug effects, including the Saskatchewan Health database, the General Practice Research Database, and various Medicaid/Medicare databases among others (Strand, Malcolm, Ray 1989; Jick *et al.*, 1984; 1991, 1997). The advantage of these databases is that they have information prospectively recorded on virtually all prescriptions used by those covered in the database. As a consequence one is not dependent on the expensive and time-consuming job of recording by hand all drugs used by an individual, as in a prospective paper-based study, nor is one relying on subject recall of drug use (as in a retrospective study), which may be of questionable validity (Klametti and Saxon, 1967). These databases also have 'complete' information on outcomes. In some databases there are only hospitalized outcomes, while others have inpatient and outpatient diagnoses. The availability of these data resources has revolutionized research in this area, making studies less expensive, faster to complete, and allowing for studies that were not previously feasible to conduct.

Analysis and interpretation of results

If a study has been designed properly the analysis is often straightforward. One must always control for confounding, as discussed above, if it has not been controled in the study design, by matching for example. It is always important to consider dose and duration in the analysis of a study. If there is only a slight increase in the overall risk of an outcome relative to a drug, it is possible that the risk is limited to those in a sub-group of the exposed such as those with long-term use, high dose exposure, or some other factor. Other subgroups should also be evaluated when relevant, such as older subjects (or younger), etc.

If a positive association is found between a drug and an exposure one has to ask if the association is causal or if it is caused by some other factor(s), such as confounding by indication, poor study design, or improper analysis. Students should understand the particular difficulty of assessing causality in conducting drug safety studies where there is often a question as to the role of the underlying disease being treated. Also of importance are questions of comparison group selection. Was the comparison group chosen properly so as to avoid selection bias? Was the analysis properly conducted? Was exposure assessed in the same way for the cases and controls? Were the exposed and non-exposed defined properly? Is there another explanation that is not causal? For example, in a study of inhaled corticosteroids and the development of cataracts, could an association with heavier use be caused by the drug or could it be that more severe asthma is itself associated with increased risk for cataract? Students should think through these possible explanations carefully.

As with all epidemiologic studies a null result must also be interpreted with the appropriate considerations, including misclassification of exposure, negative con-founding, or, as mentioned above, misclassification of the outcome. In drug studies, in particular the source of information on exposure can be more or less subject to misclassification. It is helpful to have the students think through the effects of biased and random misclassification of exposure.

Assessing students' achievements

Below are some exercises whose output provides the teacher with good information on a student's grasp of the material covered in the course. One such exercise is to pro-vide the students with several published studies on the same topic where the result is not consistent across the studies. (See the five references to papers on the risk of venous thromboembolism in users of oral contraceptives and the four references to papers on calcium channel blockers and the risk of cancer.) Have the students review each article and compare the studies across the key areas: study design, study popula-tion, exclusion criteria, exposure and outcome definitions, selection of cases and con-trols or exposed and non-exposed, data resource, control of confounding, analysis, results, and interpretation. The students who more thoroughly grasp the material will uncover more subtle and critical differences in the studies while others will demon-strate a more superficial understanding of the findings.

Another exercise is to provide a study topic and ask students to select the most appropriate database (and say why), and to design a study to best answer the question at hand. Students should indicate why they chose their particular study design. Possible topics could include studies of NSAIDs and renal stones, cholesterol lowering agents and cancer, oral hypoglycemic drugs and liver disease, or meloxicam and gastrointestinal bleeding. Each study has its own methodologic complexities that will challenge the students to employ the techniques taught in class.

References

Boston Collaborative Drug Surveillance Program. (1974) Regular aspirin intake and acute myocardial infarction. *Br Med J* i, 440–3.

Jick, H.. (1997) A database worth saving (commentary). *Lancet* **350**, 1045–6.

Jick, H., Vessey, M. P. (1978) Case-control studies in the evaluation of drug induced illness. *Am J Epidemiol* **107**, 1–7.

Jick, H., Miettenen, O. S., Shapiro, S., *et al.* (1970) Comprehensive drug surveillance. *JAMA* **213**, 1455–60.

Jick, H., Madsen, S., Nudelman, P. M. (1984) Postmarketing follow-up at Group Health Cooperative of Puget Sound. Pharmacotherapy **4**, 99–100.

Jick, H., Jick, S. S., Derby, L. E. (1991) Validation of a large general practice based data base in the UK. *Br Med J* **302** ,766–8.

Jick, H., García Rodríguez, L. A., Pérez Gutthann, S. (1998) Principles of epidemiological research on adverse and beneficial drug effects. *Lancet* **352**, 1767–70.

Jick, S. (1998) A study of the relation of exposure to quinolones and suicidal behavior. *Br J Clin Pharmacol* **45**, 77–81.

Klemetti, A., Saxen, L. (1967) Prospective versus retrospective approach in the search for environmental causes and malformations. *Am J Public Health* **57**, 2071–5.

Malcolm, E., Downey, W., Strand, L. M., McNutt, M., West, R. (1993) Saskatchewan Health's linkable databases and pharmacoepidemiology. *Postmarketing Surveillance* **6**, 175–264.

Ray, W. A., Griffin, M. R. (1989) Use of Medicaid data for pharmacoepidemiology. *Am J Epidemiol* **129**, 837–49.

Ray, W. A. (1988) Pharmacoepidemiology: is ignorance bliss? *J Clin Res Drug Dev* **2**, 67–74.

Schumacher, M., Jick, S. S., Jick, H. *et al.* (1990) Cimetidine use and gastric cancer. *Epidemiology* **1**, 251–4.

Strand, L. M. (1985) Drug epidemiology resources and studies: the Saskatchewan database. *Drug Info J* **19**, 253–6.

Vessey, M. (1998) 30th Anniversary of the Oxford-FPA Contraceptive Study. *Trends in Urology Gynaecology and Sexual Health* **3**, 26–33.

Further reading

Venous thromboembolism and oral contraceptives

Bloemenkamp, K. W. M., Rosendaal, F. R., Helmerhorst, F. M., Buller, H. R., Vandenbroucke, J. P. (1995) Enhancement by factor V Leiden mutation of risk of deep-vein thrombosis associated with oral contraceptives containing a third-generation progestogen. *Lancet* **346**, 1593–6.

Farmer, R. D. T., Lawrenson, R. A., Thompson, C. R., Kennedy, J. G., Hambleton, I. R. (1997) Population-based study of risk of venous thromboembolism associated with various oral contraceptives. *Lancet* **349**, 83–8.

Jick, H., Jick, S., Gurewich, V., Myers, M. W., Vasilakis, C. (1995) Risk of idiopathic cardiovascular death and nonfatal venous thromboembolism in women using oral contraceptives with differing progestagen components. *Lancet* **346**, 1589–90.

Lidegaard, O., Edstrom, B., Kreiner, S. (1998) Oral contraceptive and venous thromboembolism. *WHO Technical Report Series 877*. Geneva: WHO.

World Health Organization. (1995) Effect of different progestagens in low oestrogen oral contraceptives on venous thromboembolic disease. *Lancet* **346**, 1582–8.

Calcium channel blockers and the risk of cancer

Fitzpatrick, A. L., Daling, J. R., Furberg, C. D., Kronmal, R. A., Weissfeld, J. L. (1997) Use of calcium channel blockers and breast carcinoma risk in postmenopausal women. *Cancer* **80**, 1438–47.

Jick, H., Jick, S., Derby, L. E., Vasilakis, C., Myers M. W., Meier, C. (1997) Calcium-channel blockers and the risk of cancer. *Lancet* **349**, 525–8.

Pahor, M., Guralnik, J. M., Ferrucci, L. *et al.* (1996) Calcium-channel blockade and incidence of cancer in aged populations. *Lancet* **348**, 493–7.

Rosenberg, L., Sowmya, R., Palmer, J. R. *et al.* (1998) Calcium channel blockers and the risk of cancer. *JAMA* **279**, 1000–4.

Other

Derby, L., Jick, H., Henry, D. A., Dean, A. D. (1993) Cholestatic hepatitis associated with flucloxacillin. *Med J Australia* **158**, 600–2.

García Rodríguez, L. A., Jick, H. (1994) Comparison of the risk of gynaecomastia associated with cimetidine, omeprazole and other antiulcer medications. *Br Med J* **308**, 503–6.

Jick, H. (1977) The discovery of drug induced illness. *N Engl J Med* **296**, 481–5.

Jick, H. (1985) Use of automated data bases to study drug effects after marketing. *Pharmacotherapy* **5**, 278–9.

Jick, H., Watkins, R. N., Hunter, J. R., *et al.* (1979) Replacement estrogens and endometrial cancer. *N Engl J Med*; **300**, 218–22.

Tilson, H. (1989) A proactive approach to monitoring for adverse drug reactions. *J Clin Res Drug Dev* **3**, 39–51.

Chapter 14

Nutritional epidemiology

Walter C. Willett

Introduction

Diet has long been thought to have important impacts on human health. Roughly one-third of cancers and an even higher percentage of cardiovascular diseases are thought to be diet-related, but the specific aspects of diet responsible have been less clear. Many other conditions previously not thought to be diet-related, including birth defects, cataracts, renal stones, and other degenerative conditions, have also been found to have dietary etiologies. Nutritional epidemiology is a relatively new branch of epidemiology which focuses on understanding the relation between diet and long-term health and disease. Our understanding of biologic mechanisms remains far too incomplete to predict confidently the ultimate consequences of eating a particular food or nutrient. Therefore, epidemiologic studies directly relating intake of various dietary components to risk of disease among humans, complemented by laboratory investigations and mechanistic studies, will play a critical role in guiding individual food choices and public policy. In the 1980s, a major expansion of the literature in nutritional epidemiology occurred and a firmer quantitative basis for this field developed. In particular, the substantial variation in diet among individuals was quantified in many populations, standardized dietary questionnaires were developed for large epidemiologic studies, and the ability of these questionnaires to measure diet was documented. Most of the major questions about diet and disease remain unresolved, but the foundations for obtaining such information are now relatively well established. Thus, a reasonable basis exists for formal courses on the topic of nutritional epidemiology.

Any teaching activity should take into account the background and interests of the students. The basic nutritional epidemiology course that we teach assumes students have already taken introductory epidemiology and biostatistics courses, or equivalent experience. The depth is greater than would usually be appropriate for medical or MPH students, unless they have a special interest in this topic.

Among the various audiences are researchers actively engaged in studies of diet and disease, and other persons who are attempting to read and interpret published epidemiologic reports related to nutrition. Many epidemiology students whose primary interest is not nutritional epidemiology often take our courses because diet needs to be considered in almost any field, if nothing more than as a potential confounding variable or effect modifier. Potential students may include those who are simply interested in the most up-to-date knowledge about diet and health. In general, I discourage such students from taking a methodologic course in nutritional epidemiology as the substantive knowledge is changing rapidly and an emphasis is therefore appropriately given to fundamental methodologic issues. The course I have taught and will describe here specifically does not address problems of undernutrition among nutrition in developing countries. This topic has a long tradition, mainly based on anthrometric measurements, and is covered elsewhere in our School of Public Health. Nevertheless, students interested in such problems can gain much by a general course in nutritional epidemiology as the current methods can be applied to problems of undernutrition in children.

In the early 1980s a single course could almost exhaustively cover the area of nutritional epidemiology because the literature was minimal. However, as in any field, further development moves the methodologic frontier more distant from the level of knowledge needed by someone entering the field. Thus, teaching a course that serves both as an introduction and as an up-to-date account of new developments becomes increasingly challenging. For this reason, we have now begun teaching both an introductory basic course for those entering the field as well as an advanced level course that covers emerging methodologic issues in more detail.

Many epidemiology students find nutritional epidemiology to be useful in a wider epidemiologic context because a number of the issues are not traditionally covered well in basic epidemiology curricula. For example, most exposure measurements in epidemiology courses are considered as categoric variables, whereas in nutrition most exposure variables, as well as many outcome variables, are continuous. As another example, measurement error and corrections for measurement error are generally not included in our primary epidemiology curriculum. As much of the work in this area has emanated from nutritional epidemiologic problems, this topic is covered in our course, but the principles have wide application throughout epidemiology. Thus, one of the course objectives is to reinforce epidemiologic principles that apply to other areas of our broader field.

Teaching objectives

Students who complete our introductory course in nutritional epidemiology should:

1. Be familiar with the basic concepts in this field.
2. Be able to read and interpret critically published articles relating diet to disease.
3. Be able to conduct basic analyses using dietary data, including adjustment for total energy intake and de-attenuation of correlation coefficients, and interpret findings from both a statistical and biological perspective.

Format

The course we have used for nutritional epidemiology has consisted of four major components: lectures, readings, data collection experiences, and computer problem sets. The mix of these would appropriately depend on the time allotment and student background. Ordinarily, the introductory course is given as 16 two-hour periods plus individual work on data collection and computer analysis. About half of the lecture sessions are devoted to methodologic issues in the measurement and analysis of dietary data, illustrated with relevant examples. The second half of the course usually uses substantive topics in nutritional epidemiology to reinforce the principles.

As usual, a lecture format is optimal when the class size is small to allow interaction when students have done preparatory readings. For our teaching, we have used my textbook, *Nutritional Epidemiology* (Willett, 1998), as the primary material supplemented by readings of original reports. The other major textbook in this field is by Margetts *et al.* (1997).

Data collection by students has involved the keeping of multiple 24-hour recalls, diet records, and the completion of a food frequency questionnaire. Students enter and analyze their own diet record and 24-hour recall data using standard nutrient analysis software (currently the Minnesota Nutrient Analysis System). The food frequency questionnaire is scanned and analyzed by our standard procedures. Individual and summary reports for the class are returned to the students.

The computer problem sets provide students with actual experience in manipulating nutritional data; the topics relate to specific issues that are discussed in the lectures and readings. Typically, students have found this to be one of the most valuable aspects of the course as this requires the understanding of the principal issues and provides students confidence that they are able to analyze information appropriately. The major problems deal with analysis of within and between person components of variation in diet, validation of a food frequency questionnaire, examination of the relation between dietary intake and blood levels of nutrients, and correction of correlation coefficients for measurement error. These will be discussed further in the relevant topics below. Students are typically required to turn in the primary computer output and a discussion of the results incorporating both the biological and statistical considerations.

Teaching contents

In the following sections, the major lecture topics will be discussed and the most important points noted. The abridged syllabus is shown in Table 14.1.

Overview

Nutritional epidemiology is introduced as essentially a subdivision of epidemiology, with diet as the exposure and disease as the outcome. However, this field is unusually complex because of the many dimensions of diet representing many correlated variables, and likely interactions with other nutrients, genetic factors, obesity, and physical activity.

The first session is devoted to an overview of nutritional epidemiology. A brief historical background is provided. The dominant historic role of international ecological studies in nutritional epidemiology is emphasized, as well as the potentially large and often intractable problems of confounding in such studies. The further development of nutritional epidemiology was hindered by the conventional wisdom that there was no heterogeneity in diet within populations and that individuals could not remember what they had previously eaten. A large amount of this negativity arose because of the

Table 14.1 Syllabus for introductory nutritional epidemiology

Session 1	Overview of epidemiology in nutrition studies
	Sources of variation in the diet (chapters 1 and 3)
	Introduction to computer assignments
	(Hand out homework 1)
	Handouts: Beaton (1979)
Session 2	Dietary methodology: food frequency (chapters 2 and 5)
	Dietary methodology: validation (chapter 6)
	Dietary assessment assignment
	Handouts: Willett (1985; 1997)
Session 3	Body composition/anthropometry (chapter 10)
	Obesity and mortality
	Handouts: Manson (1987; 1995), Spiegelman (1992)
Session 4	Dietary methodology: 24-hour recalls and diet records (chapters 4 and 7)
	(Homework 1 due; hand out homework 2)
Session 5	Meaning and analysis of total energy intake (chapter 11)
	Handouts: Willett (1986)
Session 6	Dietary methodology: nutrient database
	(Homework 2 due; hand out homework 3)
Session 7	Introduction to regression analysis of nutrients
	Review of homeworks 1 and 2
Session 8	Correction for measurement error (chapter 12)
Session 9	Biochemical assessment of nutritional status (chapter 9)
Session 10	Data analysis and presentation in nutritional epidemiology (chapter 13)
	Handouts: Hu (1999)
Session 11	Folic acid and neural tube defect (chapter 18)
	(Homework 3 due; hand out homework 4)
Session 12	Diet and heart disease (chapter 17)
	Handouts: Shekelle (1981), Hu (1997)
Session 13	Diet and breast cancer (chapter 16)
	(Diet assessment due)
	Handouts: Holmes (1999)
Session 14	Vitamin A and cancer (chapter 15)
	(Homework 4 due)
	Handouts: Hennekens (1996), Omenn (1996), Steinmetz, Cancer Research (1993), ATBC (1994)
Session 15	Review homeworks 3 and 4
	Review of course
Session 16	Examination

Textbook: Willett, *Nutritional Epidemiology*, 2nd edition

inability to document correlations between dietary intake of cholesterol and serum cholesterol. There are several reasons for this minimal correlation, the most important being that serum cholesterol is heavily controlled by homeostatic factors and a substantial part of the between person variation appears to be under genetic control. Thus, at most very weak associations between diet and serum cholesterol should be expected. Furthermore, most studies of diet had used only a single 24-hour recall, which necessarily provides a poor assessment of usual intake because of large day-to-day variation. Thus, the focus on serum cholesterol as the criteria for validity of dietary assessment methods was highly unfortunate.

In addition to ecological studies, the importance of migrant studies and secular trends in the development of nutritional epidemiology is emphasized. Importantly, such studies indicate that the primary determinants of disease rates of cancer and cardiovascular disease are primarily due to non-genetic factors. The role of case control and cohort studies in nutritional epidemiology is also discussed. The problem of bias in case control studies of diet is particularly substantial because of the modest relative risks that are to be expected and the sensitivity of relative risks to even small degrees of bias because of differences in recall between cases and controls or unrepresentative selection of controls. Cohort studies are primarily limited by feasibility because of the large sizes and the long duration of follow-up that are typically needed.

The role of controlled trials in nutritional epidemiology is also discussed. Again, feasibility is a major issue, in part because of the problem of maintaining high levels of compliance over long periods of time, uncertainty about the relevant follow-up period, and the large sample sizes required to test most hypotheses. Because of the impossibility of testing most diet and disease hypotheses in randomized trials, the importance of sound observational study design is obvious.

Food and nutrients

In this section the complexity of human diets is examined. The foods we consume each day contain thousands of specific chemicals, some of which are known and well quantified, and others that are poorly described or not even measured. These dimensions of diets include the essential nutrients (including minerals, vitamins, lipids, and amino acids), major energy sources (proteins, carbohydrates, fats, and alcohol), additives (nitrates, salts, coloring agents, etc.), agricultural contaminants (pesticides, herbicides, fungicides, and growth hormones), microbial toxin contaminants (aflatoxin being a classic example), inorganic contaminants (including lead, cadmium, and PCBs), chemicals formed in the cooking or processing of food (various mutagens, *trans* fatty acids for example), natural toxins (including a plethora of phytochemicals that plants have developed through evolution to deter insects and diseases), and other natural compounds (for example, the constituents of normal cell structures). Available databases allow intakes to be estimated for only a small fraction of these various constituents of foods, mainly the essential nutrients and energy sources.

The value of examining both foods and nutrients in relation to disease risks is addressed. If a specific nutrient is a cause or preventive factor for disease, the most powerful relationship will be achieved by examining this nutrient. Nevertheless, confidence in causality can be increased if major food sources of that nutrient are also similarly related to risk of disease. On the other hand, an examination of foods may be revealing because the important dietary constituent may not be represented by any calculable variable. Moreover, foods are always complex mixtures and their relationship to disease risk cannot necessarily be predicted by examination of a single constituent. Because dietary advice will often be made on the basis of foods, it will be important to examine intake of specific foods directly in relation to disease risk. Thus, there is great value in examining foods and nutrients simultaneously in relation to disease outcomes.

Food composition data sources and computation systems

The calculation of nutrient intakes from data on food consumption requires a food composition database. The underlying assumption in this calculation is that the nutrient content of a specific food does not vary from one sample to another. Naturally, this is never completely true because the composition will depend on many factors, including the growing and harvesting conditions, the variety, the degree of maturity, and factors in the processing, storage, and cooking. In most cases this is not a serious problem; however, in some instances the variability may be so great that calculations become useless. Selenium is a classic example, as the content in food can vary over 100-fold depending on the soil in which the food was produced.

Considerations in selection of databases are reviewed in this session of our course. Key points are that the food composition be as accurate and up-to-date as possible, that uniformity in the determination in nutrient composition across foods is desirable for each specific nutrient, that the database is comprehensive in the scope of foods because all foods reported must be assigned nutrient values, that the specificity is adequate for nutrients that will be evaluated (for example, the composition of margarines can vary dramatically depending on the processing), and that the range of nutrients included should be as comprehensive as possible. In the US, the Department of Agriculture maintains the most comprehensive system overall, but for a number of dietary variables this will need to be supplemented with further information. For other countries, investigators will need to determine the most appropriate food composition sources.

In addition to a food composition database, computer software will be needed for the computation of nutrient intakes from dietary data. For food frequency questionnaires, investigators will generally need to assemble their own corresponding database to match the foods that are included on their questionnaire. For more open-ended methods such as 24-hour recalls or dietary records (see below), more extensive database systems are required. Fortunately, a wide variety of options are now available that can aid in the efficient analysis of dietary information.

Nature of variation in diet

An understanding of the sources of variation in dietary intake is essential for nutritional epidemiologists. In addition to the relevant chapter in *Nutritional Epidemiology*, students are asked to read the classic paper by Beaton *et al.* (1979) on this topic.

For most individuals nutrient intake varies tremendously from day to day. In some circumstances, particularly in developing countries where food availability changes dramatically by season, major seasonal variation can also exist. The most important implication is that a single 24-hour recording of food intake, no matter how accurate, will generally be a poor representation of a person's average long-term intake. Moreover, the degree of variability differs dramatically from one nutrient to another. Only for total energy intake is there potent physiologic regulation to dampen day-to-day variation. Thus, variability is lowest for total energy intake and next lowest for the major contributors to energy intake, specifically total fat, carbohydrate, and protein. Minor constituents of the diet are much less constrained; for example, the day-to-day variability in vitamin A or cholesterol can be extremely large. Because the absolute intake of nutrients is in part determined by total energy intake, the composition of diets (intakes adjusted for energy intake, discussed further in a later section) can be considerably more variable than for absolute intake.

The implications of large day-to-day variability for epidemiologic studies are also reviewed. These include that observed distributions based on single 24-hour recalls are much broader than the true distributions of long-term individual intakes. Also, measures of association such as relative risks, and correlation and regression coefficients are biased toward the null. As part of this topic, students receive a problem set with multiple days of 24-hour intake and conduct an analysis of variance to partition the within-person and between-person components of variance for several nutrients.

Short-term dietary assessment methods: 24-hour recall and food records

In this section the process of collecting 24-hour recall and diet record data is described by a dietitian experienced in these methodologies. The advantages and disadvantages of 24-hour recall and diet record methods are reviewed, a particular advantage being that there is no constraint placed on the food data and no assumptions made about ways of consuming foods or portion sizes. A strength of the 24-hour recall method is that it does not require literacy or any substantial effort on the part of participants. On the other hand, an advantage of food records is that this method does not depend on memory, and quantities can actually be measured and weighed directly at the time of recording. However, diet record collection requires a highly motivated and literate participant.

For both of these methods, the effort in collection and processing of dietary data is large, and this has generally precluded these methods in large prospective studies. Moreover, only information about current diet is obtained so that this may not be relevant for application in case control studies, where past diet is usually of interest. A major role of these short-term methods in nutritional epidemiology is for the validation of food frequency questionnaires. Also, for description of group means or for cross-cultural comparisons, 24-hour recall information may be optimal.

Food frequency methods

Because of the practical and conceptual limitations of 24-hour recalls and food records for assessing average long-term intake, most investigators have converged upon the use of food frequency questionnaires in epidemiologic studies. The underlying principles of this method were described by the British statistician, Heady, who noted that differences in nutrient intakes were primarily determined by the frequency with which foods were consumed rather than the differences in serving sizes (Heady, 1961). Also, cognitive research has documented that reporting of usual food consumption is generally easier than describing what was eaten at a specific meal.

The design of food frequency questionnaires is considered. Decisions in creating a food list are reviewed, with the most important criteria being that foods most accounting for between-person variation in nutrients of interest should be given priority. A variety of ways to identify foods for inclusion on a food frequency questionnaire are described. Decisions about the collection of frequency information are also considered, including whether open-ended responses or a multiple choice format is preferable. The multiple choice format has major advantages in making the form available for optical scanning data entry. The issue of serving size is also reviewed, including whether to ignore serving sizes and simply ask about frequency, to ask specific questions about serving size, or to specify a typical serving size. A major advantage of standardized food frequency questionnaires is that they can be self-administered and optically scanned. This has made large prospective studies feasible, in particular repeated assessments of diets. Available evidence suggests that, in a reasonably literate population, mailed self-administered questionnaires and detailed interviewer-administered questionnaires provide similar degrees of validity.

Reproducibility and validity of food frequency questionnaires

Although practical considerations greatly favor the use of food frequency questionnaires in epidemiologic studies, it is also crucial to consider in detail the degree to which such questionnaires measure true dietary intake. Reproducibility of a questionnaire is an important, but not sufficient, indicator of the value of dietary data obtained by that method. In general, validity, which involves a comparison with a superior method, will be a more important criterion. In assessing the validity of dietary assessment methods, an important consideration is whether errors in the comparison method are correlated with errors in the method under evaluation. The use of biochemical measures to assess validity has appeal in that errors are likely to be highly independent. However, they do not provide a quantitative evaluation of validity and for many nutrients no practical biochemical measure exists. Thus, most validation studies have used primarily either dietary record data or 24-hour recall data for comparisons. Dietary record data have the advantage that the cognitive processes are quite different than those for food frequency questionnaires, thus the errors are less likely to be correlated.

A large number of validation studies have now been performed in a variety of populations comparing food frequency questionnaire information with diet records or 24-hour recalls. In general, with comprehensive questionnaires, correlations of 0.6–0.7 appear to be attainable for nutrient intakes adjusted for total energy. Although this degree of validity is not perfect, it will be enough to assure that important associations will not be missed if this study size is sufficiently large. In this section, a variety of alternatives for expressing validity are described.

For this topic, a computer problem is usually included in which students are asked to analyze data from a validation study and present the results. Subsets of data for three or four nutrients from the comparison of a food frequency questionnaire with repeated diet records are used for this purpose (Willett, 1985; Rimm, 1992). To discourage use of student work from previous years, we extract different subsets of data from year to year.

Biochemical indicators of dietary intake

This section focuses on the principles underlying the use of biochemical indicators in nutritional epidemiology. A comprehensive review of available biochemical indicators is not attempted. A fundamental distinction is made between the use of a biochemical measurement as an indicator of dietary intake (which is the primary rationale in nutritional epidemiology) *versus* being of inherent interest as a predictor of disease. Serum cholesterol is used as an example that is a poor indicator of dietary intake, but is still of interest in predicting risk of coronary heart disease. Important considerations in the evaluation of a potential biochemical indicator are whether it is sensitive to intake. Many biochemical measurements, such as serum calcium or sodium, are tightly regulated and thus represent diet poorly. The ability of a biochemical measure to integrate intake over an extended period of time is also critical. It is also important to identify other non-dietary factors that influence the level of biochemical indicators; if they are known, it may be possible to adjust for these factors to eliminate them as extraneous sources of variation.

The use of biochemical indicators in epidemiologic studies is also considered. Important issues are the timing of sampling, and proper processing and storage to avoid artifacts or degradation. The use of biochemical indicators in nested case control studies is also covered, with particular attention to the avoidance of bias. In general, the usefulness of biochemical indicators of diet in epidemiologic studies can be viewed as a spectrum: at one end dietary methods perform poorly and only biochemical measurements will be useful (for example, selenium intake), in the middle both dietary and biochemical measurements may be similarly useful (e.g. beta-carotene and folic acid), and at the other end only dietary intake data is likely to be useful (such as calcium or dietary fiber intake). Particular attention is given to the monitoring of laboratory precision in epidemiologic studies as this is a frequent cause of error.

The evaluation of biochemical indicators of diet for use in epidemiologic studies is also described. Approaches include the evaluation of repeated measurements in the same individuals over time. If there is not a reasonably high correlation, a biochemical indicator will not provide useful information on long-term intake for an individual. Whether the measure is sensitive to dietary intake can be evaluated by comparisons between intake and biochemical levels in cross-sectional studies or by the manipulation of dietary intake in intervention studies. Typically, we use several examples to illustrate the use of biochemical indicators for epidemiologic applications.

For the topic of biochemical indicators of diet, students are required to analyze a dataset relating dietary intakes to blood levels of several nutrients. Specific attention is given to the effects of adding covariates on the primary association. As an example, we have used data comparing intakes of carotenoids, retinol, and vitamin E assessed by food frequency questionnaires with their corresponding blood levels (Willett, 1983), but any similar dataset would suffice.

Anthrometric measures and body composition

Anthropometric variables, particularly weight and height, are the most commonly employed measures of nutritional status in epidemiologic studies, mainly because of their simplicity and ease of collection. Measures of body dimensions and mass can be used directly, but most often combinations of weight and height have been used to estimate the relative body composition, such as fatness. Compared to other biologic measurements, height and weight can be assessed with great precision in epidemiologic studies, even by self-report within most populations. The limitation of body mass index as a measure of adiposity relates to the failure of weight to distinguish between fat mass and lean mass. In middle-aged general populations in western countries it does appear that the large majority of variation of body weight-adjusted-for-height is due to differences in fat mass. However, this assumption upholds less well in other groups, such as body builders, the elderly, and quite probably persons in developing countries where physical labor is more common.

A variety of new methods have become available for measuring body composition, including electrical impedance and dilution methods. Unfortunately, the superiority of these compared to standard anthropometric measurements has yet to be documented for epidemiologic applications. A large literature has addressed the relative value of various combinations of height and weight to assess body fatness. The use of external criteria, such as biochemical measurements sensitive to body fatness, is described as a method of evaluating relative validity. In general, the use of the simple measure of weight divided by height squared (body mass index) appears to be at least as useful as other combinations and has the virtue of being widely used and comparable across studies.

Recently, great interest has emerged in the use of measurements to assess the distribution of body fat, with the assumption that intra-abdominal fat has metabolic properties that are distinct. The use of circumference measurements alone or in combination to assess body fat distribution is discussed. Similarly, the value of skin folds is considered, although these are generally unlikely to be practical in most epidemiologic investigations. The virtue of body circumference measurements is that they can be assessed by individuals themselves with relatively good validity. As an example, the controversies regarding the setting of weight guidelines are reviewed.

Implications of total energy intake for epidemiologic analyses

Total energy intake deserves special consideration in nutritional epidemiology for several reasons. First, energy intake may be a primary determinant of disease. Second, individual differences in total energy intake produce variation in intake of specific nutrients because the consumption of most nutrients is positively correlated with total energy intake; this added variation may be extraneous to disease risk and thus a source of error. Third, when energy intake is associated with disease but not a direct cause, the effects of specific nutrients may be confounded by total energy intake.

The topic of total energy intake is introduced by a discussion of energy physiology. Notably, total energy intake is largely determined by lean body mass and level of physical activity. Thus, unless a person is willing to change physical activity or body fat substantially, total energy intake for an individual is relatively fixed. Thus, to alter intake of specific nutrients, it is necessary for an individual to do this primarily by change in the composition of their diet rather than by change in total food intake. This is fundamentally important in nutritional epidemiology because the implication is that we need to study primarily the relation of dietary composition, rather than absolute nutrient intake, to disease risk.

A number of methods to account or adjust for total nutrient intake in nutritional epidemiologic studies are described. The classical approach has been to use nutrient density (nutrient divided by calories). The inherent problem with this is that the nutrient density will remain confounded if total caloric intake is a predictor of disease. Other approaches include adding total energy intake as a covariant or utilizing the residual method to isolate variability in nutrient intake independent of total energy intake. An energy partition model can also be used, but this does not control for energy intake. Illustrations are given of situations where inadequate or inappropriate adjustment for energy intake can actually reverse the direction of associations between dietary factors and disease risk. Thus, careful attention to total energy intake is essential in nutritional epidemiologic analysis. For readings, we use Chapter 12 of *Nutritional Epidemiology* and Willett (1997).

Correction for measurement error

Forms of measurement error in epidemiologic studies are considered. The most common assumption is that measurement error for an individual is simply random within-person variation, as usually assumed for 24-hour recalls. Systematic errors can occur within individuals or groups, particularly when assessing diet using structured methods such as food frequency questionnaires. The effects of these various types of errors on associations are considered in detail.

Until recently, it has usually been simply noted that measurement error will tend to bias associations to the null. However, it is possible to measure the degree of error and utilize correction methods to obtain an estimate of association that would exist if there had been no measurement error. In our introductory course, several simple methods for correctional methods are provided. These include the correction of standard deviations for distributions of a single variable, correction of correlation coefficients, and correction of relative risks using the regression calibration approach. The effect of measurement errors in covariates and correction of these errors is also described. In addition, issues regarding the use of imperfect 'true' measurements as the standard, and the potential implications of correlated measurement errors between the standard and surrogate method, are described in principle. The topic of correction for measurement error is a rapidly expanding area in epidemiology and the current literature exceeds what can be inducted in an introductory course.

As part of this section, students are usually given a computer problem set involving the correction of standard deviations, the de-attenuation of correlation coefficients, and the correction of relative risks in a univariate context.

Analysis and presentation of dietary data

The analysis and presentation of data from epidemiologic studies is not inherently different from other aspects of epidemiology, but some topics are particularly important because of the complexity of nutritional data. A common issue is the handling of blank information on foods and outlying values. Several approaches are discussed. Advantages and disadvantages of using nutritional data in categoric or continuous forms are also addressed. Alternatives in the graphic presentation in the data are described with illustrations and discussions of advantages and disadvantages.

Temporal relationships in the study of most chronic diseases can be critical. Most frequently, we do not know the temporal relationship between diet and the diagnosis of disease, although at times we have reasons to hypothesize specific induction periods. An exploration of alternative relationships can provide information that can be inherently valuable. In addition, when no association is observed, this conclusion will be most compelling if a wide range of induction periods is evaluated. A variety of analytic strategies are discussed.

Multivariate approaches to the data analysis can be particularly important because dietary factors tend to be correlated, sometimes strongly. However, a number of serious pitfalls can exist in many situations. The inclusion of the covariate can radically alter the biologic meaning of the original variable even though the analysis might be logical from a purely statistical standpoint. In addition, the inclusion of multiple variables can dramatically reduce the remaining variation, leading to an analysis that is essentially uninformative. Another common situation arises when one or more variables are components of another, such as saturated, monounsaturated, and polyunsaturated fat, which are all components of total fat. Various options for analytic strategies are discussed that address somewhat different questions.

Interest in overall dietary patterns has generated various approaches to creating dietary scores. These factors of methods are discussed. Other topics include the analysis and interpretation of subgroups and interactions.

The use of meta-analysis for systematically summarizing results of randomized trials has become routine, but its place in epidemiology has been controversial. Meta-analysis of published data from dietary studies is particularly problematic because of the wide variety of ways that data have been analyzed and presented. The use of pooled analyses based on primary data is particularly attractive because this will allow a consistent analytic approach in studies.

Nutrition monitoring and surveillance

Monitoring and surveillance is used to discern possible subgroups within a population and trends in populations in diet or nutritional status over time. This can represent an important application of nutritional epidemiology. Epidemiologic approaches in monitoring and surveillance are described.

Substantive examples of nutritional epidemiology applications

A variety of topics are now available that can be used to illustrate and reinforce issues in nutritional epidemiology. Although applications and examples are valuable when interwoven into issues discussed throughout the course, a focused discussion of a specific topic can be valuable. Specific topics that have been used in our course follow.

Vitamin A and lung cancer

This topic has a long history in nutritional epidemiology, beginning with the early report of a protective effect of vitamin A against lung cancer by Bjelke in 1975. Interest shifted to the hypotheses that beta-carotene might be a responsible factor for the remarkably consistent inverse association between food and vegetable consumption, and risk of lung cancer. However, randomized trials of high beta-carotene did not support any evidence of benefit and suggested possible harm. This area illustrates many issues, including the use of biochemical indicators, potential pitfalls of extrapolating from data on foods to a specific nutrient, and the strengths and limitations of randomized trials for testing hypotheses.

Dietary fat and breast cancer

The relation between dietary fat and breast cancer has been a major focus in nutritional epidemiology because prospective cohort studies have not supported the hypotheses based on ecologic correlations. The possible explanations for these findings are considered, including lack of validity of dietary assessment, an inadequate range of dietary intake, and inappropriate specification of the induction period, and a true lack of association. Various means of addressing these alternative explanations are described.

Diet and coronary heart disease

This has been one of the longest standing issues in public health for the last 50 years. The original diet–heart hypothesis focused on saturated fat and dietary cholesterol, and has become a widespread belief with limited empirical support. More recent evidence suggests that this hypothesis was highly incomplete as it did not take into account the strong benefits of unsaturated fatty acids and adverse effects of *trans* fatty acids. Moreover, recent evidence has suggested that many other dietary constituents can have important impacts on coronary heart disease risk; these factors include the characteristics of dietary carbohydrate, omega-3 fatty acids, folic acid and vitamin B6, dietary antioxidants, and other micronutrients. The topic illustrates the importance of multivariate analysis in nutritional epidemiology and the integration of metabolic studies, observational epidemiology, and randomized trials.

Folic acid and neural tube defects

The relationship between folic acid intake and risk of neural tube defects has prompted a major paradigm shift in nutrition. This most clearly illustrates the enormous impact of differences in micronutrient intake without accompanying signs of clinical deficiency. The topic is a rich source of teaching material and includes contributions of randomized trials, case control and cohort studies using dietary intake data, and biomarkers. Recent data also illustrate the use of genetic polymorphisms in nutritional epidemiology and how they may greatly enhance the causal interpretation of associations. The topic also illustrates the application of nutritional epidemiologic approaches after a causal association has been established because the existence of an effect raises questions about optimal intake and public health approaches to achieve optimal levels.

Advanced topics in nutritional epidemiology

The basic material in an introductory course in nutritional epidemiology is too substantial to allow in-depth examination of current methodologic issues in this field. Moreover, for many students such an in-depth discussion is neither necessary nor appropriate. Thus, a course on advanced topics can be valuable for those who will be actively engaged in research.

An advanced topics course would appropriately include readings and discussions on current literature in the field of nutritional epidemiology, particularly focusing on methodologic issues. A large part of this literature presently involves issues regarding measurement error and correction for measurement. In our department, Drs Alberto Ascherio and Donna Spiegelman have developed computer simulation problems based on actual data from our large cohort studies and validation substudies. These problems allow students to investigate the impacts of measurement error and to use correction procedures. In addition, the advanced course can allow students to analyze diet and disease relationships using actual data.

Supervised research

As in any doctoral program, much of the actual learning process occurs in the context of supervised original research. An ideal student experience would include not just the analysis of existing data, but also participation in a full cycle of hypothesis development, grant writing, data collection, data cleaning and processing, analysis of data, and reporting of research findings in written and oral form. The complete process from beginning to end will almost always take more than the usual number of years for completion of a doctoral degree. Thus, typically we attempt to have students involved in all aspects of this work, but not necessarily with all aspects directly related to the same topic.

Assessing students' achievements

For our basic course in nutritional epidemiology student achievement is assessed by:

♦ Written reports based on homework problems.
♦ Completion of their own dietary assessments, including the analysis of diet records using a standard food composition analysis system.
♦ Classroom discussion which encourages completing the assigned readings.
♦ Final examination covering key concepts in the course.

Conclusion

In a relatively short period, nutritional epidemiology has developed into a major area of activity within the overall field of epidemiology. Nutritional epidemiology has generated methodologic work that has implications broadly across the overall field. Because of the complexity of nutritional epidemiology, training in this field will provide students with concepts and skills that can be applied in many other aspects of epidemiology. The coming years are sure to provide a major growth in available data because a number of large prospective dietary studies are only now beginning to provide results. These will provide an enormous expansion in knowledge of diet and health, and should hopefully stimulate further the refinement and development of epidemiologic methods.

References

Beaton, G. H., Milner, J., Corey, P., McGuire, V., Cousin, M., Stewart, E. *et al.* (1979) Sources of variance in 24-hour dietary recall data: implications for nutrition study design and interpretation. *Am J Clin Nutr* **32**, 2546–9.

Bjelke, E. (1975) Dietary vitamin A and human lung cancer. *Int J Cancer* **15**, 561–5.

Heady, J. A. (1961) Diets of bank clerks. Development of a method of classifying the diets of individuals for use in epidemiologic studies. *J R Stat Soc* **124**, 336–61.

Hennekens, C. H., Buring, J. E., Manson, J. E., Stampfer, M., Rosner, B., Cook, N. R. *et al.* Lack of effect of long-term supplementation with beta carotene on the incidence of malignant neoplasms and cardiovascular disease. *N Engl J Med* **334**, 1145–9.

Holmes, M. D., Hunter, D. J., Colditz, G. A., Stampfer, M. J., Hankinson, S. E., Speizer, F. E. (1999) Association of dietary intake of fat and fatty acids with risk of breast cancer. *JAMA* **281**, 914–20.

Hu, F., Stampfer, M. J., Manson, J. E., Rimm, E., Colditz, G. A., Rosner, B. A. *et al.* (1997) Dietary fat intake and the risk of coronary heart disease in women. *N Engl J Med* **337**, 1491–9.

Hu, F. B., Stampfer, M. J., Rimm, E., Ascherio, A., Rosner, B. A., Spiegelman, D. *et al.* (1999) Dietary fat and coronary heart disease: a comparison of approaches for adjusting total energy intake and modeling repeated dietary measurements. *Am J Epidemiol* **149**, 531–40.

Manson, J. E., Stampfer, M. J., Hennekens, C. H. and Willett, W. C. (1987) Body weight and longevity. A reassessment. *J Am Med Assoc* **257**, 353–8.

Manson, J. E., Willett, W. C., Stampfer, M. J., Colditz, G. A., Hunter, D. J., Hankinson, S. E. (1995) Body weight and mortality among women. *N Engl J Med* **333**, 677–85.

Margetts, B. and Nelson, M. (1997) *Design concepts in nutritional epidemiology*. Oxford University Press, Oxford.

Omenn, G. S., Goodman, G. E., Thornquist, M. D., Balmes, J., Cullen, M. R., Glass, A. *et al.* (1996) Effects of a combination of beta carotene and vitamin A on lung cancer and cardiovascular disease. *N Engl J Med* **334**, 1150–5.

Rimm, E.B., Giovannucci, E. L., Stampfer, M. J., Colditz, G. A., Litin, L. B. and Willett, W. C. (1992) Reproducibility and validity of a expanded self-administered semiquantitative food frequency questionnaire among male health professionals. *Am J Epidemiol* **135**, 1114–26.

Shekelle, R. B., Shryock, A. M., Paul, O., Lepper, M., Stamler, J., Liu, S. *et al.* (1981) Diet, serum cholesterol, and death from coronary heart disease: The Western Electric Study. *N Engl J Med* **304**, 65–70.

Spiegelman, D., Israel, R. G., Bouchard, C. and Willett, W. C. (1992) Absolute fat mass, percent body fat, and body-fat distribution: Which is the real determinant of blood pressure and serum glucose? *Am J Clin Nutr* 55, 1033–44.

Steinmetz, K. A., Potter, J. D. and Folsom, A. R. (1993) Vegetables, fruit, and lung cancer in the Iowa Women's Health Study. *Cancer Res* 53, 536–43.

The Alpha-Tocopherol Beta-Carotene Cancer Prevention Study Group (1994) The effect of vitamin E and beta carotene on the incidence of lung cancer and other cancers in male smokers. *N Engl J Med* 330, 1029–35.

Willet, W. C. (1998) *Nutritional epidemiology, second edition.* Oxford University Press, New York.

Willett, W. C., Howe, G. R. and Kushi, L. H. (1997) Adjustment for total energy intake in epidemiologic studies. *Am J Clin Nutr* 65(*Suppl*), 1220S–8S.

Willett, W. C., Sampson, L., Stampfer, M. J., Rosner, B., Bain, C., Witschi, J. *et al.* (1985) Reproducibility and validity of a semiquantitative food frequency questionnaire. *Am J Epidemiol* 122, 51–65.

Willett, W. C. and Stampfer, M. J. (1986) Total energy intake: implications for epidemiologic analyses. *Am J Epidemiol* 124, 17–27.

Willett, W. C., Stampfer, M. J., Underwood, B. A., Speizer, F. E., Rosner, B. and Hennekens, C. H. (1983) Validation of a dietary questionnaire with plasma carotenoid and alpha-tocopherol levels. *Am J Clin Nutr* 38, 631–9.

Outcome oriented epidemiology

Chapter 15

General epidemiology of infectious diseases

Dimitrios Trichopoulos and Jørn Olsen with Pagona Lagiou and Alkistis Skalkidou

Introduction

The study of outbreaks, usually of infectious diseases, established the roots of epidemiology in the middle of the 19th century. Unfortunately, this is now often forgotten in courses of modern epidemiology. Infectious disease epidemiology has its own terminology and a set of mathematical formulations to describe transmission, etc. In many ways, all of these principles had to be brought back into use once more when the AIDS epidemic appeared.

The area of chronic disease epidemiology, starting in this century, replaced much of the methodology developed to describe outbreaks of infectious diseases, but this may change. Infectious diseases play an increasingly important role and many chronic diseases may have an infection as part of the causal field leading to the disease. Several cancers, multiple sclerosis, reproductive failures, myocardial infarctions, and some of the psychiatric diseases may, for instance, have an infectious etiology. Therefore, we have devoted more space to this chapter in the book than was provided to other chapters.

Rationale

The teaching of general epidemiology of infectious diseases is a demanding undertaking. On the one hand, infectious disease specialists, as a rule, teach the course using examples that may not allow the conceptualization of the general issues to the proper depth. On the other hand, modern epidemiologists are familiar with the abstract notions, but rarely have first hand experience of infectious disease epidemiology. There are exceptions, of course, but this book is intended for the young epidemiology instructor, who may have to deal with the teaching of both epidemiologic concepts and methods, and the principles that specifically concern infectious disease epidemiology (e.g. period of communicability, transmission patterns, the carrier state, the host and the vector paradigms, and, for epidemics like AIDS, the reproductive rate). An additional problem is that most books on epidemiology of infectious diseases written by formally trained infectious disease epidemiologists belong to the era when most epidemiologists were specialists in infectious diseases (Taylor and Knowelden, 1964; Fox *et al.*, 1970; Paul and White, 1973; Sinnecker, 1976). Things have changed, however, in the last decades, with a new emphasis on infectious agents as causes of diseases such as hepatocellular carcinoma, cancer of the cervix, and AIDS.

This chapter, therefore, covers the notions behind the specific characteristics and terminology of infectious disease epidemiology, and is addressed to the young instructor who has been formally trained in epidemiology and has limited expertise and perhaps training on infectious diseases.

Teaching objectives

An infectious disease epidemiology course, according to this chapter, should make the student familiar with the concepts of this discipline. The student should be able to describe the interplay between the agent, the host, and the environment, and to understand the preventive rationale behind vaccinations at the individual and the population level.

At the end of the course, the student should be able to conceptualize preliminary investigations of the most frequent outbreaks of diseases and to discuss how infectious diseases are best controlled, taking the nature of the infectious agent, immunity, and transmission into consideration.

The student should be able to read epidemiologic papers in the field and to discuss the validity of these papers.

Teaching methods and format

The main concepts should be presented in lectures. Exercises on outbreaks or discussions of papers are best done in smaller groups. If time permits, most public health units may arrange shorter or longer stays, which allow the students to participate actively in preventive actions or in the search for determinants of outbreak. Often the search is not for the determinants, which may be well known, but rather to the specifics of a particular outbreak (deductive epidemiology).

Assessing students' achievements

Written or oral exams may be used. Some institutions, like the Center for Disease Control (CDC) have developed a set of tests which can be used at the individual or group level.

Structure of chapter

This chapter is in five sections:

+ Infectious diseases, infectious agents, and host defense
+ Herd immunity
+ Reservoir
+ Dynamics of the human–infectious agent association
+ Transmission

Infectious diseases, infectious agents, and host defense

Infectious or communicable diseases are those attributed to propagating agents or their toxic products. Infectious agents may be transmitted to humans either directly (from other infected humans or animals) or indirectly (through airborne particles, arthropod vectors, or vehicles, liquid or solid, of the inanimate environment). Infectious diseases which may be transmitted from a human to another human without the intervention of a particular vector or a specific vehicle are termed contagious. Thus, malaria is a communicable but not a contagious disease, whereas measles and AIDS are contagious as well as communicable diseases. The epidemiology of infectious diseases is peculiar in several ways, on account of the defining characteristic of all infectious agents: they are entities with reproductive potential.

Epidemics and outbreaks

Epidemics of infectious diseases, like epidemics of other origin, can last a few hours (staphylococcal food poisoning) or several decades (cholera, AIDS), and cover the area of a small military camp (meningococcal meningitis) or that of one or more continents (influenza, AIDS). Epidemic 'outbreaks' (i.e. epidemics restricted with respect to time, place, and size of affected population) are usually of infectious origin. The term endemic is also usually (but not exclusively) applied to infectious diseases, and indicates the continuous presence of sporadic cases of a particular disease in a certain geographic area or population group. Endemicity is frequently the background of major epidemics of infectious diseases. An endemic infectious disease can become epidemic following a similar epidemic in animals in the same or a neighboring area, or a disproportional increase of the density of the necessary arthropod vectors, or a disproportional increase of the susceptible (non-immune) individuals, or a critical change in other relevant variables.

Nature of infectious diseases

Infectious agents have reproductive potential and are occasionally or always disease-inducing (pathogenic). They include, in increasing order of complexity, prions, viruses, chlamydia, rickettsiae, schizomycetes (bacteria), fungi, monocellular parasites (protozoa), and multicellular parasites (metazoa). It should be noted that several parasites and many bacteria are not infectious for humans (saprophytes), and that even those which are potentially infectious do not always cause disease or even subclinical infection. On the other hand, it is now established that infectious agents are responsible for manifestations that bear little clinical resemblance to the traditional infectious diseases, including such varied conditions as Kuru, genital herpes, subacute sclerosing panencephalitis and hepatocellular carcinoma.

Epidemiologic properties of infectious agents

Several properties of the infectious agents are important epidemiologic parameters of the corresponding diseases, including the properties that concern survival of the agents, their disease-inducing potential, and their antigenic and immunogenic capacity.

The survival of a particular agent is a complex function of many factors. It depends on:

+ The viability in the free state, i.e. on the ability to withstand unidimensional or multidimensional adverse environmental conditions (extremes of temperature, dryness, radiation, etc.).

+ The growth requirements, since viruses, contrary to schizomycetes, can only grow in living cells (food poisoning is usually caused by the latter and only rarely to the former).

+ The multiplicity of the potential hosts (the broader the host range the higher the chances of survival).

+ The sensitivity to chemotherapeutics and other substances, and the ability to develop mutant forms (with reduced chemosensitivity or altered antigenic determinants).

The disease-inducing potential may be evaluated at two levels. The first level refers to 'infectivity' (or transmissability), i.e. the ability of the agent to develop, or multiply, or both, in the human host. Infectivity may be defined in terms of the minimum infective dose, but this parameter is difficult to measure. An acceptable epidemiologic alternative is the 'secondary attack rate', but this is only applicable to contagious diseases. An infection may become clinically manifest (infectious disease) or may remain inapparent. The proportion of those infected who develop the corresponding disease is termed 'pathogenicity' (or expressivity). Obviously, the number of overt cases of an infectious disease in a particular situation is a function of the product of infectivity and pathogenicity. Some diseases are characterized by relatively high values of both infectivity and pathogenicity (measles, chicken pox), others by relatively high values of infectivity but not pathogenicity (poliomyelitis, hepatitis A), others by relatively high values of pathogenicity but not infectivity (common cold, mumps, AIDS), and still others by relatively low values of both infectivity and pathogenicity (leprosy, tuberculosis). Pathogenicity is not a reliable predictor of clinical severity (e.g. chicken pox is characterized by very low proportions of both clinically inapparent and clinically severe cases).

Antigenicity is a distinctive property of most infectious agents and refers to their ability to react specifically with humoral antibodies or sensitized lymphocytes or both. Antigenicity is responsible for the specificity of the immune response and forms the scientific basis for most procedures of immunodiagnosis, as well as for the discipline of seroepidemiology. Antigenicity must be distinguished from immunogenicity; the latter refers to the potential of most infectious agents to *elicit* humoral or cellular immune response, of variable strength and duration, in their respective hosts. Immunogenicity depends on the inherent antigenicity of an infectious agent, as well as on the site of multiplication and the extent of dissemination of the agent in the host. Thus, the gonococcus bacteria and the influenza virus are much less immunogenic than the viruses of measles and hepatitis A, because the former two agents tend to multiply in the epithelial cells of the genitourinary tract and the tracheobronchial tree, respectively, whereas the latter two agents disseminate widely throughout the body.

Host defense

The occurrence of a particular infection in an individual who has been exposed to an infective dose of the corresponding agent depends on the 'susceptibility' of the individual. Susceptibility is the negative expression of 'resistance' which has two components, the inherent or natural, or non-specific resistance, and the acquired, or specific resistance, or 'immunity'.

The inherent resistance depends neither on antibodies nor on specific cellular reactions. It is determined by species and is genetically conditioned, and encompasses mechanical protection by the skin and other structures, local non-specific inflammatory reactions, non-specific phagocytic activities, and the intracellular antiviral effects of interferons. By contrast, immunity is acquired and depends on the presence of specific antibodies (humoral immunity) or specifically sensitized T lymphocytes (cellular immunity). Immunity (mainly humoral immunity) may be distinguished into 'passive immunity' (natural or artificial), and 'active immunity' (natural or artificial).

Passive immunity is caused by antibodies generated in one or more individuals other than the one who is eventually protected. Natural passive immunity is caused by the transplacental transfer of antibodies from the mother to the newborn. Antibodies of the IgM class, which characterize the primary immune response, and the 'secretory' IgA antibodies do not cross the placenta and do not convey natural passive immunity. Natural passive immunity lasts, usually, from about 3 to 5 months, depending on the antibody titer in the maternal organism. Artificial passive immunity is conferred through parenteral administration of gamma globulin, the antibody-containing fraction of pooled human plasma. When the gamma globulin originates from randomly chosen adults, it will be safe to assume that it contains a modest concentration of antibodies against most of the common infectious diseases in the corresponding population, and for this reason the gamma globulin is called immune globulin ('immune serum'). If, however, the pooled serum originates from individuals specifically chosen on the basis of their recent infection by a particular agent, it will be safe to assume that it contains a high concentration of antibodies against this particular infection, and for this reason, the gamma globulin is called hyperimmune to that particular agent ('hyperimmune serum'). Artificial passive immunity is of shorter duration than natural passive immunity, and is mainly used for short-term, postexposure prophylaxis against some viral diseases, e.g. hepatitis B. It should be noted that, occasionally, passive immunity may provide protection against clinically overt disease, but subclinical infection could occur, thus allowing the development of natural active immunity.

Active immunity is caused by antibodies or sensitized T lymphocytes generated in the immune individual him or herself. It may be due to antecedent infectious disease or subclinical, inapparent, infection (natural active immunity); it may also be the result of vaccination with a modified, attenuated, inactivated, or killed agent, or a fraction of the agent, or a modified non-toxic product (artificial active immunity). Active immunity is, in general, both strong and longlasting, the natural generally being stronger and lasting longer than the artificial.

Immunity is a quantitative rather than a categoric variable; it declines with the passage of time, it may be overwhelmed by an excessive dose of the infectious agent, and it may be affected by a concurrent infection or immunosuppressive treatment. The inability to develop an immune response, in spite of the existence of antigenic stimulation, is termed 'tolerance'; this phenomenon may be responsible for the chronic persistence of certain infectious agents in the organism, and may represent the biologic background for the congenital (transplancental) transmission of other infectious agents.

Herd immunity

The susceptibility or resistance of a population group (e.g. the residents of a military camp, a boarding school, a village or a city) against a particular infectious disease is termed 'herd immunity' or population immunity. Herd immunity depends on several factors, including the equilibrium of the reservoir system of the infectious agent. However, in most situations, the most important determinant of herd immunity is the proportion of susceptible individuals in the corresponding population group. This is particularly true in contagious diseases, since, in most of these instances, immunity protects from covert infection (and the chronic carrier state) as well as from overt infectious disease. A corollary is that, in contagious diseases, immunity tends to limit not only the number of susceptible individuals but also the number of potential sources of infection, and that, in these diseases, herd immunity is more than the sum of individual immunities (Fig. 15.1).

Herd immunity is, therefore, a critical parameter in the epidemiology of contagious diseases, and helps to explain several phenomena, including the dynamic of many epi-

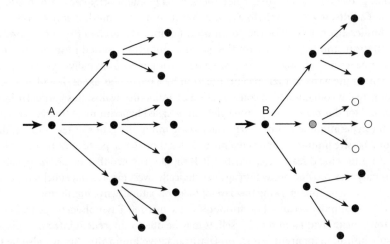

Figure 15.1 The principle of herd immunity. Black circles indicate individuals affected by a particular contagious disease, white circles individuals not affected by this disease, and the circle with the diagonal lines, the sole individual who was originally immune. The arrows indicate the direction of effective contact (transmission). In situation A, all individuals were susceptible and subsequently affected. In situation B, only one individual was immune and yet four were protected (even though three of them were, and remained, susceptible).

demic outbreaks, their periodic epidemic occurrence, and the variable effects of alternative vaccination strategies.

Dynamic of contagious epidemic outbreaks

It is difficult to immunize (actively or passively, naturally or artificially) all the individuals in a population group. In artificial immunization, it is rare to reach more than 90% of the target population. In active immunization (natural or artificial) there will always be individuals with defective immune response. In all situations the level of immunity will tend to decline with time (unless boosted by subclinical inapparent infections), while the composition of the population may change with the entry of susceptible (non-immune) individuals (infants or migrants). However, immunity of all the members of a population group is not a condition for the avoidance of an epidemic from a contagious disease, ('propagated', 'progressive' or 'contagious' epidemic), even when there are one or more sources of infection (usually infectious individuals). This can be explained. In the initial phase of a propagated epidemic many of the susceptible persons are affected, generating an exponential amplification of the epidemic wave. With the passage of time, however, the earlier affected individuals develop immunity, and become 'barriers' which prevent the transmission of the infection from the currently affected persons to those remaining susceptible.

Mathematically, the progress of a propagated epidemic is associated with a gradual reduction of the basic transmission parameter of the particular disease in the particular community. This transmission parameter (sometimes symbolized by $\hat{R}$), represents the *instantaneous* 'reproductive rate' of the contagious infection, and indicates the average number of additional cases generated directly by an infectious individual. It depends on both the 'force of infection' of the disease (reflecting, to a large extent, the infectivity of the respective agent) and the proportion of immune individuals in the community (herd immunity). When the proportion of susceptible individuals is so low that the transmission parameter becomes less than 1, the epidemic outbreak is bound for extinction and the population group may be considered as possessing adequate herd immunity against this particular disease. There may be a relatively large residual number of susceptible individuals, but they are not sufficient to sustain the necessary sequence of effective contacts for the continuation of a propagated outbreak. For example, were it not for transmission of HIV through needle-sharing, the reproductive rate of AIDS would be below 1, at least in developed countries.

It is of obvious importance to determine the 'critical proportion' of immune persons for a particular contagious disease in a particular community; that is, the level of herd immunity sufficient to limit the dispersion of the infectious agent and to prevent a major outbreak. The critical proportion depends on several factors, including:

♦ The infectivity of the infectious agent.

♦ The duration of the period of communicability.

♦ The number of infectious sources, or the frequency of introduction of the infectious agent into the population at risk.

♦ The overall density (macro-level), the crowding (micro-level), and the health attitudes and behavior of the population at risk.

+ The effect of individual immunity on the carrier state.

+ The importance of the carrier state for the transmission of the disease.

When carriers are important for the transmission of the disease, and the individual immunity does not affect the carrier state, then herd immunity plays little or no additional beneficial role, and the critical proportion of immune individuals approaches 100%.

Various approaches, including empirical studies and epidemiologic modeling, have been used to estimate the critical proportion of immune persons in various diseases under variable conditions. These proportions are said to be 90% or more for smallpox, rubella, and measles, but lower for pertussis and diphtheria. However, the applicability of these figures is questionable when there is substantial socioeconomic heterogeneity in the population at risk, since the non-immune persons are likely to cluster in particular neighborhoods, schools, or other population groups.

Periodic occurrence of epidemics

In stable populations which are not artificially immunized, most contagious diseases tend to recur periodically. This periodicity is accounted for by a similar periodicity in the level of herd immunity. Thus, after an epidemic from a highly contagious disease, there remain very few susceptible individuals who have escaped infection, and the level of herd immunity is very high. However, in almost all populations there is a continuous introduction of susceptible individuals, mainly of infants who have gone through their transient stage of natural passive immunity. After a relatively short period (usually a few years), the addition of susceptible individuals results in a reduction of the herd immunity below the critical level. The subsequent introduction of a new infectious case, or the creation of favorable conditions around an asymptomatic carrier or another source of infection, may lead to a new epidemic. In any relatively large population, one of these events is bound to happen sooner or later, closing the cycle of the periodic epidemicity.

The interepidemic period, T, is related to the mean age at acquisition of the infection, A, through the Anderson–May equation

$$T = 2\pi \sqrt{AD}$$

where π is equal to the constant 3.14 and D the disease constant 'generation time'. Generation time is the interval between effective exposure of an individual and the end of the period of communicability from that individual to others. Thus, for a disease with a generation time of 17 days (0.047 years) and a mean age at infection of 5 years, the interepidemic period would be expected to be 3.0 years.

The age at infection is an important parameter in the epidemiology of contagious diseases and is a sensitive correlate of the herd immunity equilibrium. In particular, when two infectious agents are very common and elicit strong and longlasting individual immunity, then the mean age at infection from these agents is, for obvious reasons, inversely related to their infectivity. Thus, in non-vaccinated communities, the mean age at infection from measles is lower than that from mumps, since the infectivity of the former is higher than that of the latter (the estimated secondary attack proportions are about 75% and 30%, respectively).

The inherent infectivity of an infectious agent is not the only factor that affects the potential for transmission of the corresponding contagious disease. Several other factors may contribute substantially, including population density, housing conditions, hygienic standards, health attitudes, and behavior and socioeconomic situation. These factors form an aggregate composite variable, occasionally termed 'force of infection'. This variable, in association with herd immunity, determines the actual transmission parameter $\overset{\circ}{R}$. A decrease in the force of infection of a contagious disease is usually accompanied by increases in the average age at infection as well as in the length of the interepidemic period.

The epidemic periodicity may be seriously affected by effective widespread vaccination, or, on the contrary, by the sudden inflow of a large number of susceptible individuals. Thus, in military camps of army recruits, the mixing of transient or long-term carriers with susceptible adults, under conditions of extreme crowding, suboptimal hygienic conditions, and low herd immunity, may favor the eruption of small outbreaks due to various strains of meningococcus, adenoviruses of types 4 and 7, etc.

Development and role of active immunity

Active natural immunity is a critical determinant of the descriptive epidemiology of the corresponding disease only when the infectious agent is both common and capable of eliciting an effective and longlasting immune response. The infectious agents of many zoonoses (rabies, plague, tularemia, many encephalitides from arboviruses , etc.) are so uncommon that their naturally generated immunity is rarely of major epidemiologic importance. On the other hand, in the absence of vaccination, the viruses of measles, rubella, and hepatitis A are so common, and their naturally generated immunity so effective, that herd immunity becomes of critical importance and the corresponding diseases tend to occur among the younger age groups (since adults tend to acquire protective antibodies at some earlier stage of their lives). Lastly, the infectious agents of influenza and common cold are very common, but their antigenic instability (influenza), or heterogeneity (common cold), do not permit the development of effective and lasting natural immunity, so that the corresponding diseases tend to occur in all age groups, without systematic childhood predilection.

In many infectious diseases (for example, hepatitis A and B) the development of active natural immunity is taking place through inapparent subclinical infections rather than through overt clinical disease. The ratio of subclinical infections to clinical attacks varies substantially, both 'between' infectious diseases (from less than 1:10 in smallpox to more than 100:1 in poliomyelitis) and 'within' a certain disease. In general, this ratio is higher in children than in adults, creating a paradox: in communities with higher socioeconomic conditions and hygienic standards, the incidence of some clinically apparent infectious diseases may be actually higher than in communities with lower conditions and standards. This is because, in the former, the decreased force of infection may lead to a higher average age at infection, when the proportion of clinical disease is usually higher.

Natural active immunity tends to limit not only overt clinical disease but also the carrier state, although perhaps less effectively. This is particularly important when contagious diseases are concerned, because for these control of the carrier state is a precondition for optimal function of herd immunity. A vaccine for a contagious disease is, therefore, optimal when it can mimic, in this respect, natural immunization, which generates herd immunity in addition to effective individual immunity. A comparison between the parenterically administered inactivated vaccine against poliomyelitis (Salk vaccine) and the orally administered live-attenuated (Sabin) vaccine, is instructive in this respect. Both vaccines are very effective in inducing strong and longlasting individual immunity, and in protecting the immunized individual against clinical disease. However, of these two procedures, only the Sabin vaccine can protect the alimentary tract from reinfection, thus preventing the transient carrier state, the dispersion of the infectious agents, and the multiplication of the infectious sources. Thus, only the Sabin vaccine can generate herd immunity and protect, in addition to those vaccinated, the remaining few who have not been immunized. Other vaccines which appear to limit the transmission of the corresponding infectious agents and to generate herd immunity are those against diphtheria and hepatitis B, whereas it has not been conclusively established whether the pertussis and the meningococcus vaccines have the same potential to the same degree.

Reservoir

A 'reservoir' of a particular infectious agent may be the human species, other vertebrates, arthropods (mainly insects), plants, or elements of the inanimate environment, in which the infectious agent normally lives, multiplies, and depends on for survival, reproducing itself in such manner that it can be transmitted to a susceptible host. In effect, reservoir is a simplified expression of the frequently complex and always dynamic system through which an infectious agent perpetuates its existence in nature. For many multicellular parasites (e.g. the helminths) and several unicellular parasites (e.g. the malarial parasites), perpetuation in nature requires a series of profound biologic changes (e.g. from ova to larval and mature stages, or from asexual to sexual stages), which constitute the 'biologic cycle' or 'life cycle' of the infectious agent.

When a reservoir belongs to the animal kingdom (including man, other vertebrates and arthropods), it is termed 'host'. A host may be 'biologic' (when the infectious agent multiplies or undergoes biologic development), or 'mechanical' (when the infectious agent remains alive but does not multiply systematically or undergo biologic development).

Some infectious agents may have two or more different biologic hosts. In the case of parasites which undergo a biologic cycle, it is common for the different hosts to support different and distinct stages of the life cycle of the corresponding parasite. Hosts in which the parasite attains maturity or passes its sexual stage are 'primary' or 'definitive' hosts; those in which the parasite is in a larval or asexual stage are 'secondary' or 'intermediate' hosts. Thus, for the plasmodia of malaria, the intermediate host is man, and the definitive host is the female anopheline mosquito, whereas for

Echinococcus granulosus, intermediate hosts are the sheep, other herbivores, and occasionally man, and definitive hosts are the dog and occasionally other carnivorous animals. The set of potential biologic hosts of an infectious agent has been termed 'host range'.

Some hosts may also be 'vectors', transmitting the infectious agent to the susceptible human. Vectors are usually insects (or other arthropods), and may be mechanic or biologic hosts (intermediate or definitive). Thus, the female anopheline mosquito is the primary biologic host as well as the transmitting vector for the plasmodia of malaria, whereas the rat flea *Xenopsylla cheopis* is the mechanical vector transmitting *Yersinia pestis* (the plague bacillus) from rat to man. On the other hand, domestic flies, although they are frequently transport hosts of several *Salmonella* and *Shigella* species, and are frequently responsible for the contamination of various foods and feeds, should not be considered as proper 'vectors' for these agents in human disease, since they do not transmit them directly to humans.

With the exception of a few agents which have the potential to develop biologically resistant forms in the free (inanimate) environment (e.g. *Clostridium tetani* and *Histoplasma capsulatum*), and of some others which are able to multiply in various foods and other materials (e.g. staphylococci, salmonellas, and other agents which can cause outbreaks of food poisoning or other syndromes), the maintenance in nature of most agents of human infections depends on a sequence of direct or indirect transmissions between similar or dissimilar hosts. For the majority of these agents (including HIV, the viruses of measles, rubella, and mumps, *Corynebacterium diphtheriae*, *Treponema pallidum*, and *Salmonella typhi*), man is the only host, and maintenance in nature is based on an endless chain of transmissions between humans. Sometimes the frequency of transmission is high and the duration of the infection (clinical or subclinical) is short (e.g. the viruses of common cold and rubella); sometimes the opposite may be true (e.g. the viruses of herpes simplex and herpes zoster, and the *Treponema pallidum* of syphilis); and sometimes other combinations may exist, even for the same infectious agent (e.g. the virus of hepatitis B and *Salmonella typhi*, which may be associated both with acute disease and a chronic carrier state, and *Rickettsia prowazeki*, which may be associated with both typhus fever and Brill–Zinsser disease). For another group of infectious agents, man is a necessary host but not a sufficient one, because the chain of transmission involves two or more hosts in a certain sequence (e.g. the plasmodia of malaria). For yet another group of infectious agents, man is not a necessary, but an alternative, irregular, or exceptional host, 'substituting' for another, more regular, vertebrate host (e.g. the yellow fever virus and several of the salmonellas). Finally, there is a group of infectious agents for which man is not a host in the ecologic context, but only the subject of a dead-end infection, beyond which there can be no further transmission of the infectious agent (e.g. the virus of rabies, because humans do not usually bite other humans or animals, and *Echinococcus granulosus*, because human remnants or organs are not fed to dogs or other carnivorous animals). Diseases caused by infectious agents of the last two categories are frequently called 'zoonoses' on account of their transmissability, under natural conditions, from vertebrate animals to man. It may be noted that the infectious agents of zoonoses can frequently cause disease in their respective non-human vertebrate hosts, whereas invertebrate hosts (mainly insects), whether biologic or mechanic, are rarely affected by their infection (a notable exception is the lethal infection of *Pediculus humanus humanus*, the human body louse, by *Rickettsia prowazeki*, the agent of epidemic typhus fever).

Control of reservoir is one of the three main approaches for the prevention of infectious diseases (the other two being control of transmission and regulation of the herd immunity). Control of reservoir depends on the type of the reservoir and the overall ecologic equilibrium. When the reservoir is the anopheline mosquito or the rat, extermination is desirable, if not always possible. When reservoir is a more friendly or useful animal, quarantine or vaccination may be found useful, as, for instance, has been the case for rabies control in the UK. When humans are the only reservoir, various approaches may be considered, including:

1. Vaccination (e.g. against smallpox, diphtheria, and meningococcal meningitis), which both increases the level of herd immunity and reduces the volume of the potential reservoir.

2. Chemotherapy (e.g. against tuberculosis), which shortens the period of communicability that springs from the reservoir.

3. Chemoprophylaxis (e.g. against the meningococcal and streptococcal diseases), which reduces the carrier-based reservoir for these diseases.

Dynamics of the human–infectious agent association

Exposure of a human to an infectious agent may be of no consequence when the 'dose' of the infectious agent is inadequate, or the exposure site inappropriate for the agent, or the inherent resistance insurmountable, or the specific immunity sufficient. In other instances, however, exposure may lead to infection and is termed 'effective exposure', or 'effective contact'. Infection signifies the entry and development or multiplication of an infectious agent in the body of man (or another animal). Infection may be overt (infectious disease) or covert without clinically evident symptoms or signs, but with laboratory demonstrable biologic reaction (subclinical or inapparent infection). The milder form of subclinical infection is termed 'colonization' and is characterized not only by the absence of clinical symptoms and signs, but also by the absence of any systematic biologic reaction of the host, in spite of the multiplication of the infectious agent in one or more of the exterior or interior surfaces of the body and the existing potential for dissemination (e.g. the colonization by *Staphylococcus aureus* in the nasal epithelium). The lack of systematic biologic response (e.g. production of antibodies) distinguishes colonization from other forms of subclinical infection, whereas the living nature of the colonized surfaces distinguishes colonization from contamination (the latter term refers to the transfer and potential multiplication of infectious agents in elements of the inanimate environment). The term pollution refers also to elements of the inanimate environment (e.g. the air and the sea), but is conceptually broader, encompassing physical and chemical pollutants as well as infectious agents. Finally, 'infestation' is the lodgment, development, and reproduction of arthropods (e.g. lice) on the exterior surface of the body or in the clothing.

As already mentioned, an infected person may develop overt infectious disease or subclinical, inapparent, infection. In the latter instance the infected person may become a carrier (in which case he/she becomes part of the reservoir system, empowered with the ability to disseminate the infectious agent and to transmit the disease further), or may develop latent infection (in which case he/she cannot disseminate the infectious agent and transmit the disease, and does not become part of the reservoir system). Thus, a carrier of a toxinogenic strain of *Corynebacterium diphtheriae* may be the source of infection for a new case of diphtheria, whereas individuals with latent third-stage syphilis cannot further transmit the infectious agent *Treponema pallidum*. Although both the patient with infectious disease and the carrier are components of the reservoir system and are, therefore, theoretically capable of transmitting the disease, they can only do so during a particular stage of their infection, the 'period of communicability'. During this period, the infected persons (or animals) are also infectious for other persons (or other hosts) and they may be considered as 'sources of infection'. In general, a source of infection is a person, animal or object from which an infectious agent passes directly to a host. The terms 'source of infection' and 'source of contamination' are not synonymous: the latter refers to the transfer and potential multiplication of infectious agents to elements of the inanimate environment. Thus, a cook who is a carrier of *Salmonella typhi* may become the source of contamination of a particular food, which, in turn, may become the source of infection of other humans. As another example, an inappropriately built septic tank may be thought of as a potential source of contamination of a water supply.

The carrier state

The carrier state exists for a multitude of infectious agents, including viruses, schizomycetes, and even parasites. The immunologic basis of the phenomenon is not fully understood, but epidemiologically it is one of the most important components in the ecologic equilibrium of many infectious diseases. A carrier has been defined as an infected person (or animal) that harbors a specific infectious agent in the absence of discernible clinical disease and serves as a potential source of infection for man. The carrier may be an individual in the incubation period, the convalescence, or the postconvalescence of a clinically recognizable disease (incubatory, convalescent, or postconvalescent carrier), may reflect a transient subclinical infection (inapparent infection carrier), or it may indicate a chronic situation with peculiar structural or functional host correlates (persistent carrier). The carriers of the last two categories are frequently termed 'healthy' or 'asymptomatic', in contrast to the carriers of the first composite category who do experience clinical symptoms or signs, before or after the establishment of the carrier state. The persistent carriers are usually chronic (long-term), although some are not continuously infectious (intermittent carriers). By contrast, the carriers of the other categories are usually temporary or transient (short-term). Examples of the various categories of carriers are:

1. Incubatory carriers, e.g. individuals shedding the viruses of rubella and chicken pox before the onset of the corresponding rush.

2. Convalescent or postconvalescent carriers, e.g. some individuals who have had diphtheria and streptococcal diseases.

3. Inapparent infection carriers, e.g. the majority of those infected with the virus of hepatitis A and a minority of those infected with the virus of mumps.

4. Chronic carriers, e.g. individuals harboring *Salmonella typhi* in their gallbladder and chronic carriers of hepatitis B.

As the carrier state can precede or follow the clinical infection, or appear and disappear independently of it, so can the latent infection appear or disappear independently of the other two infection states. Furthermore, the latent infection, as well as the carrier state, may lead to complete recovery or to an intermittent course characterized by clinical recurrences and reactivations. It should be noted that the re-emerging disease may or may not be similar to the original disease. Thus, *Rickettsia prowazeki* originally causes epidemic typhus and, after a variable period of latent infection, may cause the Brill–Zinsser disease, which has clinical similarities to epidemic typhus. On the other hand, latent infections with the viruses of chicken pox and measles, may re-emerge with the strikingly dissimilar clinical pictures of herpes zoster and subacute sclerosing panencephalitis, respectively.

Stages of an infectious disease

There is enormous variability in nature concerning the clinical presentation, the evolution, and the outcome of most infectious diseases. The variability is large, not only among different diseases, but also among cases of the same infectious disease. Therefore, the outline in Fig. 15.2 is only useful for didactic purposes.

The starting point of an infectious disease is the effective exposure to the corresponding infectious agent. Two important overlapping stages originate from this point: the 'latent period' (latent infection), which terminates when the period of communicability begins, and the 'incubation period' (incubation time), which terminates at the first appearance of any observable symptom or sign. During the latent period, which is usually shorter than the incubation period, the infectious agent cannot be transmitted, except in extraordinary situations. For instance, evidence suggests that, concerning AIDS, infectiousness may be high during the initial period after infection with HIV. As a general rule, the speed of spread of a *contagious* disease is inversely

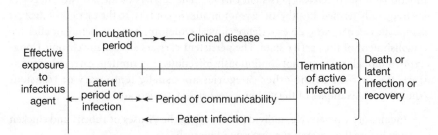

Figure 15.2 Schematic representation of the phases of an infectious disease.

related to the length of the latent period. The period of communicability lasts as long as the infectious agent can be emitted or discharged from the infected person in a manner and dose sufficient for the transmission of the disease to another host, but it has no fixed relation with the duration or termination of the clinical disease. This fact, and the usual start of the period of communicability before the appearance of any evidence of clinical disease, help to explain why the isolation of patients is not a sufficient measure for the control of most epidemics of most infectious diseases. Indeed, the eradication of smallpox became possible not only because of the availability of a very effective vaccine and the lack of an animal reservoir, but also because of the rarity of subclinical infections and the onset of the period of communicability *after* the appearance of clinical disease. An infection is considered active (patent) during either the clinical stage or the period of communicability (including the carrier state). Therefore, the active infection is terminated when both the clinical disease and the period of communicability are terminated, and the outcome may be recovery, death, or a transient or permanent stage of latency.

The period of communicability is of paramount importance for all infectious diseases, and not only for those that are contagious. Most infectious diseases are not communicable during the initial part of the incubation period, nor after the complete clinical recovery. However, in diseases in which mucous membranes are involved immediately after effective exposure (e.g. diphtheria and scarlet fever), the period of communicability may last from the actual date of exposure until the infectious agent is no longer disseminated (i.e. until the termination of the carrier state, if such a state exists). In several other diseases, including syphilis, gonorrhea, genital herpes, tuberculosis, some of the salmonelloses, and hepatitis B, the period of communicability may be very long (continuous or intermittent), because the combination of structural or functional defects with unhealed surface lesions permit the discharge of infectious agents from the skin or through one of the body orifices. Finally, for diseases which are transmitted by arthropods (e.g. malaria or leishmaniasis), the period of communicability lasts as long as the infectious agent exists in the peripheral blood or other externally accessible tissues of the infected individual in an infective form and in sufficient numbers to permit vector infection (e.g. in malaria the only infective form in the human blood is the gametocyte of the respective plasmodium). A period of communicability also exists in the arthropod vector; it is the period during which the infectious agent exists in the arthropod vector in such form, localization, and concentration as to make it infective for the human host (e.g. in malaria the female anopheline mosquito is infective when it carries a sufficiently high number of sporozoites of the respective plasmodium in the salivary glands). When the arthropod is a biologic (rather than mechanic) vector, it does not become infective immediately after effective contact with an infected and infectious host, but after passage of a certain period, which is termed the 'extrinsic incubation period'.

Patients and carriers in disease transmission

The contribution of man to the reservoir system of an infectious agent depends on the likelihood of transfer of the agent to another human or animal host, but it does not presuppose the occurrence of overt disease or the appearance of specific clinical signs or symptoms. Thus, it is possible for a patient with a particular infectious disease to be unable to transmit this disease further (e.g. patients with clinical measles or hepatitis A, when at least a week has elapsed from the first appearance of the rash or the jaundice, respectively). It is also possible for an individual with subclinical or presymptomatic infection to be a major focus of dissemination of the respective agent and an important source of infection (and subsequent disease) for many other susceptible hosts (e.g. individuals with subclinical hepatitis A infection, or those in the later part of the incubation period of clinically overt hepatitis A disease). Indeed, the fact that individuals with subclinical inapparent infections frequently represent important sources of infection and disease for other susceptible individuals helps to explain why measures focusing exclusively on patients, their contacts, and their immediate environment (e.g. patient isolation, quarantine of contacts, and disinfection of excreta and fomites) are usually ineffective for the control of most epidemics.

The relative importance of patients and carriers for the overall transmission and general dissemination of an infectious agent varies substantially from disease to disease (as well as from time to time and from place to place). In some infectious diseases, such as smallpox, measles, and chicken pox, there are very few carriers, because the pathogenicity (expressivity) of the corresponding agents is very high. For these diseases the patients themselves are by far the most important sources of new infections, and they can provide identifiable targets for effective planning of control measures. Indeed, it is the low (rather than the high) pathogenicity of an infectious agent that makes it difficult to launch effective control measures, since low pathogenicity implies many subclinical infections and, therefore, many inapparent and hidden sources of additional infections.

Several other diseases, including poliomyelitis, hepatitis A, hepatitis B, staphylococcal diseases, meningococcal meningitis, typhoid fever, and tuberculosis, are characterized by the relatively low pathogenicity of their infectious agents and, accordingly, by the relatively high ratio of covert subclinical infections to overt clinical cases. For these diseases, the relative importance of patients and carriers for overall disease transmission depends on the following parameters:

1. The average prevalence ratio of patients to carriers during the reference time period in the reference community.

2. The infectivity of carriers relative to that of the clinical cases (the degree of communicability of the clinical cases during their own period of communicability is usually higher than that of the carriers because the discharged infectious doses among the former are correspondingly higher, e.g. in staphylococcal disease, bacillary dysentery, gonorrhea, and meningococcal meningitis).

3. The duration of the period of communicability among clinical cases relative to the average duration of the corresponding period among carriers of all categories.

4. The relation of the onset of the period of communicability and the subsequent onset of clinical disease (the longer the period between the onset of communicability and the subsequent onset of clinical disease, the larger is the contribution of eventually clinical cases to the frequency of transmission).

5. The actual physical mobility of carriers relative to the corresponding mobility of patients (since patients are frequently hospitalized, they have fewer opportunities to transmit their disease further).

On the whole, in most infectious diseases characterized by moderate or low pathogenicity, the majority of transmissions are accounted for by subclinical carriers rather than by presymptomatic or clinical cases, a fact which helps to explain why:

♦ Patient isolation is not an effective measure for the control of most epidemics.

♦ Personal exposure histories cannot be relied upon for an accurate assessment of the existing level of herd immunity.

In the past, it has been suggested that a rapid increase in the prevalence of carriers is a reliable sign of an impending outbreak of clinical disease, but it appears now that this is not universally true. It has not been established why in certain situations an increase in the prevalence of carriers is associated with a substantial increase in the incidence of clinical disease, whereas in other situations the association is much weaker or completely absent. Several factors appear to be involved, including the nature of the infectious agent, the level of herd immunity, the crowding of the population, seasonal factors, and host characteristics (e.g. nasal carriers of hemolytic streptococcus are more infectious than throat carriers of the same agent).

Transmission

The transfer of an infectious agent from a source of infection to a susceptible host is termed 'transmission' – of the infectious agent as well as of the corresponding disease. There are two basic models of transmission, 'direct' and 'indirect', which may be distinguished further in more specific patterns (Table 15.1).

Direct transmission

Direct transmission refers to the immediate (in both time and place) transfer of an infectious agent from a source of infection to a receptive portal of entry of an appropriate host. It may take place by any of the following ways:

♦ By direct physical contact between two humans as in sexual intercourse, kissing, or touching.

♦ By direct projection of droplet spray on to mucous membranes of the nose, mouth, or eyes, as in coughing, sneezing, singing, or talking (transmission by droplet spread is limited to distances of no more than 1.5 meters because droplets tend to fall quickly on the ground).

♦ By direct physical contact between an infected vertebrate animal (not an arthropod vector) and a human, as in biting by a dog (rabies) and in scratching by a cat (cat scratch fever).

♦ By direct exposure of susceptible human tissue (e.g. injured exposed tissues, occasionally bare skin) to infective forms of infectious agents in the free inanimate environment, as in soil, compost or other decaying organic matter.

Table 15.1 Transmission patterns of infectious diseases

Direct transmission	
Direct contact with humans*	
Droplet spread*	
Direct contact with vertebrate animals (bites, etc.)	
Contact with agents in the free environment (soil, etc.)	
Indirect transmission	
→	
Vector-borne	mechanic
	biologic
→	
Vehicle-borne	short-range (indirect contact)*
	long-range
→	
Air-borne	droplet-nuclei*
	dust*

* Contagious diseases.

Indirect transmission

Indirect transmission refers to the indirect transfer of an infectious agent from a source of infection to an appropriate host; it may be mediated through a vector, an inanimate object or substance, or airborne particles (Table 15.1).

Vectors are arthropods (mostly insects) and may be distinguished into 'mechanic' and 'biologic'. Mechanic vectors are usually crawling or flying insects, carrying infectious agents through soiling of their feet or proboscis, or by passing them through their gastrointestinal tract. Mechanic transmission does not involve biologic development of the infectious agent and does not require its multiplication. In contrast, biologic transmission requires multiplication (propagation) of the agent, or its biologic (cyclic) development, or a combination of these, before the vector becomes infective at the end of the extrinsic incubation period. Transmission may be by saliva during biting or by deposition on the skin of feces or other material, capable of subsequent penetration through the minute wounds generated by the bite, the scratching, or the rubbing.

Vehicles are contaminated objects or elements of the inanimate environment (e.g. soiled clothes, eating utensils, water, milk, etc.), which serve as intermediate means by which an infectious agent is transported and introduced into a susceptible host through a suitable portal of entry. The infectious agent may or may not multiply or develop in or on the vehicle, before its final transfer and introduction into humans.

Vehicles may be distinguished into two main categories: 'short-range' and 'long-range'. Short-range vehicles are contaminated objects of personal use, such as handkerchiefs, clothes, bedding, cooking or eating utensils, surgical instruments, or dressings (fomites). Transmission by short-range vehicles is frequently considered as 'indirect contact' and depends, to a very large extent, on the ability of the infectious agent to survive in the free environment. Long-range vehicles include water, milk, various foods, blood and blood serum, parenteral solutions, etc. In some long-range vehicles (e.g. water) and in most short-range vehicles, the infectious agents do not multiply; as a result, the corresponding outbreaks are characterized by relatively low attack rates (because the dose of the infectious agent is small, it can cause clinical disease only to the small minority of highly susceptible individuals) and by relatively long incubation periods (because the initial dose is small, a longer time period is required for the attainment of the infectious threshold in the human body). Thus, in milk-borne outbreaks of typhoid fever, the attack rate is usually higher and the average incubation period is usually shorter than the corresponding values in water-borne outbreaks of the same disease, since *Salmonella typhi* multiplies in milk but not in water.

In most long-range vehicles, including many foods, several infectious agents of microbial (as opposed to viral) nature are able to multiply, and cause, under appropriate conditions, outbreaks of 'food poisoning'. Food poisoning is not always of infectious origin, and all food-borne diseases are not examples of food poisoning (e.g. hepatitis and bacillary dysentery). What distinguishes microbial food poisoning from other food-borne infectious diseases is that, in the former, the infectious agents themselves (or their toxins) are already present to a large extent in the consumed foods ('poisoned' foods).

Air-borne transmission is characterized by the dissemination, and eventual transfer to the respiratory tract of a susceptible individual, of microbial aerosols (particles suspended in the air and consisting, partially or wholly, of microbes or other infectious agents). The particles of the air-borne transmission have, in general, smaller dimensions and weight than the droplets of direct transmission, a fact which helps to explain why the former tend to remain suspended in the air for relatively long periods of time (sometimes gradually losing their infectivity), while the latter tend to fall quickly onto the ground. The average diameter of the air-suspended particles varies substantially (from about 0.1 micrometer to about 10 micrometers) and critically influences the fate of the inhaled particles. Relatively large particles (more than 10 micrometers) are almost wholly retained in the nose or other sites of the upper respiratory tract, and are later discharged in the environment. As the diameter of the suspended particles decreases, the probability of their penetration into the lungs and their retention there increases; particles with a diameter between 1 and 2 micrometers penetrate easily into the alveolar spaces and are retained there in a proportion that approaches 50%. Particles with a diameter between 0.25 and 1 micrometer penetrate easily but are not sufficiently retained because their small size facilitates their discharge in the environment. The situation changes again for the very small particles (diameter of less than 0.25 micrometer); for them, the Brown movement becomes important and facilitates their absorption onto the alveolar membrane.

The air-suspended particles of the air-borne transmission may be distinguished into two main types: 'droplet-nuclei' and 'dust'. Droplet-nuclei are the small residues which usually result from evaporation of fluid from droplets emitted by an infected host, and, occasionally, from artificial processes involving a variety of atomizing devices (e.g. in microbiology laboratories, abattoirs, etc.) Dust consists of particles of variable size and origin (e.g. contaminated soil, clothes, bedding, or floors) with common characteristics of the potential for long-term suspension in the air, and a (originally, and throughout) solid constitution.

Indirect air-borne transmission by droplet-nuclei is more important than has been previously assumed, and in many situations it is more important than direct droplet spread. Droplets, if they are not directly inhaled, fall quickly to the ground; however, even those which are inhaled are frequently too large for deep penetration and retention in the lungs. Furthermore, it appears that infective doses are generally smaller in air-borne transmission than in direct droplet spread. Dust, however, is important for disease transmission only when the infectious agents are resistant to dryness and other adverse conditions, and when the environment is heavily contaminated (e.g. in hospitals and other similar institutions).

The distinction between air-borne transmission by droplet-nuclei and direct droplet spread is important because control measures are very different. Because of the speed which characterizes direct droplet spread, there is no scope or utility in strategies focusing on ventilation or disinfection. More effective in this respect are measures based on control of the sources of infection, on coverage of the mouth and nose during coughing and sneezing, and on reduction of overcrowding in the living, working, and sleeping quarters. On the contrary, control of truly air-borne infections is, in principal at least, a technical problem which could be dealt with, effectively, with measures focusing on regular ventilation, air disinfection, and systematic control of dust. These measures aim at the reduction of the concentration of the infectious agents in the respired air.

References

Taylor, I. and Knowelden, J. *Principles of Epidemiology*. London, Churchill, 1964.

Fox, J. P., Hall, C. E., Elveback, L. R. *Epidemiology, Man and Disease*. New York, Macmillan, 1970.

Paul, J. R. and White, C. *Serological Epidemiology*. New York, Academic Press, 1973.

Sinnecker, H. *General Epidemiology*. London, Wiley, 1976

Suggested readings

Anderson, R. M., May, R. M. Vaccination and herd immunity to infectious diseases. *Nature* 1985; **318**, 323–9.

Anderson, R. M., May, R. M. *Infectious Diseases of Humans: Dynamics and Control*. Oxford University Press, 1991.

Benenson, A. S. (ed.) *Control of Communicable Diseases Manual*, 16th edn. American Public Health Association, 1995.

Fine, P. E. M. Herd immunity: history, theory, practice. *Epidemiologic Reviews* 1993; **15**, 265–301.

Giesecke, J. *Modern Infectious Disease Epidemiology.* Oxford University Press, 1994.

Murray, C. J. *Global Epidemiology of Infectious Diseases.* Harvard University Press, 1998.

Wilson, M. E. *A World Guide to Infections: Diseases, Distribution, Diagnosis.* Oxford University Press, 1991.

Chapter 16

Cancer epidemiology

Dimitrios Trichopoulos, Eleni Petridou, and
Jørn Olsen

Introduction

Cancer epidemiology appears to be an attractive topic to teach. It is a popular topic to
both health professionals and the lay public, there are thousands of publications and
books, and it is the most frequently discussed issue in the media. Teaching the subject,
however, presents considerable difficulties:

♦ Some students lack in-depth knowledge of molecular entities and processes that
  are essential for the understanding of carcinogenesis and eventually cancer
  epidemiology.

♦ Other students know more about molecular entities and processes than a middle
  age teacher, who may thus become insecure, evasive, or even antagonistic.

♦ For several forms of cancer the information is so limited (e.g. brain cancer) or so
  conflicting (e.g. lymphomas) that it becomes impossible for a teacher to present a
  coherent picture on the basis of the available information. The invocation of a
  coherent picture is essential for a successful presentation even when the story
  turns out to be wrong. There is nothing more unpleasant for students and teachers
  alike than to provide a list of fragmentary data that cannot be unified by even a
  working hypothesis.

♦ When teaching cancer epidemiology it is usually required that students should
  have had at least an introductory course of epidemiologic principles and methods.
  We all know, however, that understanding basic issues of epidemiology takes a lot
  more than an introductory course and students will usually welcome the presentation of methodologic issues as applied to specific aspects of cancer epidemiology.

♦ Integration of behavioral sciences, biology and, in particular, molecular biology
  with cancer epidemiology is clearly highly desirable. The epidemiologists' knowledge of molecular biology is, however, often superficial. This is not catastrophic
  unless the knowledge limitations are not recognized.

♦ Clearly, biologic plausibility is essential for the interpretation of epidemiologic
  data. Two errors can be made in this context. The first is to discard biology,
  because some 50 years ago epidemiology had changed a particular biologic perspective. Today's biology is considerably more advanced than the biology of half a
  century ago. A second error is to argue that something is biologically plausible

simply because it is conceivable. Conceivability may hinder refutation but it is not, in itself, as supportive of the hypothesis as plausibility can be. For instance, the nature of prions was clearly implausible but not inconceivable. In contrast, the cold fusion process and some epidemiologic theories should have been labeled as inconceivable as soon as it was recognized that they tend to contradict simple laws of physics or chemistry.

Goal and objectives

The goal of a 20–30-hour course of cancer epidemiology is to integrate simple principles of biology with epidemiologic characteristics so that the discipline moves beyond biostatistics into the realm of biomedical sciences. Indeed, as a distinguished epidemiologist has pointed out, the relation of epidemiology to biostatistics is similar to that between physics and mathematics. In other words, the goal of cancer epidemiology is not only to describe the principal risk factors of various forms of cancer, but to evaluate the compatibility of the risk profile of a particular cancer with alternative biologic hypotheses or combinations of hypotheses. Thus, at the end of the course the students should be able to answer questions like the following:

♦ What aspects of the natural history of carcinogenesis are more likely to be of genetic rather than epigenetic nature and vice versa (hereditary retinoblastoma may be linked to a germ cell mutation but why does cancer not develop from all tissues or organs)

♦ What are the principal stages in the natural history of neoplasias (initiation by genotoxic agents, promotion by conditions that favor cellular multiplication, progression by growth factors)

♦ What is the common characteristic of genotoxic agents (electrophilic reactants)

♦ Which type of oncogenic viruses are intimately linked to oncogenes (RNA viruses)

♦ Which is the common characteristic of infectious agents that are carcinogenic to humans (they cause chronic infection)

♦ What characteristic makes a form of radiation definitely carcinogenic (ionization)

♦ Which forms of cancer have clear long-term trends (lung cancer is increasing among women, stomach cancer is decreasing in both genders, melanoma is increasing in both genders, etc.)

♦ Why a causal factor is ranked differently depending on the use, as a criterion, of the relative or the population attributable risk (prevalence of exposure matters only for attributable risk)

♦ Why the incidence of lung cancer among women in some populations is lower in people older than 70 years than among younger people (cohort smoking phenomenon)

♦ Do sophisticated statistical techniques always remove confounding (no, because confounders may be unknown, poorly measured or follow a causal pattern that is not captured in the statistical model)

+ Can the very high mortality rate from AIDS in some African countries reduce age-adjusted cancer mortality rates in these countries (no, because rates do not compete)

+ Can the very high mortality rate from AIDS in some African countries reduce the cumulative risk for dying from cancer in these countries (yes, cumulative risks do compete)

+ Which form of cancer is most affected, in terms of relative risk, by specified exposures (e.g. squamous cancer of the urinary bladder by *Schistosoma haematobium*; stomach cancer by salt intake; corpus of the uterus by caloric excess)

+ Can magnetic fields cause cancer as initiators or as growth enhancers (impossible as initiators, conceivable but implausible as growth enhancers)

+ Which aspects of breast cancer epidemiology are not compatible with a simple effect of circulating estrogens (higher risk among Caucasians in Europe than among Chinese or Japanese in their respective countries even though these groups have comparable levels of blood estrogens; protective effect of early first pregnancy)

+ Which aspects of breast cancer epidemiology are not compatible with the hypothesis that prolactin increases the risk for this cancer (minimal or absent protective effect of the two physiologic conditions associated with substantial increase of prolactin, that is, pregnancy and lactation).

+ Which epidemiologic design is usually more appropriate for documentation of carcinogenicity of a particular occupational exposure (retrospective cohort study of an exposure group with internal reference group)

+ What are the most important achievements in cancer epidemiology from the start and during the past 10 years?

+ Which epidemiologic design is usually more appropriate for calculation of population attributable risk from an occupational carcinogen (an internally valid case control study of a representative series of cases)

+ Which prognostic indicator is appropriate for the evaluation of a randomly allocated screening program (none, because of lead time bias and length time bias).

Teaching contents

Review of biology

It is usually useful to start a course on cancer epidemiology by reviewing principles of cancer biology. This is in most situations a very difficult session because a majority of the students may have a more solid grasp of biology than their teacher and a minority will not be able to get an adequate grasp of the issues within 2 or 3 hours. It is advisable to request that, for the first session, students must have read a simple overview, such as the articles 'How cancer arises' (Weinberg, 1996) and 'How cancer spreads' (Ruoslahti, 1996) or the book *Genes and the biology of cancer* (Varmus and Weinberg, 1993). Similar review articles frequently appear in journals addressed to educated but not specialized readership.

During the first and relatively long session several issues need to be touched upon, because they need to be invoked during the teaching of cancer epidemiology. These are: the monoclonal nature of most cancers; the importance of apoptosis in carcinogenesis; antigenic and biochemical differences between normal and cancer cells; *in vitro* transformation; the cell cycle and control points; genetic and epigenetic phenomena in carcinogenesis; stages of carcinogenesis and experimental and epidemiologic evidence that cancer is a multistage process; chemical carcinogenesis; precarcinogens; ultimate carcinogen; DNA repair deficiency; nature and mode of action of oncogenic viruses; oncogenes; chromosomal aberrations, including constitutional changes (e.g. retinoblastoma); heritability of cancer predisposition (e.g. Fanconi's anemia) and chromosomal rearrangements; polymorphic systems and their importance in environmental carcinogenesis; immunologic phenomena in carcinogenesis; tolerance; short-term *in vitro* tests for carcinogen detection; rodent and other animal bioassays for carcinogen detection; the limited predictability of human carcinogens on the basis of *in vitro* tests and animal bioassays.

Cancer incidence around the world and overview of cancer causation

The second session should be devoted to an overview of cancer incidence around the world and a summary of existing knowledge on cancer causation. Data on incidence from cancer registries are regularly published by the International Agency for Research on Cancer (IARC) in the volumes *Cancer incidence in five continents* (IARC, 1992). We found it useful to present data from only eight registries, so that the generated tables covering all major sites of cancer would be more comprehensible. These registries are, for Europe: Denmark (national), Sweden (national), UK (Birmingham only), Spain (Zaragoza), and Hungary (Szabolcs); for North America: USA Surveillance Epidemiology and End Results, White and Black; for South America: Colombia (Cali); and for Asia: Japan (Osaka). Unfortunately, there are no well functioning registries in Africa. The indicated registries cover, to a considerable degree, the existing variation for cancers at different sites throughout the world.

It appears preferable to present cumulative incidence rates that can be interpreted as probabilities and are usually expressed in percentages. The cumulative incidence rates cover the age span 0–74 years and are easier to understand than standardized incidence rates. Thus, many people are able to indicate that the cumulative incidence of breast cancer among white women in the USA is more than 10%, as compared to less than 2.5% among women in Japan. In contrast, few investigators, let alone students, are able to provide reasonable figures for the world population age-adjusted incidence of breast cancer in the USA and Japan (per 100 000 women years). The students may be asked to try to explain the observed differences and the discussion is generally lively and occasionally quite insightful.

Subsequently, the teacher may wish to present a table (Table 16.1) of the occupational agents that have been judged by the IARC as being human carcinogens up to the end of 1999. The students may not recognize all of the over 40 listed occupational carcinogens, but they are always impressed that so many carcinogens have already been established – even though occupational agents in developed countries are

Table 16.1 Important occupational agents or work processes considered by IARC (WHO) as being human carcinogens

Substance of process	Site(s) of cancer
Acrylonitrile	Lung
Aluminum production	Lung, bladder
4-Aminobiphenyl	Bladder
Arsenic and certain arsenic compounds	Lung, skin
Asbestos	Gastrointestinal tract, mesothelioma of pleura and peritoneum, lung, larynx
Auramine manufacture	Bladder
Benzene	Hemopoietic tissue
Benzidine	Bladder
Beryllium and beryllium compounds	Lung
Bis(chloromethyl) ether and chloromethyl methyl ether	Lung
Boot and shoe manufacture and repair	Nasal cavity
1,3-Butadiene	Hemopoietic tissue
Cadmium and cadmium compounds	Lung
Coal gasification	Lung
Coal-tars and pitches	Skin
Coke production	Lung
Chromium and certain chromium compounds	Lung
Diesel exhaust	Lung
Dioxins	Soft tissue sarcoma, non-Hodgkins lymphoma
Ethylene oxide	Hemopoietic tissue
Formaldehyde	Nose and nasopharynx
Glass manufacture	Lung
Hairdresser or barber	Lung Bladder
Underground hematite mining	Lung
Iron and steel founding	Lung
Magenta, manufacture of	Bladder
Mineral oils, treated and mildly treated	Skin
Mustard gas	Pharynx, lung
2-Naphthylamine	Bladder
Nickel and nickel compounds	Nose and nasal sinus
Non-arsenical pesticides, spraying of	Lung

Table 16.1 Important occupational agents or work processes considered by IARC (WHO) as being human carcinogens *continued*

Substance of process	Site(s) of cancer
Painter	Lung
Petroleum refining, occupational exposure	Skin, hemopoietic tissue
Polychlorinated biphenyls	Liver, skin
Radon	Lung
Rubber industry	Bladder, hemopoietic tissue
Shale oils	Skin
Silica	Lung
Soots	Skin
Sulfuric acid mist	Nasal cavity, larynx, lung
Talc-containing asbestiform fibers	Lung
Trichloroethylene	Liver, biliary tract
Vinyl chloride	Liver
Wood dust	Nasal cavity

thought to contribute to less than 5% of all cancer deaths. It is instructive to point out to the students that the success in identifying occupational carcinogens is due to tragic exposure in the past to very high concentrations of carcinogens.

Table 16.2 presents the biologic agents judged by IARC and the wider scientific community as being carcinogenic. The teacher may wish to comment that infectious agents may account for up to 20% of all cancer deaths in the developing countries but much less in developed countries. Some researchers include *Aspergillus flavus* in this category because it contaminates stored foods (e.g. peanuts), where it produces the liver carcinogen aflatoxin.

Table 16.3 shows life style factors, excluding nutrition, established as human carcinogens. These factors account for about 30% of all cancer deaths around the world, mainly because of tobacco smoking. Table 16.4 refers to the role of diet in the etiology of various forms of cancer (Willett and Trichopoulos, 1996; World Cancer Research Fund and American Institute for Cancer Research, 1997). There are no IARC evaluations for nutritional factors and there is no adequate evidence concerning the relation with cancer of any micronutrient. Although higher estimates have occasionally been published, it appears that diet in adult life is responsible for only about 15% of all cancer deaths worldwide.

Medical products and procedures are responsible for about 1% of cancer deaths worldwide and it is generally accepted that the effectiveness of these procedures outweighs their cancer risks. Three categories of pharmaceutical agents are considered as increasing cancer risk: cancer therapeutic drugs, immunosuppressive drugs, and exogenous hormones. Among the iatrogenic processes that increase cancer risk one

Table 16.2 Biologic agents judged by IARC (WHO) as being human carcinogens

Agent	Site(s) of cancer
Hepatitis B virus	Liver
Hepatitis C virus	Liver
Helicobacter pylori	Stomach
Schistosoma hematobium	Bladder
Opisthorchis viverrini	Cholangiocarcinoma
Human papillomaviruses	Cancer of the cervix and anus
Human herpes virus 8	Kaposi's sarcoma
Human immunodeficiency virus 1	Non-Hodgkins lymphoma, anal cancer, Kaposi's sarcoma
Human T cell leukemia virus	Adult T cell leukaemia
Epstein–Barr virus	Lymphoproliferative diseases, nasopharyngeal carcinoma

also needs to consider radiotherapy and perhaps diagnostic radiation. With respect to exogenous hormones, it should be taken into account that they do not only have general beneficial effects but can also reduce the risk for some cancers (e.g. oral contraceptives reduce the risk for ovarian cancer but they may slightly increase the risk for breast cancer).

The teacher must stress that there are endogenous factors that affect cancer risk, some of them already known but others unknown and many of them uncontrolable. Reproductive factors are of critical importance for breast, ovarian, and endometrial cancers, whereas sexual activity is an important risk factor for cancer of the cervix. Perinatal factors, and particularly early growth, may affect the risk of several forms of cancer, perhaps by modulating the number of susceptible stem cells. Finally, genes need to be considered in two categories: major genes, frequently dominant with high penetrance, like *Brca1*, *Brca2*, and *Brca3*, which may be responsible for less than 5% of all cancer deaths; and genetic polymorphisms that are likely to interact with a wide

Table 16.3 Life style factors established as human carcinogens

Life style factor	Site(s) of cancer
Tobacco smoking	Lung, bladder, esophagus, mouth, larynx
Environmental tobacco smoke	Lung
Ethanol	Esophagus, larynx, mouth, pharynx, liver
Betel chewing	Mouth
Ionizing radiation	Marrow and probably all other sites
Ultraviolet light	Skin, lip

Table 16.4 Risk implications for major forms of cancer by consumption of foods in major groups, intake of energy generating nutrients, intentional dietary exposure to selected non-nutrients, and nutrition-related indicators

	Oral cavity	Naso-pharynx	Esophagus	Stomach	Large bowel	Liver	Pancreas
Major food groups							
Vegetables	reduce		**reduce**	**reduce**	reduce	reduce?	reduce?
Fruits	**reduce**		**reduce**	**reduce**	reduce	reduce?	reduce?
Red meat					**increase**		increase?
Macro-nutrients							
Protein (as animal)					increase?		increase?
Fiber					reduce?		reduce?
Saturated fat (as animal)					increase		
Mono-unsaturated fat							
Non-nutrients							
Alcohol Salt (NaCl)	**increase**	increase	**increase**	increase	increase	**increase**	
Nutritional covariates							
Height							
Obesity					**increase?**		
Physical activity					**increase** reduce		
Hot drinks			**increase**				

'?' indicates current data are only suggestive. Bold type indicates data are convincing
Source: Based on Willet W., Trichopoulos D. Nutrition and cancer: A summary of the evidence. Cancer Causes and Control 1996; 7: 178–80.

range of environmental factors in the causation of an unknown but probably large proportion of cancer cases and deaths worldwide. Students should appreciate that natural selection tends to limit the prevalence of powerful cancer-causing genes much more than it affects the prevalence of interacting alleles in polymorphic systems.

Table 16.5 shows proportions of cancer deaths in the world in the 1990s that may be attributed to environmental factors. Students should be aware that attributable fractions are, in general, non-additive because several etiologic factors act synergistically. The teacher should conclude the session by pointing out the dominant role epidemiology has played in the identification of most causes of cancer; then admit that, for at least one-third of all cancers, the causes may never be identified or may turn out to be unavoidable, possibly because they are intimately linked to natural growth phenomena.

Table 16.4 Risk implications for major forms of cancer by consumption of foods in major groups, intake of energy generating nutrients, intentional dietary exposure to selected non-nutrients, and nutrition-related indicators *continued*

	Larynx	Lung	Breast	Endo-metrium	Cervix uterine	Prostate	Urinary bladder	Kidney
Major food groups								
Vegetables	**reduce**	**reduce**	reduce	reduce	reduce	reduce?	**reduce**	reduce?
Fruits	**reduce**	reduce	reduce?	reduce?	reduce?	reduce?	reduce	reduce?
Red meat								
Macro-nutrients								
Protein (as animal)				increase?				
Fiber								
Saturated fat (as animal)		increase?		increase?		increase?		increase?
Mono-unsaturated fat			reduce?					
Non-nutrients								
Alcohol Salt (NaCl)	**increase**		increase					
Nutritional covariates								
Height								
Obesity								increase
Physical activity			**increase**			reduce?		
Hot drinks			dual reduce?					

'?' indicates current data are only suggestive. Bold type indicates data are convincing

Liver cancer

The epidemiology of no other cancer is so attractive to students as that of liver cancer. Although rare in developed countries it is very common in sub-Saharan Africa and south-east Asia, areas of the world that young and idealistic students are interested in and care about. It is the first major human cancer that was identified as having a powerful viral etiology. It is an important cancer for preventive medicine because it is virtually incurable but largely preventable with current knowledge and technology. Last, and most important, the discovery of the causes of liver cancer is ideal for a textbook in epidemiology. The discovery of the etiologic role of hepatitis B virus (HBV), in particular, follows an epidemiology textbook sequence, from case reports and geographical observations to case control studies and cohort investigations, culminating in a randomized trial for the prevention of hepatocellular carcinoma through HBV vaccine in Gambia.

Table 16.5 Non-additive proportions of cancer deaths in the world in the 1990s that may be attributed to environmental factors

Factor or class of factors	Percentage
Tobacco	25
Alcohol	2
Diet in adult life	15
Excess energy intake in early life	5
Food additives and contaminants	1
Sedentary life	1
Infectious agents	12
Reproductive factors	3
Ionizing and ultraviolet radiation	2
Occupational factors	5
Environmental pollution and industrial products	5
Medical products and procedures	1

Students should know that liver cancer is distinguished into three histologic types: by far the most common hepatocellular carcinoma, cholangiocarcinoma, and the very rare angiosarcoma. The distinction is crucial because the three histologic types have distinct etiologies. For hepatocellular carcinoma the established causes are aflatoxins, HBV, hepatitis C virus, alcoholic cirrhosis; less strongly, other forms of cirrhosis and, convincingly, although not widely recognized, tobacco smoking. For cholangiocarcinoma the established causes are *Opistorchis viverrini* and *Clonorchis sinensis*, both flukes prevalent in south-east Asia. Lastly, for angiosarcoma, thorotrast, vinyl chloride monomer, inorganic arsenic, and androgenic anabolic steroids are established causes.

Every teacher should structure the presentation on the basis of a particular text that reflects his or her own style. The chapter on liver cancer in the textbook edited by Adami and colleagues (in press) is a useful source, as are the IARC monographs on hepatitis viruses (IARC, 1994), liver flukes (IARC, 1994) and alcohol (IARC, 1988). Information on smoking in relation to hepatocellular carcinoma is well presented in a recent paper by Kuper and her colleagues (in press).

Lung cancer

Lung cancer in relation to smoking has been traditionally used as a teaching example in epidemiology. Most students, however, consider the topic somewhat boring. The teacher may reinstate their interest if the problem is presented as follows: at least half and perhaps two-thirds of the lung cancer cases around the world are caused by smoking. However, until the smoking epidemic is controlled, it would be of interest to know *who* among the smokers are likely to develop lung cancer and *why* some of the non-smokers end up developing the disease. It is also a surprise for many students to realize that lung cancer among non-smokers is a problem of comparable magnitude to that of cancer of the pancreas or ovary.

Introduction of the descriptive epidemiology of lung cancer is facilitated by presenting the figures regularly produced by the American Cancer Society and published every year in the January issue of *CA – a cancer journal for clinicians* (Landis *et al.*, 1999). These figures effectively convey the magnitude of the lung cancer problem in developed countries, in which almost one-third of cancer deaths among men and about a quarter of deaths among women are due to lung cancer.

The evidence linking tobacco smoking with lung cancer can be a fascinating story, going through population correlations to case control investigations and major cohort studies. Invocation of experimental evidence and molecular discoveries further enrich the presentation. Although everybody knows that smoking causes lung cancer, many aspects of this relation and the methodologic twists that were required for their identification are rich teaching material.

Among the issues to be addressed are: the comparative lung carcinogenicity of cigarettes, pipes and, cigars; the modifying effects of inhalation; the variable lung cancer risk in relation to number of cigarettes smoked and mouth-keeping time; the substantially higher risk among early starters of this habit; the disproportionally high effect of duration of smoking on lung cancer risk; and the consequences of introduction of low tar and filter cigarettes. This session can be concluded by pointing out the success, however limited, of smoking cessation. For more advanced classes the teacher can indicate to the students how the exposure response patterns between smoking and lung cancer risk have contributed to the estimation of the tobacco initiation and tobacco cessation lung cancer latencies; the multiple stages of the lung cancer carcinogenesis; the absence of a threshold in the exposure response curve; and other subtle and intriguing issues.

Although invocation of smoking is a reciprocal reflex in lung cancer epidemiology the teacher should also point out that many occupational carcinogens have the lung as their target. Among them asbestos, radon, and polycyclic aromatic hydrocarbons are of major and continuing interest. In the context of ionizing radiation effects, it is useful to present the comparative risks of α (alpha) particles, β (beta) particles and γ (gamma) radiation as a function of their relative biologic effectiveness. Although occupational causes of lung cancer have been well documented in the context of the conditions prevailing in plants of developed countries several years ago, they collectively explain a small and declining proportion of lung cancer cases. In contrast, the effect of a factor of potential importance for a non-negligible fraction of lung cancer cases has remained undocumented. This is air pollution, the prolonged exposure to which is very difficult to measure accurately. The conflicting evidence of ecologic and analytical epidemiologic studies and the biologic plausibility of an effect of air pollution on lung cancer risk creates a rich but complex field for methodologic explorations and biologic considerations.

There is convincing evidence that intake of fruit and vegetables reduce the risk for lung cancer but attempts to attribute this effect to vitamin A and beta-carotene have failed. Randomized trials have not supported a beneficial effect of micronutrients hypothesized to protect from lung cancer on either epidemiologic or biomedical evidence. This raises issues about the limitations of nutritional epidemiology, particularly with regard to extrapolation from foods to nutrients.

The relation of passive smoking to lung cancer risk also needs to be considered. The epidemiologic evidence linking passive smoking to lung cancer risk is only slightly stronger than the corresponding evidence linking extremely low frequency electromagnetic fields to childhood leukemia. Because, however, smoking is an established carcinogen and there is no threshold in the exposure–response association between smoking and lung cancer risk, it is reasonable to assume that passive smoking has some effect on lung cancer risk. Whether the excess risk for lung cancer among individuals exposed to environmental tobacco smoke (ETS) is 30%, 50% or higher, in comparison with those not exposed to ETS, has been the subject of an interesting controversy involving both epidemiologic evidence and biomedical plausibility (Trichopoulos, 1994).

The chapter on lung cancer in the textbook edited by Adami and his colleagues (in press) is a useful source of information for a prospective teacher, but there are many other good reviews of lung cancer epidemiology and etiology (Schottenfeld and Fraumeni, 1996).

Breast cancer

After the presentation in distinct sessions of two success stories of epidemiology with respect to liver and lung cancer, the students should share with their teacher the reality of failure, all too frequent in real life. Indeed, given the overall stability of breast cancer mortality rates over time around the world, it would be difficult to disagree with the statement of a fellow scientist: 'for no disease have so many researchers worked so long for so few practical results'. Because the overall situation is at present so fluid, teachers generally follow the approach they feel more comfortable with.

The approach that follows reflects, to a certain extent, the context in which the authors of this chapter are currently working, which may or may not be similar to the context in which other investigators are working.

Established breast cancer risk factors

The epidemiology of breast cancer has been reviewed by many investigators and the following factors are generally recognized (Kelsey *et al.*, 1993; Adami *et al.*, 1998):

+ Breast cancer is about 100 times more common among women than among men.
+ The incidence of breast cancer increases with age with a characteristic inflection around the age of menopause.
+ An earlier age at menarche is associated with increased breast cancer risk.
+ An earlier age at menopause is associated with reduced breast cancer risk.
+ For a given age of menopause, a surgically induced one conveys more protection than a naturally occurring one.
+ The earlier the age of the first full-term pregnancy the lower the risk for breast cancer.
+ Subsequent full-term pregnancies have similar but quantitatively much weaker effect.

+ After the age of approximately 35 years, occurrence of a pregnancy increases rather than reduces breast cancer risk.

+ Prolonged lactation conveys some protection against breast cancer risk, but the effect is small and may be limited to premenopausal breast cancer.

+ Height is positively associated with breast cancer risk.

+ Obesity is inversely related to breast cancer risk among premenopausal but positively among post menopausal women.

+ Caucasian women in Europe and North America have a more than fivefold risk compared to women in Asia or Japan.

+ A high density mammogram indicates an almost fourfold risk in comparison to a low density mammogram.

+ Breast cancer tends to be slightly more common among women of higher socioeconomic status.

+ Breast cancer tends to be more common among urban than among rural residents.

+ At least four genes that convey increased susceptibility to breast cancer have been identified (*Brca1, Brca2, p53* and *AT*), but these genes are responsible for less than 5% of breast cancer cases overall.

+ Current or recent use of oral contraceptives slightly increases the risk for breast cancer.

+ Current or recent use of long-term hormone replacement therapy increases the risk for breast cancer.

+ Ionizing radiation is an established cause of breast cancer, but of limited quantitative importance.

+ Consumption of alcoholic beverages increases breast cancer risk.

+ Adult life diet and physical activity have limited effect on breast cancer risk.

+ There is no compelling evidence that exposure to organochlorines or electromagnetic fields affect breast cancer risk.

An etiologic model

A synthesis of existing hypotheses has four key components (Adami *et al.*, 1998):

1. The likelihood of breast cancer occurrence depends on the number of cells at risk (Trichopoulos and Lipman, 1992). This proposition is supported by theoretical arguments and empirical data, such as follows:

   • Mammographic density, which expresses the mammary gland mass as a fraction of total breast area, is a strong predictor of breast cancer risk.

   • Women with small mammary gland mass who were motivated to have augmentation mammoplasty were found to have inherently reduced breast cancer risk.

2. The number of target cells and their responsiveness to hormonal stimulation is partially determined early in life, perhaps even *in utero*.

- There is substantial experimental evidence in support of this hypothesis (Hilakivi-Clarke *et al.*, 1997).

- In large studies a positive association was found between birth weight and breast cancer risk (Adami *et al.*, 1998).

3. The long-term effect of a pregnancy is considered to convey protection against breast cancer through terminal cellular differentiation in the mammary gland (Russo *et al.*, 1992).

   - There is substantial experimental evidence in support of this proposition.

   - A pregnancy transiently increases breast cancer risk by hormonally stimulating the replication of already initiated cells but in the long term it has a definitive protective effect.

4. In adult life oestrogens and other mammotropic hormones in conjunction with their receptors affect the rate of expansion of initiated clones.

   - In case control and cohort studies estrogen levels have been positively associated with breast cancer risk.

   - Estrogen α (alpha) receptor expression is much lower among Japanese women who are at low risk for breast cancer than among Caucasian women who are at high risk for breast cancer (Lawson *et al.*, 1999).

The teaching process

The composite hypothesis presented above does not contradict any of those that are currently dominant and is a synthesis rather than an original construct. Its advantage in a teaching process is that it provides biologic underpinnings for the whole spectrum of empirical evidence and specifies targets for refutation, in line with the mainstream Popperian approach.

Diet and cancer

Cancer epidemiology has been generally successful, from the discovery of tobacco smoking and HBV as the most important cause of two common forms of cancer, to the identification of asbestos and several other carcinogens in various occupational settings. This has created optimism in the scientific community and the general public about the prospects of clarifying the role of nutrition in the etiology of several other common cancers. However, in their successful efforts, epidemiologists were trying to assess the effects of single, easily identifiable factors. Furthermore, these effects were large in the relative sense, either inherently (HBV) or because the exposure levels in particular settings were extreme (asbestos in insulation workers). In contrast, it is difficult to assess nutritional factors over a long period of time; it is *a priori* difficult to indicate whether food items, food groups, particular nutrients, or nutritional patterns are more important, and the relative risk associated with any particular nutritional factor is likely to be small (extreme contrasts can be found only with respect to supplemental micronutrients and their effects are likely to be either protective or null). Indeed, the widely held assumption that a large proportion of human cancers is caused by nutritional factors is not based on direct evidence but is derived by exclusion. Thus, for several common cancers, the large interpopulation variation or evidence from migration studies cannot be attributed to genetic factors and cannot be accounted for by other established environmental factors or personal attitudes.

In the session dedicated to the nutritional epidemiology of cancer the emphasis should be on the methodologic complexities of epidemiologic studies in this field. The validity of long-term diet ascertainment is known to be limited. This has long been recognized but it has usually been assumed that it would generally lead to findings indicating that there are no associations when actually there would be real, although small ones (false-negative results). However, given the extensive intercorrelation between food items and food groups, extensive mutual confounding should also be expected and residual confounding can cause both false-negative and false-positive results. Furthermore, even without confounding, extensive misclassification can reduce the statistical power to such an extent that the predictive power of a particular 'positive' finding will be minimal (the $-$alpha-β error would be large, so that findings due to $-$beta-α error would dominate the results of the study). The situation can be further complicated when the latencies of particular nutritional factors are different or operationally non-definable, or when thresholds must be invoked. These conditions are particularly relevant when promoting or growth-enhancing agents are considered.

Another complex issue focuses on the components of variability of particular nutrient intakes (intraindividual, interindividual and time-dependent variability). Important work has recently been undertaken in this field (Willett, 1998), but many problems remain unresolved. Additional complexity is introduced by the dependence of the relative risk associated with a particular nutritional factor on the presence of other nutritional component causes in the same or in different etiologic complexes, and by the need to integrate, for operational reasons, converging effects of several foods or nutrients into unidimensional indicators.

Current knowledge on the nutritional etiology of human cancer has been carefully compiled and summarized in a large volume that has been prepared by the World Cancer Research Fund and the American Institute for Cancer Research (1997). This is a reference book but it also provides summary tables for nutritional factors in the etiology of various forms of cancer.

A flexible session

The seventh session may be a flexible one and depends on the background and interest of the students. If several students have had difficulty in following the course, the session could be dedicated to reviewing the material covered, enriched with additional methodologic issues or substantive information.

For students who are interested in methodology or have a strong background in physics, it might be useful to consider the evidence concerning the alleged carcinogenicity of extremely low frequency magnetic fields. In this area, the empirical evidence is conflicting but the methodologic issues are of particular interest because they emerge from efforts to distinguish between null effects distorted by chance, confounding, and bias, and weak effects attenuated by poor exposure ascertainment and latency mis-specification. A useful discussion of these methodologic issues, slightly colored by opposition to the hypothesis that magnetic fields are potentially carcinogenic, is given in a chapter of the Oak Ridge Associated Universities Report on the health effects of extremely low frequency magnetic fields (Trichopoulos, 1992).

For students with a strong background in biology it might be preferable to discuss the epidemiology of colorectal cancer because several epidemiologic findings are well documented and there is also an adequate understanding of the molecular events that underlie the natural history of this cancer. A useful reference is the relevant chapter in the book edited by Adami *et al.*(in press), or the corresponding chapter in the book edited by Shottenfeld and Fraumeni (1996).

Another alternative is to discuss the epidemiology of prostate cancer, a tumour about which little is known and for which study design issues are complicated by the expanding use of screening for prostate-specific antigen (PSA) and by the large fraction of cases in which the histologically indistinguishable disease tends to remain latent and subclinical. Another attractive topic is to discuss the interplay of environment and genes in the etiology of skin cancer, including melanoma.

Occupational cancer

The epidemiology of occupational cancer is a topic rich in substantive knowledge. Indeed, most established causes of cancer have been identified through epidemiologic studies done in settings where extremely high exposures have generated very high excess risks for specific forms of cancer. It is again better to devote most of the available time on methodologic issues and discuss only briefly the principal occupational carcinogens and their associated cancers, as indicated, for example, in Table 16.1.

Because situations leading to the documentation of a particular agent, mixture, or process as carcinogenic represent the outcome of tragic 'natural experiments', it is useful to compare genuine experimental studies in laboratory animals with observational studies involving humans and being harvested by occupational epidemiologists. The advantages of animal experiments are:

1. The detailed definition of exposure and of possibly interacting factors.

2. The careful establishment of outcome.

3. The free use of randomization without methodologic or ethical constraints.

4. The exploitation of animal inbreeding that tends to produce animals that are genetically similar and thus have a smaller variability that, in turn, leads to smaller standard errors in the various estimates.

Against these advantages animal experiments also have considerable disadvantages. Because the animal populations cannot be very large, exposures have to be unrealistically high, further complicating the already substantial biologic barriers for interspecies extrapolations.

Most studies of occupational epidemiology are by definition relevant to humans, except when working conditions have changed so rapidly and so substantially as to make the results of the occupational epidemiologic studies irrelevant. However, occupational epidemiologic studies are not as straightforward as they are generally thought to be for various reasons:

1. Occupations appear and disappear, work tasks change and are often not comparable over time or between countries, and there may be questionable correspondence between occupational titles and actual exposures.

2. It is difficult to know whether short-term peaks or time-weighted averages are more important.

3. There may be limited comparability between exposed and non-exposed individuals, particularly when an outside population is used for the calculation of expected cases.

4. Outcome data may be of questionable quality or limited to death certificates.

5. Information on confounders, except gender and age, is usually missing.

6. Actual measurements of the exposures under consideration are rarely available so that duration of exposure is used as a proxy for exposure quantification. In this instance, however, time is counted in two different ways, one for estimating cumulative exposure level and another for estimating the total person time at risk.

Given the complexity of these issues and the considerable obstacles in undertaking a sound epidemiologic study it may be surprising that occupational epidemiologic studies have been so successful. This is for two reasons: first, the effect estimate (e.g. relative risk) is so high as to override any concern about confounding and bias, and, second, the carcinogenic effect is so specific as to leave very little doubt about the underlying validity (e.g. the causation of mesothelioma after asbestos exposure is very difficult to explain in terms of confounding and bias). Several other methodologic issues need to be addressed even in a medium level course. The student should understand that retrospective cohort studies with internal or external comparison groups are the only realistic option for the calculation of relative risk, unless an exposure, however rare in the general population, dominates the histories of patients with a particular tumour (e.g. again, history of asbestos exposure among patients with mesothelioma). Students should also be warned that confounders can rarely generate confounded rate ratios of more than 50% and that confounding can also be assessed through sensitivity analyses or with external data.

Occupational epidemiology provides the best context for learning the applicability and the interpretability of exposed attributable rates (or risks) and for understanding the legal implications of an exposed attributable rate higher than 2 (it is more likely than not that a particular exposure was the cause of the relevant outcome in an exposed person). The student should also recognize that although rate ratios and exposed attributable rates (or risks) can be estimated in retrospective cohorts, this design can rarely generate population attributable rates (or risks), because the latter effect parameter requires an unbiased estimate of the exposure prevalence and the average rate ratio (relative risk) in the corresponding population. These issues are considered in the dated but still relevant report by Doll and Peto (1981).

The issue of the proportion of cancer cases in a population that can be attributed to occupational exposure has been estimated in developed countries to be about 5%. It may be smaller, however, because conditions in the workplace improve over time in

most countries. It may also be higher if occupational carcinogens have not been identified because the hazard has been unsuspected, the rate ratio (or relative risk) is
small, there are few exposed individuals in relevant working places, and the latency of
the particular cancer is long. Little is known about occupational cancers in the developing countries.

The epidemiology of occupational carcinogenesis is a complex topic, mainly
because time is considered in several dimensions (person–time at risk, proxy for
cumulative exposure, latency indicator, etc.) but also because the quality of data is
rarely satisfactory. The students should realize that relative risks below 1.5, when generated from inherently poor studies, can rarely be interpreted with confidence. They
should also realize that, whenever they accept an unsubstantiated elevated risk at face
value because workers should have the benefit of the doubt, they may actually harm
them by failing to identify the true cause of the excess risk.

A helpful source of information for the prospective teacher is the relevant chapter
in the textbook by Schottenfeld and Fraumeni (1996).

Screening for cancer

Whatever the duration and the content of a cancer epidemiology course, it is proper
to conclude it with the principles of screening. Screening is an unusual process in that
philosophically it belongs to prevention and methodologically it relies on epidemiology, but it cannot be implemented without some form of effective intervention which
has the hallmarks of therapeutic activity. Screening is in the epicentre of all secondary
prevention activities although, when screening is focused on risk factors, it may also
be thought of as a primary prevention process. Screening activity has been defined as
the presumptive identification among healthy people, with simple means, of those
who are likely to be diseased. The screening activity should not be confused with the
screening test, which is simply a test that is applied without clinical indication.
Screening activity should also be distinguished from the timely recognition of cancer
symptoms or signs, which is a manifestation of good clinical practice and has as an
objective the recognition of cancer at an earlier but already clinical stage. Application
of screening tests in a hospital population is generally considered as 'case finding'
because the population is not strictly speaking healthy.

The philosophy of screening can be operationalized by invoking the 'concept' of the
critical point. The critical point is that point in the natural history of cancer beyond
which the disease becomes essentially uncontrolable; for example, because metastases
have taken root. If the critical point is beyond the clinical time of diagnosis, there is
no scope for screening because the disease can be effectively treated even after the
appearance of clinical disease, e.g. non-melanoma skin cancer. Screening is also
pointless when the critical point occurs before the screening generated diagnosis, as
for example, in screening for lung cancer or hepatocellular carcinoma. In contrast,
screening is valuable when clinical diagnosis occurs after the critical point, whereas
screening diagnosis may take place before that point. The latter situation exists for
screening of colorectal, cervical, and breast cancer. Indeed, in about 25% of breast
cancer cases, the critical point lies between the point of clinical diagnosis and the

point of screening diagnosis, so that one-quarter of women may be prevented from dying from breast cancer with proper application of screening procedures.

Application of screening requires some conditions that are linked to the disease under consideration, some conditions that are linked to the available screening test, and some conditions that refer to the overall organization of the screening program. Conditions that should be fulfilled by the disease are that the disease should be frequent, sufficiently serious, and have a detectable preclinical phase during which the critical point is frequently located. The screening test has to be simple, quick, inexpensive, safe, and acceptable by the population, and be characterized by high repeatability as well as high validity, the latter requiring high values of both sensitivity and specificity. Finally, a crucial program condition is that the detectable preclinical phase of the disease under consideration has a relatively high prevalence. This is because, for given values of sensitivity and specificity of a test, the prevalence of the detectable preclinical stage is a crucial determinant of the all-important predictive value of the test under the program conditions. Program conditions also include the compliance of the population, the availability of resources, a competitive cost-effectiveness ratio, and health consequences of false-positive and false-negative test results.

For the evaluation of a screening program there are several necessary *but not sufficient* criteria, including the yield of preclinical cases and prognostic indicators, such as the stage distribution and the fatality of the screening detected disease. Shifting the stage distribution to the left and reducing the fatality ratio of screening detected cancer cases are necessary but cannot in themselves document the effectiveness of a screening program. To establish this, the mortality rate from the disease under consideration needs to be reduced, because neither lead bias nor length bias, the two biases that compromise the prognostic indicators, can possibly affect mortality.

Only mortality rate is a valid outcome, but a valid design is also needed to generate a sound outcome. This requires randomization of the total population, because nonrandom distribution carries the risk of bias generated by the tendency of screening volunteers to have a favorable cancer stage distribution, quick response to disease warnings, and good compliance and independent classification of causes of mortality, blinded to the screening practice.

These days most students already have some knowledge of the principles underlying screening for cancer, so that the session on screening is, in terms of topic complexity, a decrescendo. It should be made clear to students, however, that screening is one of the most complex medicosocial undertakings and that those who want to specialize on the epidemiologic aspects of screening should be ready for major intellectual challenges.

For an introductory session of cancer screening one may wish to look at some early papers (Cole and Morrison, 1980), whereas recent, more extensive but still simple material can be found in the book of the late Alan Morrison (1992).

Assessing students' achievements

A series of multiple choice questions distributed to the students for self-evaluation after the fourth, sixth and eighth sessions, and subsequently discussed in class serves two purposes:

+ To allow students to evaluate their progress.

+ To repeat the material covered, to refresh knowledge, and facilitate understanding.

A subsample of these multiple choice questions, perhaps ten questions out of a total of between 60 and 100, may be given to the students during the final examination which may be oral or written. In the best case, students should have developed the skills to respond to these questions. In the worst case, they may have memorized the answers. In the end, it is up to the students to choose. The authors of this chapter do not believe in policing education, at least for graduate students.

References

Adami, H. O., Signorello, L. B., Trichopoulos, D. Towards an understanding of breast cancer etiology. *Semin Cancer Biol* 1998; **8**, 255–62.

Adami, H. O., Hunter, D., Trichopoulos, D. (eds). *A Textbook of Cancer Epidemiology.* Oxford University Press, New York, (in press).

Cole, P., Morrison, A. S. Basic issues in population screening for cancer. *J Natl Cancer Inst* 1980; **64**, 1263–72.

Doll, R., Peto, R. The causes of cancer: quantitative estimates of avoidable risks of cancer in the United States today. *J Natl Cancer Inst* 1981; **66**, 1191–308.

Hilakivi-Clarke, L., Clarke, R., Onojafe, I., Raygada, M., Cho, E., Lippman, M. A maternal diet high in n-6 polyunsaturated fats alters mammary gland development, puberty onset, and breast cancer risk among female rat offspring. *Proc Natl Acad Sci USA* 1997; **94**, 9372–7.

IARC. *Cancer Incidence in Five Continents,* Vol. VI. Edited by Parkin, D. M., Muir, C. S., Whelan, S. L., Gao, Y. T., Ferlay, J. and Powell, J. Vol 120, IARC, Lyon, 1992.

IARC. Hepatitis viruses. *IARC monographs on the evaluation of carcinogenic risks to humans.* Vol. 59, IARC, Lyon, 1994.

IARC. Schistosomes, liver flukes and *Helicobacter Pylori.IARC monographs on the evaluation of carcinogenic risks to humans.* Vol. 61, IARC, Lyon, 1994.

IARC. Alcohol drinking. *IARC monographs on the evaluation of carcinogenic risks to humans.* Vol. 44, IARC, Lyon, 1988.

Kelsey, J. L., Gammon, M. D., John, E. M. Reproductive and hormonal risk factors: reproductive factors and breast cancer. *Epidemiologic Reviews* 1993; **15**, 36–47.

Kuper, H., Tzonou, A., Kaklamani, E. *et al.* Hepatitis B and C viruses in the etiology of HCC; a study in Greece using third generation assays. *Cancer Causes Control* 2000; **11**, 171–5.

Landis, S. H., Murray, T., Bolden, S., Wingo, P. A. Global Cancer Statistics. *CA Cancer J. Clin.* 1999; **49**, 8–32.

Lawson, J. S., Field, A. S., Champion, S., Tran, D., Ishikura, H., Trichopoulos, D. Low oestrogen receptor –alpha-α expression in normal breast tissue underlies low breast cancer incidence in Japan. *Lancet* 1999; **354**, 1787–8

Morrison, A. S. *Screening in Chronic Diseases,* 2nd edn. Oxford University Press, New York, 1992.

Ruoslahti, E. How cancer spreads. *Scientific American* 1996; **275**, 72–7.

Russo, J., Rivera, R., Russo, I. H. Influence of age and parity on the development of the human breast. *Breast Cancer Res Treat* 1992; **23**, 211–18.

Schottenfeld, D., Fraumeni, J. F. (eds). *Cancer Epidemiology and Prevention.* Oxford University Press, New York, 1996.

Trichopoulos, D. Epidemiologic studies of cancer and extremely low-frequency electric and magnetic field exposures. In: *Health Effects of Extremely Low Frequency Magnetic Fields.* Oak Ridge Associated Universities, Washington D.C., 1992.

Trichopoulos, D. Risk of lung cancer from passive smoking. Principles and Practice of Oncology. *PPO Updates* 1994; **8**, 1–8.

Trichopoulos, D., Lipman, R. D. Mammary gland mass and breast cancer risk. *Epidemiology* 1992; **3**, 523–6.

Varmus, H., Weinberg, R. A. *Genes and the biology of cancer.* Scientific American Library. New York 1993.

Weinberg, R. A. How cancer arises. *Scientific American* 1996; **275**, 62–70.

Willett, W. C. *Nutritional Epidemiology,* 2nd edn. Oxford University Press, New York, 1998.

Willett, W. C., Trichopoulos, D. Summary of the evidence: nutrition and cancer. *Cancer Causes Control* 1996; **7**, 178–80.

World Cancer Research Fund and American Institute for Cancer Research. *Food, nutrition and prevention of cancer.* World Cancer Research Fund and American Institute for Cancer Research, Menasha, USA, 1997.

Chapter 17

A course in psychiatric epidemiology

Rebecca Fuhrer

Introduction

The present chapter is intended to serve as a guide for developing a course in psychiatric epidemiology; that is, epidemiologic methods applied to the study of psychiatric disorders rather than the epidemiology of specific psychiatric disorders. Methodologic issues particularly relevant for these pathologies are emphasized, leaving the delineation of the substantive content of different mental disorders to the instructor's interests and expertise. This course does not need to assume prior training in psychiatry or psychopathology, and can be oriented to students at different educational levels. It is expected that students enrolled in this type of course have an interest in public health or medicine or psychology.

Epidemiology of psychiatric disorders covers the same methods as epidemiology of other diseases, but it also has additional methodologic challenges that need to be made explicit from the outset[1]. These methods are relevant both at the design and analysis phases of epidemiologic research. References to epidemiologic studies of specific pathologies are included that are particularly illustrative of certain important methodologic points. The evolution of research in this application of epidemiology should be reviewed first, followed by methodologic issues that have been the focus of research in psychiatric epidemiology. These include measurement, i.e. case definition and case identification, psychometric properties, study design and samples, and theoretical models of environmental and genetic origins of psychopathology. Methodology can be taught in a general course, but should be reminded in the context of this area of application. The subject matter is best communicated in the context of small classes or seminar groups, where there is active teaching for approximately half the session, and then interactive exchange based on the taught material and critical analysis of well selected published work or case studies.

Psychiatric epidemiology has evolved rapidly in the second half of the 20th century. Earlier work in this field relied on data from mental health providers and facilities, and the limitations of these sources should be explained. Subsequent research endeavours, often community based, frequently defined psychopathology along a continuum from impairment to mental health[2,3]. The emphasis then shifted to rates of specific diagnoses in community-based samples using clinical diagnoses at first[4] and then structured interviewing methods with clinicians[5] and lay interviewers[6,7]. These various methodologies should be contrasted for the student to gain an understanding of the strengths and weaknesses of each approach. Furthermore, studies in children and adolescent samples have increased considerably[8].

While the number of researchers in psychiatric epidemiology has grown, the 'workforce' remains limited when compared to those working in the fields of cancer or cardiovascular diseases, despite the magnitude of the frequency of the disorders, their impact on quality of life, health services utilization, and economic burden. The level of epidemiologic literacy among psychiatrists varies and there are few training programs that are specifically oriented towards psychiatric epidemiology. However, the potential usefulness of this approach is often insufficiently addressed during clinical training and, if the students are primarily clinicians, the relevance of epidemiology to clinical practice needs to be discussed.

Teaching objectives

The course can be oriented towards two types of students. The first group would consist of students with a background and training in psychiatry, psychology or some other mental health specialty. For these students, the instructor would focus more on bringing the methodologic issues to bear on the analysis and interpretation of scientific reports. The students should come away from such a course with a sound ability to critically analyze study designs and instruments. Ideally, they should be able to design a study to respond to a specific hypothesis and be able to discuss the constraints that their study has to incorporate, as well as the resultant limitations of their findings. Although this group would be knowledgeable about psychiatric and psychological disorders, some emphasis should still be placed on diagnostic entities both in clinical and community-based samples, their validity, and measurement reliability[9,10].

The second group of students would consist of general epidemiology students, be they general medical students or established physicians or other students with public health interests. They would differ from the first group in that they would be lacking the expertise in the psychiatric disorders and therefore the instructor would wish to spend some additional time teaching the general notions of psychopathology, different theories of etiology, the symptomatic and diagnostic terminology, and treatment options and efficacy. The students would also need to learn about the prevalence and known risk factors for various mental disorders, in part so that they understood the magnitude and relative importance of this category of health problems. This type of course needs more sessions to meet its objectives, with the psychological and psychiatric content taught in a lecture format, complemented with the methodologic content as described above.

Teaching content

The general topics of epidemiology, methods, and analysis are covered elsewhere in this volume. Although students may come to such a course with no prior experience or knowledge of psychiatric disorders, the instructor should keep in mind that notions of mental health and mental illness are part of the general culture. Every one may think that they know what 'depression' is; however, this conception of depression will not necessarily be the same as depressive disorders that will be seen by clinicians or identified in epidemiologic studies. These general notions need to be discussed and used as a stepping stone to a scientific approach to the definition of pathology[11-14]. A course in psychiatric epidemiology would do well to include some discussion on a general definition of psychopathology as well as to topics covered in this chapter, such as case definition, measurement, and study design, that are important to the conception, execution, and interpretation of epidemiologic studies in psychiatry[1]. If the focus of the course is the epidemiology of psychiatric disorders, presentation of epidemiologic data should be reviewed while emphasizing the methodologic innovations and/or shortcomings that have contributed to that knowledge[15]. An introductory course would do well to include several different types of psychopathology. The following mental disorders, and associated references, provide good teaching material: psychotic disorders such as schizophrenia (which is relatively infrequent and stable in occurrence across cultures and time)[16,17], affective disorders such as depression (which is frequent and hypothesized to be increasing)[13], and has diverse etiologies, including genetic factors[18], and a developmental disorder such as autism for child psychiatry[19].

The issues raised in this chapter are not necessarily unique to psychiatry, but partially reflect the present state of knowledge about psychopathology and the concomitant problems of diagnosis and disease classification. For the most part, psychiatric epidemiologists work primarily on the identification of risk factors, a prerequisite to the determination of causal relationships. Once risk factors are identified, other scientific methods of enquiry, as well as epidemiology, can be employed to understand the specific mechanism(s) associated with the increased risk and thereby demonstrate whether a statistical relationship may be shown to be a true cause[20]. However, the instructor should also focus on the fact that knowledge about risk factors can be useful in and of itself, for planning of treatment facilities, and for preventive measures.

Measurement issues

For the students with knowledge and training in psychiatric disorders, the following can be covered by focusing more on the lack of consensus and issues of diagnostic reliability[13]. However, these points should be taught effectively, as most clinical psychiatrists and mental health providers believe that there is diagnostic agreement and are surprised to observe the contrary when studies demonstrating differences are presented. The instructor must emphasize that, without diagnostic consensus, all estimates and associations are erroneous at worst, or attenuated at best. Furthermore, it is important to differentiate diagnostic accuracy for clinical and treatment purposes, in contrast to research purposes[21].

Case definition

The *indices* that are usually employed in epidemiology, prevalence and incidence, are based on the assumption that every individual can be classified according to a dichotomous variable: *case* or not[11]. This implies that the boundary between the normal and the pathological can be distinguished with a sufficiently high level of accuracy. In psychiatry, the validity of the definitions used is more questionable than in other fields of medicine and reflects the limits of current theories of psychopathology. Unlike other branches of medicine, psychiatry presently has no external criteria that can be used to verify clinical judgements; a 'gold standard' does not exist. Thus, a definition of a disease or disorder can only be arrived at by consensus.

There are two types of approaches to classification of a case: one is the categorical approach and the other is the dimensional approach. The categorical approach defines psychopathology in a way that results in presumably discrete diagnostic entities. Important examples of the categorical approach are the manuals of disease classification. The most widely used system for classifying psychiatric disorders is the *International Classification of Diseases* 10th revision (ICD-10)[22]. Psychiatry is the only medical specialty for which a glossary exists that defines each diagnostic category, including guidelines for arriving at a diagnosis. This addition paralleled the American experience with the DSM system (*Diagnostic and statistical manual – mental disorders*, 3rd revised, 4th edition)[23], which is the classification and coding system used in the US. The instructor should stress the multiaxial classification system of the DSM that allows the clinician to evaluate and record information that may be of value in diagnosis, in planning treatment, and in predicting outcome. At present, in epidemiology little usage has been made of the axes that evaluate severity and psychosocial functioning.

The use of diagnostic criteria is important because it enhances diagnostic concordance, or reliability, a problem that has always been particularly acute in psychiatry. The advantages and drawbacks of these systems should be addressed and students must be reminded that the usefulness of the categorical approach to case definition in general population studies is uncertain, because the diagnostic nomenclatures were mostly developed from experience with populations that seek care, especially hospital and specialist care. Attention should be drawn to several papers that have evaluated the use of these definitions in community surveys, and have found discrepant findings between who is judged to be a 'psychiatric case'[24]. Such definitions may not be appropriate for individuals whose configuration of symptoms and signs may differ in terms of duration, co-occurrence, intensity, and impairment. The National Comorbidity Survey in the US attempted to resolve the case definition problem by allowing multiple diagnoses if the criteria were met[7]. They obtained high rates of disorders, both for individual disorders and for comorbidity. This could be interpreted as being accurate, or that there are multiple manifestations of the underlying constructs and that separating them into several pathologies is artificial.

The dimensional approach defines psychopathology in relative terms, i.e. an assessment of the degree of psychopathology or impairment on a continuum. Clinical status is assessed on a particular dimension of psychopathology, such as anxiety, depression, and so forth, or of general psychopathology or psychological well being. Based on symptom counts, sometimes combined with symptom severity, the addition of item scores calculates a value which varies along a continuum that taps the supposed construct of interest.

Case identification

Once a definition of a case has been established, the problem remains to identify or measure it in a heterogeneous group of individuals. To expose the student to the wide range of instruments available for identifying 'psychiatric cases', the instructor can use a volume edited by Thompson[25] that provides a comprehensive compendium of the many instruments that are available for psychiatric research, or Robins' summary of instruments for psychiatric epidemiology[26] or any of a number of psychology text-books and the National Institute of Mental Health (NIMH) website that refer to and archive instruments that use a dimensional approach.

The methodology of scale construction should be included in the program. It should be made clear to the student that clinical observation, theory on psychopathology, and prior research results, combined with consensual processes, lead to the identification and selection of items that are associated with the constructs under study. It is then preferable to use multivariate data analytic techniques to select empirically those signs and symptoms that cluster together best to represent a construct of psychopathology or diagnostic entity. Latent variable modeling methods are useful and pertinent to scale development, and the student should understand what these methods do.

It is of interest to introduce a historical perspective on the evolution and development of psychiatric instruments so that students can better comprehend how and why the instruments that are available now came into being[27,28]. The literature during the 1960s and 70s was replete with references to the lack of reliability in clinical judgement when using the categorical approach for case definition[9]. Studies have shown that diagnostic reliability among psychiatrists, even among those who are experienced and have the same theoretical orientations, was far from satisfactory. The reliability issue was aggravated when cross-national studies were carried out, as shown for adult schizophrenia[29] and for hyperkinetic syndromes in children[30].

Several sources of variance have been identified in the diagnostic process. Patients seen at different examinations may present with different clinical profiles and the symptomatic features are also likely to vary with the evolution of their disorders. Clinicians also vary in their methods of obtaining information about a subject, in their skills as interviewers, and as observers of the signs presented by a subject. Moreover, clinicians rely heavily on their personal rules and criteria in the way they use information, i.e. the interpretation of signs and symptoms, and the subsequent organization of these stimuli into a coherent construct or diagnostic category. A useful exercise would include viewing several clinical interviews, asking students to rate or code the responses and arrive at one, or multiple, diagnoses. The students could then compare and calculate diagnostic concordance[31]. A similar exercise could use computerized diagnostic interviews.

In their search for solutions to this problematic situation, psychiatric researchers have developed two complementary approaches. One approach is to design a structured method to obtain information about an individual. These structured interviews should result in comparable information for each subject. It should also be noted that interviews can be observer- or respondent-based, that is, either the interviewer judges the sign to be present or the respondent reports the presence or absence of the symptom. Another approach is to establish a set of rules and criteria that help the user arrive at a diagnosis in a consistent fashion. Then, by applying the rules or criteria to the obtained data, one should arrive at the same diagnosis regardless of the interviewer. Again, a historical perspective would be most useful at this point. For example, the Present State Examination (PSE)[32] and the Schedule for Affective Disorders and Schizophrenia (SADS)[33] are two early examples of structured interviews (interviewer-based) developed for use by clinicians with psychiatric experience, and now the Schedules for Clinical Assessment in Neuropsychiatry (SCAN)[34] appears to be its modern successor for epidemiologic studies.

The Diagnostic Interview Schedule (DIS)[35] was developed for use by lay interviewers in epidemiologic surveys, and is a respondent-based interview, i.e. the data collected is based on what is actually reported by the respondent. Algorithms and rules were developed to apply the diagnostic criteria to the data collected. Other instruments exist and continue to be improved. The Composite International Diagnostic Interview – Version 2.1 (CIDI)[36] is the culmination of many years of effort and represents the different clinical traditions because it combines elements of the DIS and the PSE, and can generate diagnoses based on either the ICD or the DSM traditions. The CIDI has been subjected to intense psychometric scrutiny and exists in many languages.

When the dimensional approach is used for defining pathology, case identification habitually entails the use of rating scales[37]. Scales can be used by trained observers or may be self-administered instruments. They are usually short, symptom checklists that assess a certain level of symptomatology along a given dimension, such as depression or anxiety. These types of measures should not be used to arrive at a diagnosis unless they were developed intentionally with that purpose in mind, which is rarely the case. They are usually intended as screening instruments or as methods to assess change in treatment evaluations. Rating scales may be used by psychiatrists or other clinical personnel within clinical settings based on the clinician's assessment of the items. Other rating scales, more appropriate to epidemiologic surveys, may be self-report, either completed by the subject or an interviewer, such as the General Health Questionnaire (GHQ)[38] or the Center for Epidemiologic Studies-depression scale (CES-D)[39].

The students should always be reminded that, when choosing an instrument, it is important to ascertain that it has been validated for the context in which its use is planned. Instruments developed for use with patients may be quite irrelevant when used in the general population, and the opposite situation may provide instruments that are completely uninformative when used to discriminate among patients. A set of symptoms observed in a clinical context may not signify the same underlying pathology in community samples. In fact, in both contexts, the constellation may represent valid underlying entities, albeit not the same.

Psychometric issues

The development and use of measures of psychopathology is the subject of numerous books and articles, and it merits detailed discussion. Key psychometric concepts should be clarified. Students might be referred to the work of Nunnally[40] as a classic text and guide to other material. There are two basic issues to be addressed in the development of any measure, be it physical or psychological: reliability and validity. Measurement error affects both the estimates of incidence and prevalence, and will attenuate or inflate the association between a risk factor and the disorder. Therefore, the link between measurement error and risk assessment should be explained and the sources of measurement error, their correction, and control should be stressed.

Errors in the data collected may be a consequence of poor reliability and/or inadequate validity of the instruments used. Emphasis should therefore be placed on the necessity to assess these properties in all measures used in a study. Reliability, which refers to the reproducibility or repeatability of measurement, is concerned mainly with chance or random errors due to the observers, the situations, and the instruments. Different ways of assessing reliability should be introduced. Some basic approaches include: interrater reliability, intrarater reliability, test–retest reliability, split-half method, and internal consistency. Statistical techniques appropriate for analysing this type of data should be taught: Cronbach's alpha, a cumulative item correlation index, for measuring internal consistency[40], the Kappa coefficient as an index of agreement for categorical data[31,41], and the intraclass correlation coefficient for continuous variables[41] are three important examples. Multiple measures of the same constructs help to reduce measurement error, though it can increase respondent burden.

Reliability is a necessary but not a sufficient condition for most forms of validity, and its assessment should be an integral part of all empirical studies. Validity refers to the extent to which an instrument in fact measures what it is intended to measure, and is a function of systematic error. The different types of validity should be presented and emphasis should be placed on the relative importance of each type in view of a study's objective. Validation efforts should include construct validity, face validity, content validity, and criterion validity[40]. Content validity refers to the appropriate selection of items from the universe of all observable characteristics of the same latent trait to be included in an instrument.

Criterion validity may be concurrent or predictive, and only the temporal availability of the criterion (present or future) differentiates the two. In psychiatry, criterion validity is usually evaluated in comparison with an 'expert' judgement or a previously validated instrument. Construct validity refers to the relationship between variables that are measured and the particular trait that they are supposed to tap. Because it links empirical indicators to abstract or theoretical concepts, this type of validity is more difficult to measure. The multimethod, multitrait matrix was one of the first empirical approaches to assess construct validity, and may serve as a basis to study this issue[42]. Factor analysis and other multivariate techniques, such as cluster analysis, multidimensional scaling, etc. are central to all types of validity, and their contribution to assessing construct validity should be emphasized. Refinements of statistical techniques proposed four decades ago[43], that is the use of latent trait models[44], have improved instruments in psychiatric epidemiology[45–48].

Given the reality that few tests are perfect, one needs to determine the instrument's sensitivity and specificity, and their correlates, the positive and negative predictive value. Students should be reminded of the effect that the prevalence of a disorder has on the predictive values, as well as on the 'true disease' classification. The determination of the aforementioned attributes of any test is discussed in great detail in chapter 19.

Study design

Measures of disease frequency

Some of the problems inherent in the definition and identification of psychiatric cases have already been addressed. The problems of disease onset, duration, relapse, and recurrence are central to the estimation of point prevalence, period prevalence, and incidence rates. Because of the difficulties intrinsic to the assessment of the incidence of psychiatric disorders, for example, identifying the moment of onset and duration, the notion of period and lifetime prevalence have been employed. Lifetime prevalence is the proportion of individuals in the population that have ever been ill and are alive on a given day. It differs from lifetime risk, which attempts to measure the occurrence of a disease in a birth cohort. Both of these indicators rely heavily on retrospective assessment of disease occurrence, which is far from reliable and produces biased estimates of disease rates and risk ratios. Despite the most recent and sophisticated efforts to design appropriate techniques and instruments, the resulting estimates are probably biased recall problems. The importance of information and recall bias, and their effects on risk assessment, should be discussed in detail.

Design

The different types of study design, such as the case control study, the cross-sectional study, or the cohort study, can all be and have been used in psychiatric research. Twin studies, adoption studies, and cross-rearing studies can be thought of as special cases of the aforementioned designs. These designs are one way of studying genetic factors, but so are family pedigree studies[49,50]. Molecular genetics now provides tools for assessing candidate genes, though the likelihood of identifying single genes for such complex disorders remains doubtful.

Numerous studies have used twin and adoption designs, especially in countries that have good case registers and the possibility of linking datasets, such as adoption files in the Scandinavian countries. The choice of a given design depends upon the objective of the study, the rarity of the disease and the putative cause, and the resources available. However, each design introduces the potential for different types of bias, some of which are particularly thorny in psychiatry, and different problems for the interpretation of the study result. The usual form of the case control study for risk factor research is used infrequently in psychiatry, particularly because of the issue of recall bias. Denial, repression, negation, screen memories, and rationalization are common defense and coping mechanisms which impede the storage and retrieval of past events in one's psychological life. Reciprocally, individuals who have had personal or familial experience with a mental disorder are often involved in a continuous search for explanatory causes. This factor, combined with persistent feelings of guilt, is likely to influence recall falsely and identification of causes. Among many examples of the extent of this phenomenon, one may cite Stott's comparative study, which showed an increased rate of stressful events during pregnancy, suggesting a psychological etiology to Down's syndrome[51].

Samples

Early studies of mental disorders used samples of people treated in psychiatric facilities, in particular those admitted to mental hospitals. This raised the issue of two potential sources of bias. First, the types of pathology seen were more likely to be severe cases of psychotic disorders. Second, the characteristics associated with health-care seeking behaviour (sex, urbanicity, social class, culture, etc.) were often the variables under study rather than those associated with the pathology. The weight of cultural factors in illness recognition and care should be emphasized within a given country and sociocultural context. These factors vary considerably from one country to another, thereby making cross-cultural comparisons or study replications more difficult. Nevertheless, these facility-based samples may be appropriate, especially for the study of the rarer disorders, such as schizophrenia, or other psychosis, or autism[16].

Choosing community samples is an alternative sampling strategy. The third generation studies from the 1980s onwards have been carried out on community samples and have used representative samples of the general population in a country, city, region or country, thereby excluding individuals residing in institutional settings, or they have used complete populations such as the Isle of Wight studies[8], which were conducted on children within a given age range, or the Stirling County study[5]. The epidemiologic catchment area (ECA)[6] studies carried out in five areas in the US included institutionalized and general population samples, and oversampled certain groups considered at higher risk for psychiatric disorders. Several reviews of psychiatric epidemiology studies and their designs are included in the bibliography and, again, a historical perspective can provide insight for the students[52]. As for all types of epidemiologic studies, the sample size is determined by the frequency of the pathology or the risk factor, or the expected impact of an intervention in an evaluation study. It should be emphasized to the students that the study design has potential effects on the estimates of the rates, and especially on the estimates of the variance. The importance of incorporating sampling weights to adjust for the design effects should be stressed. Even a short course ought to include an overview of these correction factors and the errors that can occur if they are overlooked[53].

Psychiatric case registers can also be a source of data for epidemiologic studies[54]. Their contribution to research and evaluation studies must be differentiated. The comprehensiveness of the geographical population and facilities covered should be discussed in view of the cost of registers. The reliability and validity of the diagnostic and associated data collected on a routine basis need to be examined for the student to gain a critical understanding of where and when this data source has and can contribute to the description of the occurrence of certain disorders. The student must be made aware of the requisite minimum size of the population covered to detect sufficient numbers of the rarer disorders, and the potential for underestimations or biased associations if the inclusion of providers is not comprehensive. They should understand that the utility of registers is clearly linked to the organization of healthcare services and the type of reimbursement mechanism, and their existence is dependent on the local or national laws on computer files and data linkage. Discussion could address the type of questions that case register data can be used to answer, and the type of questions for which that data source would be inadequate. Case registers could be used in conjunction with some of the usual study designs, and this too should be elaborated for the students, while reminding them of the limitations.

Assessing students' achievements

The material taught in this type of course is best evaluated with coursework, such as requiring the students to write a mini-proposal, or to review a manuscript that would be submitted to a journal that publishes psychiatric epidemiology articles, or designing a study to assess validity or reliability of an instrument. Short examinations cannot glean the understanding that one hopes the student will have acquired.

Conclusion

This chapter has focused on the important methodological aspects to be covered in a course in psychiatric epidemiology. The orientation has been historical, so that students can learn about what has been done in the past and how to progress and improve in the future. In addition, the methodological challenges that are more acute in this specific branch of epidemiology have been highlighted for the instructor, as the general topics are discussed by other authors in the book. Psychiatric disorders, in fact, cover a wide spectrum of pathologies of diverse origins and different degrees of functional impairment. The instructor will choose the specific pathologies to make his or her methodological points. Clearly, the breadth of ill-health spanned by psychiatry and psychology cannot be covered in one epidemiology course, although many of the important research issues can be addressed.

Etiologic research of psychiatric disorders has always battled over the 'nature *versus* nurture' dilemma. Adoption and twin studies have been used to disentangle the dilemma, but results have often been difficult to interpret. Recent advances in genetic epidemiology and molecular biology using linkage analysis, segregation analysis, and the study of large pedigrees are promising and tend to support the multifactorial etiologic models of psychiatric disorders. Epidemiologic research protocols in biological psychiatry should improve the present situation of that discipline.

To date, epidemiologic research in psychiatry has helped to identify factors associated with certain disorders and has contributed to improving diagnostic reliability and validity. Future research endeavours need to incorporate multidisciplinary approaches, including biological markers, social risk, and protective factors. The contributions of developmental psychology and sociology to the understanding of social support as well as to chronic and acute stress, as factors in the occurrence of illness, psychological and physical, need to be understood and encouraged. Research on the etiology of specific disorders will only progress once hypotheses and models of the causal and mediating factors, their relationships to the disorder and to each other are made explicit, tested, and rejected or not. Elaborating such causal relationships, designing the appropriate studies, and employing the proper analytic procedures, should be the goal of the next generation of research in psychiatric epidemiology.

References

1. Tsuang, M. T., Tohen, M., Zahner, G. E. P. (1995) *Textbook in psychiatric epidemiology*. New York: Wiley-Liss.

2. Hollingshead, A. B., Redlich, F. C. (1958) *Social class and mental illness*. New York: Wiley.

3. Srole, L., Langner, T. S., Michael, S. T., Opler, M. D., Rennie, T. C. (1962) *Mental health in the metropolis: the midtown Manhattan study* vol. I. New York: McGrawHill.

4. Hagnell, O. (1966) *A prospective study of the incidence of mental disorders. The Lundby report*. Stockholm: Svenske Bokforlaget, Norstedts.

5. Leighton, D. C., Harding, J. S., Macklin, D. B., Hughes, C. C., Leighton, A. H. (1963) Psychiatric findings of the Stirling Country study. *American Journal of Psychiatry* **119**, 1021–6.

6. Eaton, W. W., Kessler, L. G. (ed.) (1985) *Epidemiologic field methods in psychiatry: the NIMH epidemiologic catchment area program*. London: Academic Press.

7. Kessler, R. C., McGonagle, K. A., Zhao, S. *et al.* (1994) Lifetime and 12-month prevalence of DSM-III-R psychiatric disorders in the United States: Results from the National Comorbidity Survey. *Archives of General Psychiatry* **51**, 8–19.

8. Rutter, M. (ed.) (1988) *Studies of psychosocial risk. The power of longitudinal data*. Cambridge: Cambridge University Press.

9. Spitzer, R. L., Fleiss, J. L. (1974) A reanalysis of the reliability of psychiatric diagnosis. *British Journal of Psychiatry* **125**, 341–7.

10. Wing, J. K., Bebbington, P., Robins, L. N. (1981) *What is a case? The problem of definition in psychiatric community surveys*. London: Grant McIntyre.

11. Copeland, J. R. M. (1981) What is a 'case'? A 'case' for what? In: Wing, J. K., Bebbington, P., Robins, L. N., eds. *What is a case: the problem of definition in psychiatric community surveys*. London: Grant McIntyre.

12. Dohrenwend, B. P. (1990) The problem of validity in field studies of psychological disorders revisited. *Psychological Medicine* **20**, 195–208.

13. Hirschfeld, R. M. (1994) Major depression, dysthymia and depressive personality disorder. *British Journal of Psychiatry* (**Suppl. 26**), 23–30.

14. Wittchen, H.-U., Ustun, T. B., Kessler, R. C. (1999) Diagnosing mental disorders in the community. A difference that matters. *Psychological Medicine* **29**, 1021–7.

15. Robins, L. N., Regier, D. A. (1991) *Psychiatric disorders in America*. New York: The Free Press.

16. Sartorius, N., Jablensky, A., Korten, A. *et al.* (1986) Early manifestations and first-contact incidence of schizophrenia in different cultures: a preliminary report on the initial evaluation of the WHO collaborative study on determinants of outcome of severe mental disorders. *Psychological Medicine* **16**, 909–28.

17. Tsuang, M., Simpson, J. (1988) *Nosology, epidemiology and genetics of schizophrenia*, vol. 3: Amsterdam: Elsevier.

18. Horwath, E., Weissman, M. M. (1995) Epidemiology of depression and anxiety disorders. In: Tsuang, M. T., Tohen, M., Zahner, G. E. P., eds. *Textbook in psychiatric epidemiology*, New York: Wiley-Liss.

19. **Fombonne, E.** (1999) The epidemiology of autism: a review. *Psychological Medicine* **29**, 769–86.

20. **Robins, L. N.** (1978) Psychiatric epidemiology. *Archives of General Psychiatry* **36**, 697–702.

21. **Regier, D. A., Kaelber, C. T., Rae, D. S.** *et al.* (1998) Limitations of diagnostic criteria and assessment instruments for mental disorders: implications for research and policy. *Archives of General Psychiatry* **55**, 109–15.

22. World Health Organization (1993) *The ICD-10 Classification of Mental and Behavioural Disorders – Diagnostic Criteria for Research.* Geneva: WHO.

23. American Psychiatric Association. (1994) *Diagnostic and Statistical Manual of Mental Disorders (4ᵗʰ Edition) (DSM-IV).* Washington, DC: APA.

24. **Brugha, T. S., Bebbington, P. E., Jenkins, R.** *et al.* (1999) Cross validation of a general population survey diagnostic interview: A comparison of the CIS-R with SCAN ICD-10 diagnostic categories. *Psychological Medicine* **29**, 1029–42.

25. **Thompson, C.** (1989) *The instruments of psychiatric research.* Chichester: John Wiley.

26. **Robins, L. N.** (1995) How to choose among riches: selecting a diagnostic instrument. In: Tsuang, M. T, Tohen, M., Zahner, G. E. P., eds. *Textbook in psychiatric epidemiology*, New York: Wiley-Liss.

27. **Kessler, R. C.** (2000) Psychiatric epidemiology: selected recent advances and future directions. *Bulletin of the World Health Organization* **78**, 464–74.

28. **Eaton, W. W., Merikangas, K. R.** (2000) Psychiatric epidemiology: progress and prospects in the year 2000. *Epidemiologic Reviews* **22**, 29–34.

29. **Cooper, I. E., Kendell, R. E., Gurland, B. J., Sharpe, L., Copeland, J. R. M., Simon, R.** (1972) *Psychiatric diagnosis in New York and London. (US-UK diagnostic project).* Oxford: Oxford University Press.

30. **Prendergast, M., Taylor, E., Rapoport, J. L.** *et al.* (1988) The diagnosis of childhood hyperactivity: a US–UK cross national study of DSM-III and ICD-9. *Journal of Child Psychology and Psychiatry* **29**, 289–300.

31. **Cohen, J.** (1960) A coefficient of agreement for nominal scales. *Educational and Psychological Measurement* **20**, 37–46.

32. **Wing, J. K., Cooper, J. E., Sartorius, N.** (1974) *The measurement and classification of psychiatric symptoms.* Cambridge:Cambridge University Press.

33. **Spitzer, R. L., Endicott, J.** (1978) *NIMH clinical research branch collaborative program on the psychobiology of depression. Schedule for affective disorders and schizophrenia, lifetime version*, (3rd edn). New York: New York State Psychiatric Institute.

34. World Health Organization. (1993) *SCAN: Schedules for Clinical Assessment in Neuropsychiatry*, Version 2.0. Geneva: Psychiatric Publishers International.

35. **Robins, L. N., Helzer, J. E., Croughan, J., Ratcliff, K. S.** (1981) National Institute of Mental Health Diagnostic Interview Schedule: its history, characteristics and validity. *Archives of General Psychiatry* **38**, 381–9.

36. World Health Organisation. (1997) *The Composite International Diagnostic Interview (CIDI)*, Version 2.1. Geneva: WHO.

37. **Murphy, J. M.** (1995) Diagnostic schedules and rating scales in adult psychiatry. In: Tsuang, M. T., Tohen, M., Zahner, G. E. P, eds. *Textbook in psychiatric epidemiology*, New York: Wiley-Liss.

38. **Goldberg, D. P.** (1978) *Manual of the general health questionnaire (GHQ).* NFER-Nelson, Windsor.

39. **Radloff, L. S.** (1977) The CES-D Scale: a self-report depression scale for research in the general population. *Applied Psychological Measurement* **1**, 385–401.

40. **Nunnally, J. C., Bernstein, I. H.** (1994) *Psychometric Theory*. 3rd edn. New York: McGraw Hill Higher Education.

41. **Fleiss, J. L.** (1981) *Statistical methods for rates and proportions*, 2nd edn. New York: John Wiley & Sons.

42. **Campbell, D. T., Fiske, D. W.** (1959) Convergent and discriminant validation by the multi-method-multi-trait matrix. *Psychological Bulletin* **56**, 81–105.

43. **Rasch, G.** (1960) *Probabilistic models for some intelligence and attainment tests*. Copenhagen: Danish Institute of Educational Research.

44. **McCutcheon, A. L.** (1987) *Latent class analysis*. Sage University Paper series on Quantitative. Applications in the Social Sciences, 07-001. Beverly Hills: Sage Publications.

45. **Duncan-Jones, P. P., Grayson, D. A., Moran, P. A. P.** (1986) The utility of latent trait models in psychiatric epidemiology. *Psychological Medicine* **16**, 391–405.

46. **Bentler, P. M., Stein, J. A.** (1992) Structural equation models in medical research. *Statistical Methods in Medical Research* **1**, 158–81.

47. **Muthen, B. O.** (1996) Psychometric evaluation of diagnostic criteria: application to a two-dimensional model of alcohol abuse and dependence. *Drug and Alcohol Dependence* **41**, 101–12.

48. **Pickles, A.** (1998) Psychiatric epidemiology. *Statistical Methods in Medical Research* **7**, 235–51.

49. **Risch, N., Merikangas, K. R.** (1996) The future of genetic studies of complex human diseases. *Science* **273**, 1516–17.

50. **Sullivan, P. F., Neale, M. C., Kendler, K. S.** (2000) Genetic epidemiology of major depression. Review and meta-analysis. *American Journal of Psychiatry* **157**, 1552–62.

51. **Stott, D. H.** (1958) Some psychosomatic aspects of casualty in reproduction. *Journal of Psychosomatic Research* **3**, 42–55.

52. **Tohen, M., Bromet, E., Murphy, J. M., Tsuang, M. T.** (2000) Psychiatric epidemiology: review. *Harvard Review of Psychiatry* **8**, 111–25.

53. **Kessler, R. C., Little, R. J. A., Groves, R. M.** (1995) Advances in strategies for minimizing and adjusting for survey non-response. *Epidemiologic Reviews* **17**, 192–204.

54. **Ten Horn, G. H. M. M., Giel, R., Gulbinat, W., Henderson, J. H.** (1986) *Psychiatric case registers in public health. A world wide inventory 1960–1985*. Amsterdam: Elsevier.

Chapter 18

Neurologic diseases

C. A. Molgaard, L. M. Frazier, and A. L. Golbeck

Introduction

Neuroepidemiology has traditionally been defined as the study of the distribution and determinants of neurologic diseases and injuries, whether of a chronic (Alzheimer's disease, stroke), infectious ('mad cow disease', poliomyelitis), or toxic nature (Minamata's disease, lead poisoning). A number of textbooks in the area have been published in the last decade (Molgaard, 1993; Gorelick and Alter, 1994; Anderson and Schoenberg, 1991; Batchelor and Cudkowicz, 1999).

The teaching of this subfield of epidemiology is important because of the large public health burden neurologic diseases and injuries represent at the population level. Its importance also lies in that neuroepidemiology spans a large range of medical, social, botanical, geographic, and behavioral sciences. The result has been the sharing of interests and concepts across disciplinary boundaries in the common language of epidemiology, and the elucidation of new notions of disease risk and disease progression.

The classic example of the latter in neuroepidemiology is the work of Carleton Gadjusek beginning in the late 1950s on a disease called Kuru found among the Fore tribe of the New Guinea highlands. For his elucidation of the mechanisms for the origin and dissemination of a neurologic disease caused by a slow virus, Gadjusek received the Nobel Prize in Medicine in 1976. His research was unique in that it integrated anthropology, neurology, epidemiology, genetics, and statistics in solving a highly different type of neurologic disease outbreak (Molgaard, 1981).

Research and teaching models of neuroepidemiology have changed through time. Historically, the paradigm has been a population laboratory approach to neurologic diseases and injuries that emphasized the etiologic importance of geographic isolates. A geographic isolate is defined as a population that may be inbred, remote, isolated or otherwise distinct, and is of interest because a high incidence of a new disease or a high prevalence of a common disease in such a population may reveal etiologic clues that would otherwise be obscure (Kurland, 1978; Kurtzke and Hyllested, 1979). This paradigm originally came out of the field of geographic pathology. Other specific research foci then evolved within this context (Table 18.1). These included:

Table 18.1 Current model of neuroepidemiology used in teaching and research

Disease surveillance emphasized	Geographic isolates used to elucidate etiology
Methodologic in orientation	Individual and social risk factors used to describe disease patterns
'Slow' virus and 'slow' toxin models of exposure accepted	Collaboration across disciplines

+ Population surveillance: this involves tracing trends in neurologic diseases and injuries; for example, development of stroke registries for defined populations (Rothrock *et al.*, 1993).

+ Development of improved research methodologies: an example would be refining and validating research instruments to screen populations for Alzheimer's disease (Hough *et al.*, 1993; Prince, 1998), or the use of population-based records linkage systems, such as that of the Mayo Clinic, to study neurologic disease (Kurland and Molgaard, 1981).

+ Social and behavioral applications: research is oriented to individual and group risk factors for neurologic injury and disease. An example would be studies of the association of tobacco use by individuals and increased risk for stroke (Parra-Medina *et al.*, 1993), or a higher level of occupational exposures among low-income parents and increased risk of birth defects (Frazier and Hage, 1998).

+ International applications: an example would be research on the global patterns of neurologic disease and injury of such illnesses as multiple sclerosis, with its highly characteristic north–south gradient of higher to lower incidence (Kurtzke *et al.*, 1993; Kurtzke, 2000), or of the current controversies surrounding beef consumption and Creutzfeldt–Jacob disease (CJD) in Great Britain and other countries of western Europe (Molgaard and Golbeck, 1992; Pollack, 1999).

However, this paradigm is changing (Goldman and Kodura, 2000; Tilson, 2000). There have been major theoretical advances and the addition of new exploratory concepts from environmental health and toxicology that deserve attention in a class on neuroepidemiology, or in a segment on neurologic diseases that is a part of a general class on epidemiology (Table 18.2). Most of these concepts relate to the programming hypothesis, which holds that critical windows of exposure exist for children in terms of developmental toxicants, and that these early exposures can lead to late neurodegenerative effects.

Many etiologic exposures are now understood to be *in utero*, involving both acute and delayed effects, and exhibiting both structural and functional defects (Adams *et al.*, 2000). In essence, the relationship between environmental exposures and structural and neurobehavioral effects has become more complicated, more common, and much earlier than previously suspected (Frazier and Molgaard, 2000).

Teaching objectives

The overall teaching goal of this orientation to neuroepidemiology is to create an understanding of the complexity of the issue of exposure. Environmental exposures not only

Table 18.2 Emerging model of neuroepidemiology used in teaching and research

- Disease surveillance still a priority, but based on Internet (e.g. ProMed) as well as government reporting and surveys.
- Increased methodologic orientation to genetics, nutrition, and developmental neurotoxicity than in the past.
- Geographic isolates of less importance.
- Individual and social risk factors more clearly related to major theories of psychology, sociology, and anthropology, as well as behavioral toxicology.
- Collaboration across disciplines
- 'Slow' models of exposure extended to *in utero* and postnatal periods.
- 'Chain of causation' requires evaluation of new theories, including current animal models relating to critical periods of environmental exposures *in utero* and during development.

may be very slow, but they may be very early in the lifespan and deeply modified in impact by the genome. A good analogy comes from cardiovascular disease, where intrauterine growth restriction and low birth weight are known to be associated with a higher risk for hypertension, coronary artery disease, and diabetes in adult life (Osmond and Barker, 2000). Practically, this means that the student needs to gain an appreciation for the fact that each particular type of defect is associated with a specific window of vulnerability, and that developmental toxicants can include true teratogens, embryotoxins, and fetotoxins as they apply to neurologic structure and process (Adams *et al.*, 2000).

Learning objectives

For practical classroom purposes, it is important to emphasize key concepts of programming with specific human diseases as well as animal models. While it is clear that extrapolating from animal data to humans is often fraught with peril, it also often provides a means of thinking in new ways about exposure and outcome that can be highly stimulating. In essence, the teacher needs to achieve buy-in from students on the following research strategy:

Learning objective 1 – A good neuroepidemiologic research strategy is team-based and is devised from previous empirical research that is a combination of a) clinical, b) animal, and c) epidemiologic studies.

Accomplishing this buy-in can be difficult. However, there are multiple examples in the medical and public health literature that can drive the point home. One of the most useful approaches is to illustrate the learning objective with major public health victories that are clearcut. The eradication of smallpox, for example, is always good in general, while a more neuroepidemiologic example relates to polio and the development of the Salk and Sabin vaccines.

Learning objective 2 – Theoretical epidemiology needs to include models that are beyond mere statistical association, instead including a better understanding of molecular and cellular processes that underlie induction of disease and variable latency periods.

In neuroepidemiology, we may find a number of examples of this in terms of vulnerable periods in the development of the central nervous system (brain and spinal cord). The vulnerability of the CNS is dependent on two issues (Rice and Barone, 2000). First, does an agent or its active metabolite(s) reach the developing nervous system; second, what was the period of exposure? Here we are reaching an overlap with much of the work in molecular epidemiology from the early 1990s (Schulte and Perera, 1993). The difference is that our knowledge of the developing nervous system has improved to the point that there is recognition that, first, the developing nervous system is qualitatively different from its adult analogue and, second, that exposure before or after an organ develops is less perturbing in a system's sense than if exposure occurs during development of the organ *per se* (Rice and Barone, 2000).

> Learning objective 3 – Developmental neurotoxicity may have small effects on the individual, but if the impact occurs across an entire population as well as across the life span of individuals, the societal impact in terms of public health burden can be massive.

The cause of most neurodevelopmental disabilities – perhaps more than 75% – is unknown. Those that we do understand in terms of etiology to some extent include dyslexia, attention-deficit hyperactivity disorder, mental retardation, and autism. In terms of magnitude, approximately 3–8% of all births in the US (4 million babies a year) are affected by these disorders. Yet another one million children in the US still suffer from the effects of elevated blood lead levels with its attendant impact on neurobehavioral functioning and intellectual activity (Weiss and Landrigan, 2000).

Students need to come away from this course understanding that even a decrement in function that is within the normal range, if exposure is widespread in a society, can have an enormous impact. An example related to lead is loss of IQ. Even a small loss of perhaps five points in many lead-exposed individuals would shift the tails of the normal distribution dramatically – doubling the number of those with IQs below 70 who require greater educational and social resources from a society (Rice and Barone, 2000). There would also be a reduction of the numbers of those with high IQs (greater than 130). Considerable research has been carried out in this area by Murray (Murray, 1997). A historical example of this process that students might enjoy is the theory that one of the reasons for the decline and fall of the Roman Empire was the ubiquitous nature of lead in Roman drinking vessels and plates during the late empire, with social decay and lack of leadership being associated with widespread lead poisoning and intellectual impairment.

Teaching content, method, and format

Format depends to some extent on whether one is teaching an entire class on neuroepidemiology or a segment of a larger, introductory class. Our belief is that in teaching a specialty epidemiology, it works better to use a mixed lecture–seminar–student presentation mode, and that this mode then also applies to a module within a larger, introductory class.

The approach here is to lead off with several orienting lectures where the teaching goal and associated learning objectives are specified with multiple examples. The classic teacher's litany of, 'I am now going to tell you about x, I am now telling you about x, I have now told you about x,' is a basic principle of higher adult education that can be very useful at this point.

Content should be of two types. The first is to orient the student to a number of key concepts related to neurogenesis and programming, including neural proliferation, migration of recently proliferated cells, differentiation of neuroblasts to a terminal phenotype, synaptogenesis, gliogenesis, myelination, apoptosis, neurotransmitters, and neurotrophic signaling (Rice and Barone, 2000).

The second type of content should then relate to eight key questions relating to risk estimation in neuroepidemiology. These are:

1. In terms of vulnerability in the development of the nervous system, which time periods carry the greatest risk.

2. Are there cascades of developmental disorders in the nervous system.

3. Can critical windows of vulnerability suggest the most susceptible subgroups of children by geographic area, socioeconomic status, race, sex, or other demographic/social parameters.

4. What data gaps exist regarding the endpoints of an environmentally altered nervous system.

5. What are the best ways to examine exposure–response relationships and estimate exposures during critical periods of development.

6. What other exposures during development may interact with and alter exposures of concern.

7. How well do laboratory animal response data parallel human response data.

8. How can this type of data be used in risk assessment and public health (Adams *et al.*, 2000).

Having introduced these concepts, each student should then be assigned a specific area of neurogenesis (myelination, for example). The student then needs to research this area in terms of the scientific literature in neurology, epidemiology, and neurotoxicology for specific disease examples that are related to this aspect of development. Emphasis should be placed on both library and internet sources of information, and the student should be encouraged to use the world wide web to contact scientists directly who work in a given area and then ask questions that are relevant to the topic and the scientists' current ideas and research.

The research effort should end with a student presentation to the entire class of what was found. The presentation should try to follow the eight conceptual areas outlined by Adams *et al.* (2000) as closely as possible, but be specific to one disease. Following the presentation and discussion in a seminar-type style, the student should write a report summarizing his findings for the disease noted during the research effort, and include feedback from the rest of the class and the instructor regarding the one specific disease presented for discussion to the class.

If we return to the myelination example, a student might be encouraged to examine what we currently know about critical periods of myelin development and possible neurotoxic environmental hazards in terms of the unique north–south distribution of multiple sclerosis. We now know that myelination begins in the late prenatal period (around months five or six), and continues during the postnatal period for different systems up to the age of 10 years. We also know that, when people migrate, age at migration determines multiple sclerosis risk. Those who leave a high risk northern latitude after age 15 years take the higher risk for developing this disease with them to the low risk southern latitudes, and vice versa. Is the completion of myelination at age 10 years related to this unique risk factor profile? What environmental risk factors are suspect given the period of vulnerability for myelination and its pathologic involvement in multiple sclerosis?

During the seminar section of the class, the instructor should revisit the three key learning objectives repeatedly. Other topics, such as examining childhood development in contaminated urban and rural settings (Guillette, 2000), or discussing the impact of environmental agents (ethanol, barbiturates, etc.) in triggering massive apoptotic neurodegeneration during the last trimester of pregnancy and first several years after birth (Olney *et al.*, 2000), can be introduced at this time.

Summary

In this paper we have defined the field of neuroepidemiology, presented several examples of research paradigms used in this subfield of epidemiology, presented concepts from developmental neurotoxicology of relevance to teaching in this field, and offered suggestions for their integration into the teaching protocol used for a course in neuroepidemiology. The main epidemiologic emphasis for the teacher is the concept of programming as related to critical windows of exposure and vulnerability for the developing nervous system.

Within neuroepidemiology the standard research paradigm in the past has been one of focusing on neurodegenerative diseases as an adjunct of the normal ageing process. Seminal research during the 1950s and 1960s introduced the notion of slow viruses with extremely long latency periods between exposure and onset of neurodegenerative disease. This notion was extended to slow toxins, for example, in the case of Western Pacific ALS and the use of the cycad nut as a source of food and medicine among the Chamorro population on the island of Guam. The cycad nut is now believed to contain several neurotoxins responsible for this endemic pattern of disease on Guam.

Recent research in developmental neurotoxicity has further extended this concept of extremely long-term (often *in utero*) exposure and onset of neurodegenerative disease much later in adult life. Diseases such as Parkinson's disease, lead toxicity, methyl mercury toxicity, schizophrenia, dyslexia, epilepsy, and autism, as well as many others, are thought to be examples of this process. Two explanatory theories are posited. In the first, the development of a specific function in an organism normally occurs late, and the display of pathologic function is not obvious until that point in development is reached. In the second, developmental structural or functional damage is masked by neural plasticity so that effects are transient until much later during the lifespan (Rice and Barone, 2000).

The interaction with the processes of ageing with neurotoxic exposures is now thought to be a common event. In normal ageing, the brain loses cells in some regions, as well as suffering declines in neurotransmitters and repair mechanisms. Neurotoxic exposures of long latency can accelerate such events and increase functional disability. As populations in industrialized countries continue to age in the US, Canada, and Europe, the effect of such interaction may have significant economic and social impact on already overburdened public health systems. Research and teaching agendas in neuroepidemiology should also reflect these aspects of developmental neurotoxicity.

References

Adams, J., Barone, Jr., S., LaMantia, A. *et al.* (2000). Workshop to Identify Critical Windows of Exposure for Children's Health: Neurobehavioral Work Group Summary. *Environmental Health Perspectives*, 108 (Suppl. 3), 535–44.

Anderson, D. W. and Schoenberg, D. G. (1991). *Neuroepidemiology: a tribute to Bruce Schoenberg*, (ed. D. W. Anderson), CRC Press, Boca Raton.

Batchelor, T. and Cudkowicz, M. E. (1999). *Principles of neuroepidemiology*, (eds T. Batchelor, M. E. Cudkowicz), Butterworth–Heinemann, Boston.

Frazier, L. M. and Hage, M. L. (1998). *Reproductive Hazards of the Workplace.* Van Nostrand Reinhold, New York.

Frazier, L. M. and Molgaard, C. A. (2000). *Primer on Children's Diseases and Environmental Health,* in press. Environmental Protection Agency, Washington DC.

Goldman, L. R., and Kodura, S. (2000). Chemicals in the Environment and Development Toxicity to Children: A Public Health and Policy Perspective. *Environmental Health Perspectives*, 108 (Suppl. 3), 443–50.

Gorelick, P. B. and Alter, M. (1994). *Handbook of neuroepidemiology*, M. Dekker, New York.

Guillette, E. A. (2000). Examining Childhood Development in Contaminated Urban Settings. *Environmental Health Perspectives*, 108 (Suppl. 3), 389–93.

Hough, R. L., Kolody, B., and Du Bois, B. (1993). The Epidemiology of Alzheimer's Disease and Dementia among Hispanic Americans. In: *Neuroepidemilogy: theory and method*, (ed. C. A. Molgaard), pp. 352–65. Academic Press, San Diego.

Kurland, L. T. (1978). Geographic isolates: their role in neuroepidemiology. *Advances in Neurology*, **19**, 69–81.

Kurland, L. T. and Molgaard, C. A. (1981). The Patient Record in Epidemiology. *Scientific American*, **245**, 54–63.

Kurtzke, J. F. (2000). Multiple sclerosis in time and space-geographic clues to cause. *Journal of Neurovirology*, **6**, 134–40.

Kurtzke, J. F. and Hyllested, K. (1979). Multiple sclerosis in the Faroe Islands. I. Clinical and epidemiologic features. *Annals of Neurology*, **5**, 6–21.

Kurtzke, J. F., Hyllested, K., and Heltberg, A. (1993). Multiple Sclerosis in the Faroe Islands. In: *Neuroepidemiology: theory and method*, (ed. C. A. Molgaard), pp. 24–50. Academic Press, San Diego.

Molgaard, C. A. (1981). Review of Kuru: Early letters and field notes from the collection of D. Carleton Gajdusek, (eds J. Farquhar and D. Gajdusek), In: *Mayo Clinic Proceedings*, 56, 529–30. Raven Press, New York.

Molgaard, C. A. (1993). *Neuroepidemiology: theory and method*, Academic Press, San Diego.

Molgaard, C. A. and Golbeck, A. L. (1992). Mad cows and Englishmen: bovine spongiform encephalopathy (BSE). *Neuroepidemiology*, **9**, 285–6.

Murray, C. (1997). The Bell Curve. Quoted in Holden C. Random samples. *Science*, **276**, 1651.

Olney, J. W., Farber, N. B., Wozniak, D. F., Jevtovic-Todorovic, V., and Ikonomidou, C. (2000). Environmental Agents That Have the Potential to Trigger Massive Apoptotic Neurodegeneration in the Developing Brain. *Environmental Health Perspectives*, 108 (Suppl. 3), 383–8.

Osmond, C. and Barker, D. J. P. (2000). Fetal, Infant, and Childhood Growth Are Predictors of Coronary Heart Disease, Diabetes, and Hypertension in Adult Men and Women. *Environmental Health Perspectives*, 108 (Suppl. 3), 545–53.

Parra-Medina, D. M., Kenney, E., and Elder, J. P. (1993). Cerebrovascular Disease and Smoking. In: *Neuroepidemiology: theory and method*, (ed. C. A. Molgaard), pp. 166–78. Academic Press, San Diego.

Pollack, M. P. *PRO/AH>BSE – UK: Chronology*, http://www.healthnet.org/programs/promed.html. Accessed 14 July 1999.

Prince, M. (1998). Is Chronic Low-Level Lead Exposure in Early Life an Etiologic Factor in Alzheimer's Disease? *Epidemiology*, **9**, 618–21.

Rice, D. and Baron Jr, S. (2000). Critical Periods of Vulnerability for the Developing Nervous System: Evidence from Humans and Animal Models. *Environmental Health Perspectives*, 108 (Suppl. 3), 511–33.

Rothrock, J. F., Lyden, P. D. and Brody, M. L. (1993). The Utility of Stroke Data Banks in the Epidemiology of Cerebrovascular Diseases. In: *Neuroepidemiology: theory and method*, (ed. C. A. Molgaard), pp. 287–305. Academic Press, San Diego.

Schulte, P. A. and Perera, F. P. (1993). *Molecular Epidemiology Principles and Practices*, Academic Press, San Diego.

Tilson, H. A. (2000). New Horizons: Future Directions in Neurotoxicology. *Environmental Health Perspectives*, 108 (Suppl. 3), 439–42.

Weiss, B. and Landrigan, P. J. (2000). The Developing Brain and the Environment: An Introduction. In: *Environmental Health Perspectives*, (eds P. Landrigan, B. Weiss, L. Goldman, D. O. Carpenter, W. Suk). National Institutes of Health, National Institute of Environmental Health Sciences. 108 (Suppl. 3), 373–4.

Chapter 19

Clinical epidemiology

John A. Baron

Introduction

Although the term 'clinical epidemiology' has been interpreted in various ways, the core of the discipline has generally been accepted to be the application of epidemiologic and biostatistic techniques to clinical problems. In contrast to chronic disease epidemiology, which focuses on the discovery of the determinants of disease on a population level, clinical epidemiology aims to help clinicians conduct the daily work of caring for individual patients. Thus a typical clinical epidemiology course will consider medical measurement, research design, the interpretation of clinical tests, screening/prevention, and probably expected value decision analysis. Many of these elements are part of 'evidence-based medicine', which seeks to encourage 'the conscientious, explicit and judicious use of current best evidence in ... the care of individual patients, ... [by] integrating individual clinical expertise with the best available external clinical evidence from systematic research' (Sackett *et al.*, 1996; 1998). This practical goal of illuminating and aiding the practice of clinicians is a central theme of clinical epidemiology.

Teaching objectives

As in any quantitative course, the topics covered in a clinical epidemiology course will necessarily depend on the level and context in which it is taught. Some students will be clinicians seeking to better understand the medical literature or to improve their clinical practice; others will be investigators who want to develop skills for clinical research. Whatever the students' interests, the course should enable them to use the concepts of clinical epidemiology to help solve and understand clinical issues, and to understand the medical literature about those issues. A basic course should provide the students with an appreciation of the quantitative approaches that characterize clinical epidemiology, and include most of the following topics:

- Basic concepts of probability and statistics as they apply to clinical problems.
- Basic aspects of medical measurement, the sources of variation in medical measurements, and the consequences of that variability.
- The basic principles of prognosis, including survival analysis.
- Basic research design, including the strengths and weaknesses of various designs, and the concepts of bias and confounding.

- The interpretation of clinical tests.
- The rationale, structure, and interpretation of expected value decision trees.
- Quantitative aspects of screening and prevention.

More advanced topics include:

- The use of basic statistical techniques and the understanding of more advanced statistical concepts.
- The construction and validation of clinical scales and prediction rules.
- Research regarding clinical test measurements.
- Receiver operating characteristic curves, and the statistics involved in their interpretation.
- The observational assessment of screening.
- The basis of cost-effectiveness analysis, and the assessment of the efficacy of screening and prevention.

Teaching contents

Quantitative concepts

It is almost impossible to teach most of clinical epidemiology without the basic concepts of probability and statistics. Most clinical students will not have a solid grounding in these topics, and some will exhibit frank phobia of math. The basics of biostatistics are often included as part of the curriculum, typically taught in a block (often at the beginning of the course). Whenever introduced, these topics will be more compelling if they are taught alongside other elements of the course, as illustrated in this discussion.

For students starting off, the statistical teaching can be largely conceptual, focusing on the motivation and interpretation of the statistical constructs rather than on detailed derivation or computation. Most importantly, the probabilistic nature of biologic associations should be stressed throughout. Even for a strong risk factor (e.g. smoking and lung cancer), only a minority of patients with the risk factor will have or get the associated disease, and not everyone without the risk factor will necessarily escape the disease (Baron, 1989; Rose, 1981); no clinical test is perfect, and no decision process can be completely free of some error.

The concept of risk is easily presented as a natural extension of probability, with the addition of a time horizon. Estimation of risks requires a well defined numerator which corresponds appropriately to its denominator, as well as consideration of censoring. Prevalence and incidence are easily presented, but a detailed discussion of rates (and their relationships with risks) (Elandt-Johnson, 1975; Morgenstern *et al.*, 1980) may be left to more advanced courses.

Traditional (etiologic) epidemiology generally uses relative measures of association, a group of statistics that will need to be discussed conceptually, if not statistically. Clinical epidemiology, with its focus on clinical impact, often requires absolute risks, attributable risks, numbers needed to be treated, etc. The distinction between the difference measures of association and the relative measures is a fundamental one that deserves emphasis: each group of measures has appropriate uses and interpretation. After this foundation is laid, the distinction between the various types of relative risks (rate ratios, risk ratios, odds ratios, prevalence ratios, etc.) can be touched on, or left to a second course. The concepts of life expectancy and years of life lost (or gained) (Naimark *et al.*, 1994; Wright and Weinstein, 1998) are relatively subtle issues that could also be discussed in general terms.

Medical measurement

Components of sickness; concepts of biostatistics

The distinction between disease, illness, and setting (or 'predicament') (Taylor, 1979) is an excellent introduction to medical measurement, since these different dimensions of sickness illustrate many fundamental measurement issues. The disease (the physiologic or psychologic disturbance underlying the sickness) often has associated numeric measurements (e.g. blood pressure, the area of a stenotic valve). In contrast, the illness (the patient's experience of the disease) and the setting (the social and ecologic situation of the patient) are often measured with ordinal or nominal assessments. The relationship between disease and associated illnesses has always been imperfect (Stein *et al.*, 1987; Williams and Hadler, 1983) and, with molecular methods of disease detection, the distinctions are likely to become even wider (Black and Welch, 1993). A discussion of labeling (Alderman and Lamport, 1990) will reinforce the importance of the differences between disease and illness.

If statistical concepts are part of the course, this could be a time to introduce methods appropriate to each type of data, i.e. means and variance (standard deviation) for numeric data, medians and ranges for ordinal data, and categorization (e.g. contingency tables) for nominal data. The basics of estimation and testing can follow and be reinforced in discussions of comparisons of measurements. It will be useful to emphasize the distinction between statistical significance and clinical significance in the introductory courses.

Accuracy and precision; measures of agreement and disagreement

Discussion of accuracy, precision, and hard *versus* soft data can be used to reinforce the concepts of bias and variability. Discussion of the limitations of data that are traditionally considered 'hard' is worthwhile – for example, illustrating the difficulties with examples that can lead up to stage migration (the 'Will Rogers phenomenon') (Black and Welch, 1993; Feinstein *et al.*, 1985).

Understanding the strengths and weaknesses of clinical measurement involves issues of agreement and disagreement between two measurements (Bland and Altman, 1995; Brennan and Silman, 1992). These topics can force a review of some quantitative concepts, and can also be the occasion for the introduction of new statistics, e.g. κ. Although the rationale for this measure is fairly easy to explain, its interpretation is not clear when there are more than two observers or if the measurement is not dichotomous (Maclure and Willett, 1987). The continuous counterpart, the intraclass correlation (Bartko, 1966), is usually not included in starter courses, but can be mentioned briefly as a correlation between two measurements in the same subjects. In more advanced settings, this statistic can also be interpreted as the ratio of the between-person variance to the total variance, and as a kappa-like statistic. If statistical methods are being woven into the course, then discussion of linear regression can be introduced as an expression of the association between two continuous measures.

This statistical development can lead into a discussion of the sources of variation in clinical data (between- and within-person variation, biologic variation, measurement variation, etc). Several papers have summarized the data regarding the repeatability of various clinical measures (Elmore and Feinstein, 1992; Feinstein, 1985). Regression toward the mean (Ederer, 1972; McDonald et al., 1983) illustrates some further effects of variability and will also force consideration of the effects of subject selection and the need for controls, a topic that can be returned to later.

After the theme of variability is developed, issues of normal ranges of clinical measurements can be discussed. The term 'normal' carries several implications (Sackett et al., 1998) that can usefully be explored: Gaussian distribution, usual value, and desirable value. The idea of a normal test value can be picked up later, during discussion of clinical testing.

Clinical scales

Discussion of clinical scales (Guyatt et al., 1993) involves many of the preceding measurement issues. Often clinical scales will address the illness dimension of sickness; their validation will require statistics to describe scale coverage, reliability, validity, responsiveness/sensitivity, and calibration (McDowell and Newell, 1996; Testa and Simonson, 1996). Validation also brings in concepts such as face validity, criterion validity, and construct validity. Scales of particular interest may include functional status (quality of life) scales (Guyatt et al., 1993; Applegate et al., 1990), utilities (Froberg and Kane, 1989; Sox et al., 1988; Torrance, 1987), or symptom scales. Consideration of construction of scales (Kirshner and Guyatt, 1985; Streiner and Norman, 1989) will probably best be left to an advanced course. Clinical prediction rules (Laupacis et al., 1997; Wasson et al., 1985) are closely related to diagnosis, but can be mentioned at this juncture, with consideration of predictive efficacy discussed later, with testing theory.

Research design

Prognosis

The most useful teaching of prognosis reinforces quantitative concepts previously taught, and previews concepts that will be considered later in the course. Since a prognosis is essentially a set of probabilities of various outcomes over time, the fundamental language of prognosis is naturally that of risk. Concepts and techniques of survival analysis will need to be introduced, reviewed, or assumed to be understood:

- ◆ The concept of risk as a probability for a person, assessed by the average risk (measured in a group).
- ◆ The dependence of event probabilities on the length of follow-up.
- ◆ Censoring.

- The limitations of describing survival only over one time interval (e.g. a 5-year survival rate)
- The need to consider prognosis from a defined point in the course of the disease, preferably at the time of incidence (i.e. the formation of an inception cohort).
- The desirability of blinded follow-up to avoid ascertainment biases.
- The need to compare the outcomes for patients having a certain disease with some familiar 'benchmark'. This leads naturally to the concept of controls and cohort studies.

Because many of these issues are shared with other research designs, prognosis studies can provide an excellent entrée into research design, a topic presented elsewhere in this volume (see section on Research Design, Chapter 4). This discussion will consider only aspects that are particularly relevant for teaching clinical students.

Discussion of research design is facilitated by the use of examples that focus on clinical (rather than etiologic) issues. Relevant examples include studies that compare clinical tests, prognostic investigations, and outcome studies of clinical treatments. Although all of the classic epidemiologic research designs may be encountered in clinical discussions, their relative importance is somewhat different than in etiologic epidemiology. For example, ecologic studies are seldom encountered in clinical epidemiology, apart from a role in health services research (e.g. variation in procedure rates in various geographic areas). Cross-sectional studies are not particularly valued for etiologic inference, but are widely used to investigate clinical measurements, and so are much more valuable for the clinical epidemiologist than the disease epidemiologist.

Cohort studies are essentially elaborations of prognostic investigations using a diverse group of individuals. Fair (i.e. unbiased) follow-up will be needed for effective comparison of the exposure groups. Case control studies can now be considered as alternative designs toward assessing the same exposure/outcome association. The limitations of these observational designs need to be considered, including issues of chance, confounding, and bias. The fact that exposures are interrelated in real life sets up the conditions for confounding; case-mix is a well recognized clinical example.

Clinical trials (Peto et al., 1976; 1977) are often omitted from etiologic epidemiology courses, but deserve special emphasis in a clinical epidemiology course because of their importance in clarifying clinical issues of treatment and prevention. Trials can be seen as a special type of cohort study, with random assignment of the exposure and a highly organized follow-up. Randomization has an important role as statistical protection against confounding, even against potential confounding factors that are not identified. This powerful role cannot be duplicated by the techniques available to observational studies, such as matching or adjustment. The value of an intention-to-treat analysis and a low drop-out rate follows directly: preservation of the randomized groups is needed to take advantage of the randomization.

Blinding is the second procedure that provides important advantages for clinical trials, these being avoidance of bias in the assignment of treatments and in the assessment of endpoints. Blinding of endpoint assessment is also possible in cohort studies, a feature that reinforces the relationship between trials and cohort studies. The organized follow-up of trials (stipulated endpoint measurements at predetermined times) can also be shared by cohort studies and is important for the avoidance of biased ascertainment of endpoints.

Clinical trials, particularly multicentered trials, are typically relatively formal investigations. For example, such a trial will often have:

+ Publicized pre-study hypotheses.

+ A very detailed protocol and operations manual.

+ Several clinical centers as well as laboratory and/or pathology centers.

+ Numerous study committees, including a blinded endpoint committee.

+ Procedures for monitoring data quality at clinical sites.

+ An independent safety and data monitoring committee.

These formalisms can seem bureaucratic and unnecessary unless their role in preserving the validity of the associated study is made clear. This effort will then serve to reinforce many of the basic principles of clinical trial research.

By tradition (though certainly not necessity), several topics of general importance are often presented in the context of clinical trials, including data dredging, generalizability (internal *versus* external validity), subgroup analyses, and meta-analyses. A discussion of these issues can serve to review important aspects of research design and interpretation for virtually all types of studies.

Diagnosis and testing

Diagnosis *versus* testing

The diagnostic process should occupy a significant proportion of most clinical epidemiology courses, since here the consequences of uncertainty are well known and the advantages of quantitative understanding quite obvious (Sackett *et al.*, 1991; Sox *et al.*, 1988).

A categorization of various styles of diagnosis has been advanced (Sackett *et al.*, 1991):

+ Gestalt (pattern recognition).

+ Branching algorithm (following a specified decision tree).

+ Exhaustive testing.

+ Hypotheticodeductive approach.

Formal testing theory addresses the last of these, but only partially. Diagnosis requires assembling a list of diseases to consider, ordering the list as to which are important or likely, choosing appropriate tests and the order in which to do them, and finally interpreting their results. In contrast, testing typically assumes that a particular disease is being considered, and that a particular test has been chosen. It is much more limited than diagnosis, and only a partial depiction of the complexity of clinical reality.

The basic starting point of a discussion of testing – the 2 by 2 table (test-positive or -negative; with or without the target disease) – is relatively easy to understand, but brings a few possible points of confusion. One issue is that there are three types of probabilities that need to be distinguished:

+ Prior probabilities (obtained from one of the margins of the 2×2 table).
+ Posterior probabilities (obtained from within the 2×2 table).
+ Test operating characteristics.

Another ambiguity is the different sampling schemes which can generate a 2×2 table: selection of diseased and non-diseased patients, or selection of those who are test-negative and others who are test-positive. If diseased and non-diseased subjects are sampled, then the sensitivity and specificity of the test can be studied. These parameters describe the inherent ability of the test to distinguish diseased from non-diseased subjects and should be carefully differentiated from the probabilities that clinicians need in dealing with a patient: posterior probabilities such as the positive predictive value (PPV) and the negative predictive value (NPV).

Bayes rule can be presented as a way of combining sensitivity and specificity with the prior probability and the test result (positive or negative) to yield posterior probabilities. In contrast to etiologic studies, confounding is irrelevant to test measurements, since they are risk markers. What matters is the performance of the test, not whether the measurement reflects a causal association. The computational aspects of probability revision are relatively unimportant and usually uninformative, and therefore the details of Bayes formula need not be emphasized. More helpful are devices such as a branching diagram, which can be used as a computational crutch, and also a device to illustrate how a formula actually works (Fig. 19.1).

A fundamental fact that should be emphasized is that the PPV and NPV depend on the prior probability, and are not inherent features of the test (as are, to a first approximation, sensitivity and specificity). This point bears repeating, using examples in which the disease prevalence is varied and the PPV or NPV vary with the prior probabilities. This variation in the posterior probabilities with the prior probability may be confusing to clinical audiences. To clarify why this variation occurs, it is often helpful to demonstrate what occurs in the branching diagram (Fig. 19.1) as disease prevalence changes. This variability in the posterior probabilities is expected unless the test involved has perfect sensitivity and specificity.

There are several distinct clinical settings in which the interpretation of a test may be relevant: screening, ruling out disease, and ruling in disease. These tend to have different ranges of pre-test probabilities, and different consequences resulting from false-positive and false-negative errors. The final message is that, to rule out disease, a negative result of a very sensitive test will be needed, while to rule in disease, a positive result on a relatively specific test will be required.

Extensions of the basics of testing theory

Basic testing theory will need to be extended to tests with multiple possible values. As a first step, the practice of dichotomizing a more complex measurement into normal and abnormal ranges can be examined; this will necessarily involve consideration of the choice of the cut-off and the tension between sensitivity and specificity. The particular value of sensitive tests to rule out a disorder (with a negative result) and of specific tests to rule in a disorder (after a positive result) can be reinforced at this point.

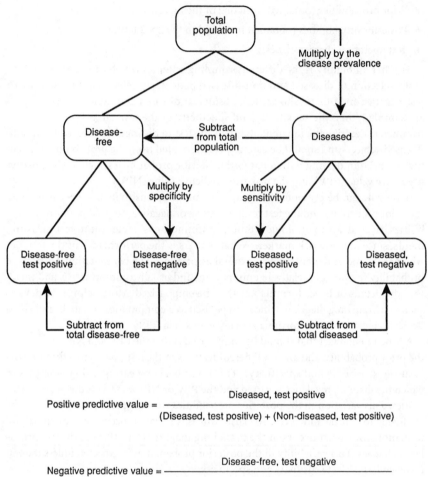

Figure 19.1 Branching diagram version of Bayes' Theorem.

Likelihood ratios (Albert, 1982; Sox *et al.*, 1988; van der Helm and Hische, 1979) incorporate test measurements with multiple values; they are the most convenient way of expressing the implications of a particular test measurement on the probability of disease. In situations with multiple test measurements, Bayes rule can most easily be considered in the odds ratio format:

posterior odds = prior odds × likelihood ratio.

With a dichotomous disease state (i.e. present or absent), multiple values also lead naturally to consideration of receiver operating characteristic (ROC) curves (Sox *et al.*, 1988; Zweig and Campbell, 1993), which express all possible trade-offs of sensitivity and specificity for the test measurement. The area under the curve expresses the inherent ability of the measurement to distinguish the diseased from non-diseased patients. Sophisticated students can be led to the construction of ROC curves, estimation of the area under the curve and the testing of differences in the areas for two different test measurements (Campbell, 1994; Centor, 1991; Hanley and McNeil, 1982).

Additional advanced topics include consideration of:

+ The lack of constancy of sensitivity and specificity (Begg and McNeil, 1988; Rozanski *et al.*, 1983).

+ Uninterpretable tests (Begg *et al.*, 1986; Simel *et al.*, 1987).

+ Research regarding the estimation of operating characteristics and ROC curves, including verification bias, associations between the test measurement under investigation and the reference ('gold standard' test), and errors in the reference test (Begg, 1987; Boyko *et al.*, 1988; Campbell, 1994; Panzer *et al.*, 1987).

+ Mathematical aspects of Bayesean testing (Baron, 1994; Begg, 1986).

Screening and prevention

At the onset of a discussion of screening (Black and Welch, 1993; Morrison, 1992), a distinction from diagnostic testing needs to be made: screening is not ordinarily intended to rule in or rule out a disease. None the less, screening can be introduced as the use of a test measurement when the prior probability is low, a situation that will naturally lead to potential problems with false-positive findings. The distinction between a screening test and a screening program is also important: the screening program includes a definition of who should be screened at what frequency, plus systems for bringing individuals to screening, resolving the diagnosis of those that screen positive, and treating those with the target disorder.

A systematic consideration of the components of a screening program and its evaluation will be important. Important points include:

+ The target of the screening: illness in the preclinical detection phase. Pseudo-disease is a related concept that will directly relate to the discussion of the risks and benefits of screening. The need for effective treatment – better applied in the preclinical phase than later – is another important point.

+ The screening test itself. In the screening situation (typically low prevalence of the target lesion), the tension between sensitivity and specificity will be an important issue, often with no crisp resolution. In longer, or more advanced courses, the difficulties of even defining the sensitivity and specificity of a test in a screening situation can be discussed.

+ The expected pattern of events after screening. The almost inevitable improvement in observed case survival will force consideration of selection into screening, lead time and length-biased sampling.

+ The effectiveness of screening. Among the students there is likely to be an assumption that a program of early detection will necessarily be beneficial and even necessarily save money. The potentially negative impact of screening on those who falsely screen negative or those who falsely screen positive will need to be illustrated, as will the possible harms from ineffective treatment. This discussion can lead naturally to cost-effectiveness analysis and expected value decision techniques.

In advanced courses, the observational assessment of screening can be discussed, as well as the computation of the operating characteristics of screening tests. Case control investigation of screening (Morrison, 1992; Weiss *et al.*, 1992) is a particularly challenging issue that combines many quantitative topics.

Prevention requires only a few additional concepts, including the distinction between primary, secondary, and tertiary prevention. Otherwise, much of the basics of prevention can recapitulate analogous discussions of screening regarding target population and effectiveness. The students will probably enter with biases regarding the inevitable benefits of prevention, and arguments similar to those used for screening can be used to discuss these. On a population level, the fact that most cases of many diseases will accrue from individuals at low or moderate risk points to the 'prevention paradox', that interventions beneficial on a population level will provide relatively small benefits to any one individual. Those with the most to gain from prevention often contribute little to the population burden of the target disease (Rose, 1981).

Expected value decision analysis and economic analyses

Expected value decision analysis (Detsky *et al.*, 1997a, b; Krahn *et al.*, 1997; Naglie *et al.*, 1997; Sox *et al.*, 1988) is often encountered in research regarding clinical policies, although its role in formulating treatments for individual patients is not so clear. It has value in teaching students a systematic approach to decisions which are uncertain, and so may aid students to think clearly even if the technique is not explicitly used clinically.

As it is usually presented, expected value decision-making is prescriptive (showing how decisions could rationally be made) rather than descriptive (showing how decisions are actually made). The approach is highly modeled, including:

- Identification of the possible actions the clinician can take, and the possible outcomes of these actions.
- Structuring of the relationships of these choices and outcomes (the decision tree).
- Quantification of the relationships in the decision tree (transition probabilities and utilities of outcomes).
- Computation leading to the identification of a preferred decision.
- Examination of the stability of the choice against perturbations of the assumptions and data used (sensitivity analysis).

Economic analyses incorporate cost issues into expected value decision analyses (Detsky and Naglie, 1990; Drummond *et al.*, 1987; Eisenberg, 1989; Sox *et al.*, 1988). New concepts that are involved include discounting, direct *versus* indirect benefits, the perspective of the analysis, and the role of marginal (incremental) analyses. Cost-effectiveness analysis is more commonly encountered than cost-benefit analyses, and merits corresponding greater emphasis.

Teaching method and format: assessment of students

Clinical students and clinicians may be borrowing clinical time for a clinical epidemiology course. Beeper interruptions tend to be common, and students may not be able to attend all sessions because of responsibilities for patient care. The optimum is to require that students turn off beepers and attend virtually all sessions. The reality is that this optimum may be impossible. As a consequence, building some redundancy into the course is useful: material presented in class can be obtained with readings, etc.

Once the readings have been assigned and the theory is presented, application of the concepts in clinical problems should be stressed. Much of the material taught in a clinical epidemiology course has the potential for clinical use, and so exercises that are drawn from clinical practice or simulate clinical practice are particularly effective. As a preliminary, however, simple exercises that review the basic concepts might be introduced, including simple true or false questions about the concepts, etc. The bulk of the exercises could then include clinical scenarios or critique of articles.

Discussion of the limitations of 'naive' (non-quantitative) approaches to clinical problems are important for three reasons: to reinforce the quantitative concepts themselves, to highlight the clinical relevance of the discipline, and to help motivate students from purely clinical backgrounds. Examples of these discussion points include errors or confusion engendered by:

♦ Reliance on numerator data alone for conclusions that require risks or rates.

♦ Confusion between relative and attributable risks.

♦ Confusion between statistical and clinical significance.

♦ Lack of adjustment for important confounding factors.

♦ Failure to anticipate a low positive predictive value in the setting of low disease prevalence.

Several media sources can provide relevant teaching materials. The American College of Physicians (ACP) Journal Club (provided with the *Annals of Internal Medicine*) and Evidence-Based Medicine (from the *British Medical Journal* and the American College of Physicians) provide abstracts and critiques of recent articles. These can be used as teaching examples, or (without the critiques) as exercises. A coordinated handbook (Sackett *et al.*, 1998) and workbook (Straus *et al.*, 1998) in the Evidence-Based Medicine Literature may also provide useful examples and exercises. Two series of articles in *JAMA* provide considerable material in the same vein (Oxman *et al.*, 1993; Sackett, 1992).

Several web sites have been developed that incorporate potentially useful material. These include:

♦ SHARR. *http://www.shef.ac.uk/uni/academic/R-Z/scharr/ir/netting.html*, a site with links to many other web sites very relevant to clinical epidemiology.

♦ Oxford Centre for Evidence-Based Medicine. *http://cebm.jr2.ox.ac.uk* a site with on-line summaries of many clinical epidemiology topics, and some useful examples.

♦ ACP Journal Club and Evidence-Based Medicine. *http://www.acponline.org/journals/acpjc/jcmenu.htm* and *http://www.acponline.org/journals/ebm/ebmmenu.htm.*

♦ The Epidemiology 'Supercourse' *http://www.pitt.edu/~super1/.* This site contains complete lectures (with slides), some of which address topics in clinical epidemiology.

Evaluation of learning in a clinical epidemiology course can proceed through a variety of paths. Particularly useful are critiques of articles dealing with the concepts covered, or solutions to clinical scenarios. Advertisements in medical journals often provide interesting and timely examples of material for interpretation in these exercises.

Summary

Clinical epidemiology can include much of the field of epidemiology in general, and this breadth is one of the challenges that confront teachers in this field. The backgrounds of the students may leave the instructor with additional challenges: some courses may involve both clinicians who have little quantitative background and epidemiologists or statisticians with almost no clinical experience. In this situation, it may be particularly difficult to keep the different types of students challenged and interested, and not overwhelmed or bored. A focus on the clinical part of clinical epidemiology will help motivate clinical students while the technical concepts appropriate for students with quantitative backgrounds is discussed.

References

Albert, A. (1982). On the use and computation of likelihood ratios in clinical chemistry. *Clinical Chemistry*, **28**, 1113–19.

Alderman, M. H. and Lamport, B. (1990). Labelling of hypertensives: a review of the data. *Journal of Clinical Epidemiology*, **43**, 195–200.

Applegate, W. B., Blass, J. P. and Williams, T. F. (1990). Instruments for the functional assessment of older patients. *New England Journal of Medicine*, **322**, 1207–14.

Baron, J. A. (1989). The clinical utility of risk factor data. *Journal of Clinical Epidemiology*, **42**, 1013–20.

Baron, J. A. (1994). Uncertainty in Bayes. *Medical Decision Making*, **14**, 46–51.

Bartko, J. J. (1966). The intraclass correlation coefficient as a measure of reliability. *Psychological Reports*, **19**, 3–11.

Begg, C. B. (1987). Biases in the assessment of diagnostic tests. *Statistics in Medicine*, **6**, 411–23.

Begg, C. B. (1986). Statistical methods in medical diagnosis. *Critical Reviews in Medical Informatics*, **1**, 1–22.

Begg, C. B., Greenes, R. A. and Iglewicz, B. (1986). The influence of uninterpretability on the assessment of diagnostic tests. *Journal of Chronic Diseases*, **39**, 575–84.

Begg, C. B. and McNeil, B. J. (1988). Assessment of radiologic tests: control of bias and other design considerations. *Radiology*, **167**, 565–9.

Black, W. C. and Welch, H. G. (1993). Advances in diagnostic imaging and overestimations of disease prevalence and the benefits of therapy. *New England Journal of Medicine*, **328**, 1237–43.

Bland, J. M. and Altman, D. G. (1995). Comparing two methods of clinical measurement: a personal history. *International Journal of Epidemiology*, **24**, S7–14.

Boyko, E. J., Alderman, B. W. and Baron, A. E. (1988). Reference test errors bias the evaluation of diagnostic tests for ischemic heart disease. *Journal of General Internal Medicine*, **3**, 476–81.

Brennan, P. and Silman, A. (1992). Statistical methods for assessing observer variability in clinical measures. *BMJ*, **304**, 1491–4.

Campbell, G. (1994). Advances in statistical methodology for the evaluation of diagnostic and laboratory tests. *Statistics in Medicine*, **13**, 499–508.

Centor, R. M. (1991). Signal detectability: the use of ROC curves and their analyses. *Medical Decision Making*, **11**, 102–6.

Detsky, A. S., Naglie, G., Krahn, M. D., Naimark, D. and Redelmeier, D. A. (1997a). Primer on medical decision analysis: Part 1 – Getting started. *Medical Decision Making*, **17**, 123–5.

Detsky, A. S., Naglie, G., Krahn, M. D., Redelmeier, D. A. and Naimark, D. (1997b). Primer on medical decision analysis: Part 2 – Building a tree. *Medical Decision Making*, **17**, 126–35.

Detsky, A. S. and Naglie, I. G. (1990). A Clinician's Guide to Cost-Effectiveness Analysis. *Ann Intern Med*, **113**, 147–154.

Drummond, M. F., Stoddart, G. L. and Torrance, G. W. *Methods for the Economic Evaluation of Health Care Programmes*, p. 182, Oxford University Press, Oxford (1987).

Ederer, F. (1972). Serum cholesterol changes: effects of diet and regression toward the mean. *Journal of Chronic Diseases*, **25**, 277–89.

Eisenberg, J. M. (1989). Clinical Economics. *JAMA*, **262**, 2879–2886.

Elandt-Johnson, R. C. (1975). Definition of rates: some remarks on their use and misuse. *American Journal of Epidemiology*, **102**, 267–71.

Elmore, J. G. and Feinstein, A. R. (1992). A bibliography of publications on observer variability (final installment). *Journal of Clinical Epidemiology*, **45**, 567–80.

Feinstein, A. R. (1985). A bibliography of publications on observer variability. *Journal of Chronic Diseases*, **38**, 619–32.

Feinstein, A. R., Sosin, D. M. and Wells, C. K. (1985). The Will Rogers phenomenon. Stage migration and new diagnostic techniques as a source of misleading statistics for survival in cancer. *New England Journal of Medicine*, **312**, 1604–8.

Froberg, D. G. and Kane, R. L. (1989). Methodology for measuring health-state preferences–II: Scaling methods. *Journal of Clinical Epidemiology*, **42**, 459–71.

Guyatt, G. H., Feeny, D. H. and Patrick, D. L. (1993). Measuring health-related quality of life. *Annals of Internal Medicine*, **118**, 622–9.

Hanley, J. A. and McNeil, B. J. (1982). The meaning and use of the area under a receiver operating characteristic (ROC) curve. *Radiology*, **143**, 29–36.

Kirshner, B. and Guyatt, G. (1985). A methodological framework for assessing health indices. *Journal of Chronic Diseases*, **38**, 27–36.

Krahn, M. D., Naglie, G., Naimark, D., Redelmeier, D. A. and Detsky, A. S. (1997). Primer on medical decision analysis: Part 4 – Analyzing the model and interpreting the results. *Medical Decision Making*, **17**, 142–51.

Laupacis, A., Sekar, N. and Stiell, I. G. (1997). Clinical prediction rules. A review and suggested modifications of methodological standards. *JAMA*, **277**, 488–94.

Maclure, M. and Willett, W. C. (1987). Misinterpretation and misuse of the kappa statistic. *American Journal of Epidemiology*, **126**, 161–9.

McDonald, C. J., Mazzuca, S. A. and McCabe, G. P., Jr. (1983). How much of the placebo 'effect' is really statistical regression? *Statistics in Medicine*, **2**, 417–27.

McDowell, I. and Newell, C. *Measuring Health: A Guide to Rating Scales and Questionnaries*, 2nd edn, p. 342, Oxford University Press, New York (1996).

Morgenstern, H., Kleinbaum, D. G. and Kupper, L. L. (1980). Measures of Disease Incidence Used in Epidemiologic Research. *International Journal of Epidemiology*, **9**, 97–104.

Morrison, A. S. *Screening In Chronic Disease*, Oxford University Press, New York (1992).

Naglie, G., Krahn, M. D., Naimark, D., Redelmeier, D. A. and Detsky, A. S. (1997). Primer on medical decision analysis: Part 3 – Estimating probabilities and utilities. *Medical Decision Making*, **17**, 136–41.

Naimark, D., Naglie, G. and Detsky, A. S. (1994). The meaning of life expectancy: what is a clinically significant gain? *Journal of General Internal Medicine*, **9**, 702–7.

Oxman, A. D., Sackett, D. L. and Guyatt, G. H. (1993). Users' guides to the medical literature. I. How to get started. The Evidence-Based Medicine Working Group. *JAMA*, **270**, 2093–5.

Panzer, R. J., Suchman, A. L. and Griner, P. F. (1987). Workup bias in prediction research. *Medical Decision Making*, **7**, 115–19.

Peto, R., Pike, M. C., Armitage, P. *et al.* (1976). Design and analysis of randomized clinical trials requiring prolonged observation of each patient. I. Introduction and design. *British Journal of Cancer*, **34**, 585–612.

Peto, R., Pike, M. C., Armitage, P. *et al.* (1977). Design and analysis of randomized clinical trials requiring prolonged observation of each patient. II. analysis and examples. *British Journal of Cancer*, **35**, 1–39.

Rose, G. (1981). Strategy of prevention: lessons from cardiovascular disease. *British Medical Journal Clinical Research Ed.*, **282**, 1847–51.

Rozanski, A., Diamond, G. A. *et al.* (1983). The declining specificity of exercise radionuclide ventriculography. *New England Journal of Medicine*, **309**, 518–22.

Sackett, D. L. (1992). A primer on the precision and accuracy of the clinical examination. *JAMA*, **267**, 2638–44.

Sackett, D. L., Haynes, R. B., Guyatt, G. H. and Tugwell, P. *Clinical Epidemiology: A Basic Science For Clinical Medicine*, 2nd edn, p. 441, Little, Brown and Company, Boston (1991).

Sackett, D. L., Richardson, W. S., Rosenberg, W. and Haynes, R. B. *Evidence-based Medicine: How to Practice and Teach EBM*, p. 250, Churchill Livingstone, Edinburgh (1998).

Sackett, D. L., Rosenberg, W. M., Gray, J. A., Haynes, R. B. and Richardson, W. S. (1996). Evidence based medicine: what it is and what it isn't. *BMJ*, **312**, 71–2.

Simel, D. L., Feussner, J. R., DeLong, E. R. and Matchar, D. B. (1987). Intermediate, indeterminate, and uninterpretable diagnostic test results. *Medical Decision Making*, **7**, 107–14.

Sox, H. C., Blatt, M. A., Higgins, M. C. and Marton, K. I. *Medical Decision Making*, Butterworth Publishers, Stoneham (1988).

Stein, R. E., Gortmaker, S. L., Perrin, E. C. *et al.* (1987). Severity of illness: concepts and measurements. *Lancet*, **ii**, 1506–9.

Straus, S. E., Bradenoch, D., Richardson, W. S., Rosenberg, W. and Sackett, D. L. *Practising Evidence-based Medicine: Learner's Manual*, 3rd edn, p. 206, Radcliff Medical Press Ltd, Oxford (1998).

Streiner, D. L. and Norman, G. R. *Health Measurement Scales: A Practical Guide to their Development and Use*, p. 175, Oxford University Press, Oxford (1989).

Taylor, D. C. (1979). The components of sickness: diseases, illnesses, and predicaments. *Lancet*, **ii**, 1008–10.

Testa, M. A. and Simonson, D. C. (1996). Assesment of quality-of-life outcomes. *New England Journal of Medicine*, **334**, 835–40.

Torrance, G. W. (1987). Utility approach to measuring health-related quality of life. *Journal of Chronic Diseases*, **40**, 593–603.

van der Helm, H. J. and Hische, E. A. (1979). Application of Bayes's theorem to results of quantitative clinical chemical determinations. *Clinical Chemistry*, **25**, 985–8.

Wasson, J. H., Sox, H. C., Neff, R. K. and Goldman, L. (1985). Clinical prediction rules. Applications and methodological standards. *New England Journal of Medicine*, **313**, 793–9.

Weiss, N. S., McKnight, B. and Stevens, N. G. (1992). Approaches to the analysis of case-control studies of the efficacy of screening for cancer. *American Journal of Epidemiology*, **135**, 817–23.

Williams, M. E. and Hadler, N. M. (1983). The illness as the focus of geriatric medicine. *New England Journal of Medicine*, **308**, 1357–60.

Wright, J. C. and Weinstein, M. C. (1998). Gains in life expectancy from medical interventions–standardizing data on outcomes. *New England Journal of Medicine*, **339**, 380–6.

Zweig, M. H. and Campbell, G. (1993). Receiver-operating characteristic (ROC) plots: a fundamental evaluation tool in clinical medicine. *Clinical Chemistry*, **39**, 561–77.

Chapter 20

Perinatal epidemiology

Lowell Sever

Introduction

My approach to perinatal epidemiology is to consider the biologic and developmental events occurring between conception and birth, the genetic basis of those events, risk factors that can perturb them, and some of the effects of these factors that are evident in childhood. Since conditions present at birth, and events occurring during the neonatal period, play such major roles in infant mortality rates, it is important to consider other contributors to such mortality rates as well. Some investigators extend this to considering the impact of perinatal factors on health conditions during adulthood as well.

With respect to disease (altered states of health), I believe the key aims of epidemiology are to:

+ Describe distribution.

+ Explain determinants.

+ Predict populations at risk.

+ Prevent occurrence.

The discussion of the topics of the course is organized based on these aims, with a strong public health focus, stressing the importance of understanding the distribution and determinants of diseases for prevention. My approach is directed toward helping students to 'think epidemiologically' about selected perinatal topics to address two questions integral to disease prevention and health promotion: 'Are we doing the right things?' and 'Are we doing things right?' This involves understanding etiology and risk factors, translating this information into preventive interventions, and then evaluating intervention programs. In the course this is often framed in terms of two of the core public health functions, assessment and assurance, and the importance of epidemiology in evaluation. Others may take a more clinical approach to the subject.

The focus of this course, therefore, is on epidemiologic and public health aspects of selected perinatal problems and methods for studying them (Wilcox and Marks, 1994). Developing an understanding of the use of epidemiologic information for prevention is central to this. The course begins by considering basic issues in normal and abnormal development (Sever and Mortensen, 1996), epidemiologic methods (Hogue *et al.*, 1991; Pless, 1994; Weinberg and Wilcox, 1998), data sources (Kleinman, 1991), and surveillance of adverse reproductive outcomes (Sever and Mortensen, 1996; Yeargin-Allsopp *et al.*, 1992). With this background, the course then covers selected perinatal outcomes from the perspectives of their public health significance, descriptive epidemiology, methodologic issues in studying them, etiology, and prevention.

The perinatal epidemiology course is appropriate both for advanced undergraduate students who have some background in human biology and for graduate students in public health-related disciplines. In organizing the course, all of the students are assumed to have a basic knowledge of human biology, particularly genetics, as well as an understanding of epidemiologic concepts and methods, particularly study designs. In the introductory sessions, the spectrum of events necessary for successful human reproduction and epidemiologic principles are reviewed as they apply to the topics of the course. This includes an overview discussion of methodologic issues specific to the outcomes and exposures covered later in the course, where these are considered in more detail.

Teaching objectives

By the end of the course, the student should:

◆ Be familiar with the sources of data used in perinatal epidemiology and their strengths and weaknesses (Kleinman, 1991).

◆ Have a basic understanding of the epidemiologic methods and problems that are relevant to perinatal epidemiology (Hogue *et al.*, 1991; Pless, 1994; Weinberg and Wilcox, 1998).

◆ Understand the goals, major design elements, and applications of surveillance for adverse reproductive outcomes (Sever and Mortensen, 1996; Yeargin-Allsopp *et al.*, 1992).

◆ Be familiar with the basic principles of teratogenesis as they relate to the design and conduct of epidemiologic studies of adverse reproductive outcomes (Sever and Mortensen, 1996).

◆ Understand the basic epidemiology of selected perinatal problems and risk factors that contribute to their etiology (Adams *et al.*, 1991; Hertz-Picciotto, 1998; Hoffman and Hillman, 1992; Kallen, 1988; March of Dimes, 1997; Sever, 1988, 1994; Sever *et al.*, 1993).

◆ Be familiar with the different types of low birthweight and their risk factors (Alberman, 1994).

◆ Understand the public health significance of major perinatal problems, such as birth defects, infant mortality and developmental disabilities, and the importance of epidemiologic studies in developing prevention strategies (Alberman, 1991; Botto *et al.*, 1999; Fryers, 1991; Kleinman and Kiely, 1991; Krause and Bulterys, 1991; Leck, 1994; Niswander and Kiely, 1991; Richardson and Kuller, 1994; Stanley and Blair, 1994; US Public Health Service, 1992; Wallace, 1994; Watkins, 1998).

Teaching contents

The course is based on establishing background issues and basic concepts and methods followed by consideration of individual outcomes and selected exposures.

Outcomes are selected based on a combination of public health significance and the possible relationship of the outcome to a variety of exposures. In selecting specific exposures an attempt is made to include those of particular scientific, public health, or community concern. At the end of the course we discuss a variety of policy-related issues where there are controversies or new approaches to study.

Background and methods

The course begins with an introduction to perinatal epidemiology that reviews three key areas: basic epidemiologic methods, with examples of applications to perinatal epidemiology; the spectrum of events that occur during reproduction and development; and adverse health outcomes of interest and their public health significance. This is followed by discussion of data sources and approaches to data collection in perinatal epidemiology, considering both existing data sources and primary data collection methods.

Because epidemiology is largely a comparative science, it is important to discuss the rates, ratios, and proportions commonly used to describe perinatal events. This includes a review of basic concepts and formulas. In discussing incidence and prevalence, I have found that a model of pregnancy loss developed by Stein *et al.* (1975) helps students to understand some of the key aspects of 'counting' pregnancy outcomes.

The 'risk approach for maternal and child health care', developed by the World Health Organization (Backett *et al.*, 1984), provides a useful framework for looking at various adverse pregnancy outcomes and their risk factors, particularly in developing countries. My experience has been that by working through the principles of the risk approach, students develop an understanding of how relatively simple data can be collected and used for informed public health decision-making.

Since an important focus of my approach to perinatal epidemiology is understanding the role that exogenous agents play in effecting human development *in utero*, I provide an introduction to teratology. In the course we discuss the principles of teratology (developmental toxicity), and the relationships between epidemiology and developmental toxicity. We also consider developmental toxicity risk assessment and the comparative strengths and weaknesses of epidemiologic studies and studies of laboratory animals. This leads into a discussion of the importance of surveillance, not only for identifying new potential teratogens but also for responding to community concerns about clusters and evaluating prevention efforts.

The final general epidemiologic methods and public health aspects of perinatal epidemiology we cover are screening programs for mothers, fetuses, and babies. Basic concepts of screening are discussed and examples are given of the importance of screening for identifying, from within a population, those persons thought to be at increased risk for disease. The discussion includes criteria and guidelines for screening programs, along with ethical and legal issues that need to be considered.

Perinatal problems

Following this background, selected adverse outcomes of pregnancy and perinatal problems are considered. In discussing each of these a consistent format is followed, based on the 'aims of epidemiology' model discussed earlier. We begin with a discussion of the definition of the outcome, its public health impact, and, if relevant, related national health objectives. This is followed by a consideration of the descriptive epidemiology (estimates of frequency and differences between populations) of the outcome, recognized risk factors, and any special epidemiologic methods related to studying and analyzing the outcome. Finally, possible prevention interventions are discussed.

Exposures

Because of complexities in assessing exposures in epidemiologic studies, and the fact that some exposures lead to multiple outcomes, a series of lectures are included with an exposure-based approach. An attempt is made to follow a consistent format here as well, including reasons for concern regarding developmental effects of the exposure, methodologic issues related to exposure assessment, timing and quantification of exposure, and potential outcomes related to the exposure.

Issues

In the final section of the course we consider, from multiple perspectives, selected broad issue-related topics in perinatal epidemiology. Alternative positions are discussed and explored in dealing with points that are potentially controversial.

Teaching method and format

Substantive course content

Background and methods

This introductory section of the course develops a base upon which the subsequent topics of the course can expand. The major points considered include the following:

1. Defining reproductive and perinatal epidemiology
   - The hazards of being a fetus
   - The spectrum of reproductive and developmental events
   - Basic concepts in embryology and development
2. Outcomes of public health significance
3. Common epidemiologic concepts and methods
   - Basic epidemiologic study designs – review with applications to perinatal problems
   - Analytic issues relevant to perinatal outcomes
   - Rates, ratios, and proportions: revisiting incidence and prevalence
4. Perinatal data sources – strengths and limitations
   - Vital statistics
   - Vital records

- Medical records
- Longitudinal studies and record linkage
- Clinical epidemiologic databases
- Primary data collection: survey instruments and questionnaires

5. The WHO risk approach for maternal and child healthcare
6. Basic principles of teratology (developmental toxicity)
   - Teratogenic principles
   - Mechanisms of teratogenesis
7. Epidemiology and developmental toxicity
   - Recognition of a new teratogen
   - Developmental toxicity risk assessment
     Epidemiologic studies
     Animal studies
8. Surveillance for adverse reproductive outcomes
   - Basic principles of surveillance
   - Birth defects surveillance
     CDC
     State-based programs
   - Developmental disabilities surveillance
9. Screening programs
   - Basic principles of screening in public health
   - Maternal serum screening for neural tube defects and Down syndrome
   - Heterozygote screening in high-risk populations
   - Newborn screening
   - Ethical and legal issues associated with genetic screening.

Perinatal problems

The specific outcomes and some of the major points considered include the following:

1. Time to pregnancy and early pregnancy loss
2. Spontaneous abortion
   - Paradigms for studying spontaneous abortions
   - Problems of ascertainment
3. Fetal deaths
   - Issues in reporting
4. Congenital malformations
   - Genetic causes of birth defects
     Single gene defects
     Chromosomal abnormalities

- Teratogenic agents

    Recognized teratogens: drugs, viruses, chemicals, and physical agents

    Contrasting models of teratogenesis

    Thalidomide *versus* alcohol

    Methyl-mercury *versus* lead

- Gene–environment interactions
- Unknown ('multifactorial') etiology

    The epidemiology and etiology of neural tube defects

    The role of folic acid in preventing neural tube defects

5. Low birthweight
    - Assessment of gestational age
    - Preterm birth
    - Small for gestational age
6. Developmental disabilities
    - Cerebral palsy
    - Mental retardation
7. Infant mortality
    - International comparisons
    - Neonatal and post-neonatal mortality rates
    - Cause of specific infant mortality and trends over time
    - Sudden infant death syndrome.

Exposures

In the section of the course that is exposure-based the topics include:

1. Alcohol and illicit drugs
    - Problems of reporting
    - Sources of population-based data
2. Prescription and over the counter drugs
    - Accutane
    - Thalidomide II
3. Occupational exposures
    - Retrospective exposure assessment
    - The use of job exposure matrices
    - Reproductive and developmental effects of male occupational exposures
    ♦ Reproductive hazards of the workplace: the conceptus
    ♦ Legal and ethical issues related to occupational reproductive hazards
4. Environmental exposures

+ Exposure assessment methods
+ Hazardous waste sites.

Issues

The following policy-related topics are considered:

1. Health policy and core public health functions
2. Program evaluation and intervention strategies
3. Race, ethnicity, and pregnancy outcome
4. Prenatal care: assessment and its impact on pregnancy outcome.

Course schedule

The course, as described, consists of 45 contact hours based on a 15-week calendar with 3 contact hours per week. The schedule is as follows:

Background and methods	3 weeks
Perinatal outcomes	6 weeks
Exposures	4 weeks
Issues	2 weeks

The topics for each week's lectures and discussion can be outlined as follows:

Background and methods

> Week 1
>> Reproduction
>> Epidemiology
>> The risk approach
> Week 2
>> Principles of teratology
>> Epidemiology and developmental toxicity
> Week 3
>> Surveillance
>> Screening

Perinatal problems

> Week 4
>> Time to pregnancy and early loss
>> Spontaneous abortion and fetal deaths
> Week 5
>> Congenital malformations I
> Week 6
>> Congenital malformations II

Week 7

   Low birthweight

Week 8

   Developmental disabilities

Week 9

   Infant mortality

   Exposures

Week 10

   Alcohol and illicit drugs

Week 11

   Prescription and over the counter drugs

Week 12

   Occupational exposures

Week 13

   Environmental exposures

   Issues

Week 14

   Health policy and core public health functions

   Program evaluation and intervention strategies

Week 15

   Race, ethnicity and pregnancy outcome

   Prenatal care.

Depending on the time available for the course, the substantive topics covered in the last three sections, perinatal problems, exposures, and issues, can be modified relatively easily. For example, it is possible to discuss the major topics from either an outcome- or exposure-based perspective, weaving in the issue-related topics the instructor considers of particular interest or concern. This approach would be particularly applicable to a course for medical students where an introduction to concepts and methods could be followed by selected case studies illustrating their application.

Instructional resources

There is no 'textbook' I consider appropriate for my perinatal epidemiology course. Instead, I develop a short reading list for each class session. In selecting the readings, which the students are advised to read before the lecture/discussion of the topic, an attempt is made to identify review or overview papers on epidemiologic, methodologic, and public health aspects of the subjects. Many of these are included in the References section at the end of this chapter. Here are listed some of the reports, textbooks, and compilations of papers that provide readings suitable for a perinatal epidemiology course. I also identify individual papers that have been useful in preparing for and teaching the course. Finally, some of the professional journals that frequently have relevant papers are listed. There are, of course, many other journals that publish epidemiologic studies or reviews.

Instructional methods

The approach I take to teaching this course utilizes a didactic lecture format which relies heavily on the use of visual materials. Questions and discussion are encouraged. A structured discussion is part of the class session for some topics, using a series of questions provided in advance to stimulate the discussion.

The heterogeneous backgrounds and experiences of the students allows them to ask questions or contribute information from diverse perspectives. This adds to the richness of the course, providing opportunities to look at topics from different perspectives as well as for the class to benefit from the participants' expertise.

Assessing students' achievements

In a course like this it is difficult, if not impossible, to define a common subset of information students should master. In my opinion, evaluation should be based on an integration and application of the concepts and methods of epidemiology to a perinatal topic of particular interest to each student. Therefore, students are required to develop a proposal based on defining a research question of personal interest. This research question must be translated into a conceptual hypothesis that includes a discussion of the relevant background literature. The conceptual hypothesis must, in turn, be converted into a study hypothesis. Based on this study hypothesis, the student writes a proposal to carry out a study to test it. The proposal includes a consideration of specific aims, methods, and the strengths and limitations of the proposed study. This provides an opportunity for students to explore how research could be conducted on a topic in perinatal epidemiology of personal interest.

References

Books and reports

Backett, E. M., A. M. Davies, and A. Petros-Barvazian. *The Risk Approach In Health Care.* Public Health Paper No.76. Geneva, World Health Organization, 1984.

Barron, S. L., and A. M. Thomson, eds. *Obstetrical Epidemiology.* New York, Academic Press, 1983.

Bracken, M. B., ed. *Perinatal Epidemiology.* New York, Oxford University Press, 1984.

Center for the Future of Children. Low Birth Weight. *The Future of Children,* 5 (1), Spring 1995.

Kallen, B. *Epidemiology of Human Reproduction.* Boca Raton, Florida, CRC Press, 1988.

Kiely, M., ed. *Reproductive and Perinatal Epidemiology.* Boca Raton, Florida, CRC Press, 1991.

Kline, J., Z. Stein, and M. Susser. *Conception to Birth: Epidemiology of prenatal development.* New York, Oxford University Press, 1989.

March of Dimes Birth Defects Foundation. *March of Dimes StatBook: Statistics for monitoring maternal and infant health.* White Plains, New York, March of Dimes Birth Defects Foundation, 1997.

Pless, I. B., ed. *The Epidemiology of Childhood Disorders.* New York, Oxford University Press, 1994.

Robins, L. N., and J. L. Mills, eds. Effects of In Utero Exposure to Street Drugs. *Am. J. Public Health,* 83 (Suppl.), December 1993.

Wilcox, L. S., and J. S. Marks, eds. *From Data to Action: CDC's public health surveillance for women, infants and children.* Atlanta, US Department of Health & Human Services, Public Health Service, Centers for Disease Control and Prevention, 1994.

Papers

Adams, M. M. *et al.* The Pregnancy Risk Assessment Monitoring System: design, questionnaire, data collection and response rates. *Paed. Perinatal Epidemiol.,* 5, 333–346, 1991.

Alberman, E. The cerebral palsies. In *Reproductive and Perinatal Epidemiology,* M. Kiely, ed. Boca Raton, CRC Press, pp. 206–17, 1991.

Alberman, E. Low birthweight and prematurity. In *The Epidemiology of Childhood Disorders,* I. B. Pless ed. New York, Oxford, pp. 49–65, 1994.

Botto, L. D., C. A. Moore, M. S. Khoury, and J. D. Erickson. Neural–tube defects. *NEJM* **341,** 1509–18, 1999.

Fryers, T. Pre- and perinatal factors in the etiology of mental retardation. In *Reproductive and Perinatal Epidemiology,* M. Kiely, ed. Boca Raton, CRC Press, pp. 171–204, 1991.

Hertz-Picciotto, I. Environmental epidemiology. In *Modern Epidemiology,* 2nd edn, K. J Rothman and S. Greenland. Philadelphia, Lippincott–Raven. pp. 553–83, 1998.

Hoffman, H. J., and L. S. Hillman. Epidemiology of the sudden infant death syndrome: Maternal, neonatal, and postneonatal risk factors. *Clinics in Perinatology,* **19,** 717–37, 1992.

Hogue, C. J. R., E. Rubin and K. Schulz. An introduction to epidemiologic methods. In *Reproductive and Perinatal Epidemiology,* M. Kiely, ed. Boca Raton, CRC Press, pp. 3–25, 1991.

Kleinman, J. C., and J. L. Kiely. Infant Mortality. *Healthy People 2000 Statistical Notes* Vol. 1, No.2. Hyattsville, USPHS, CDC, NCHS, 1991.

Kleinman, J. C. Methodological issues in the analysis of vital statistics. In *Reproductive and Perinatal Epidemiology,* M. Kiely, ed. Boca Raton, CRC Press, pp. 447–68, 1991.

Krause, J. F., and M. Bulterys. The epidemiology of sudden infant death syndrome. In *Reproductive and Perinatal Epidemiology,* M. Kiely, ed. Boca Raton, CRC Press, pp. 219–49, 1991.

Leck, I. Structural birth defects. In *The Epidemiology of Childhood Disorders,* I. B Pless ed. New York, Oxford, pp. 66–117, 1994.

Niswander, K. and M. Kiely. Intrapartum asphyxia and cerebral palsy. In *Reproductive and Perinatal Epidemiology,* M. Kiely, ed. Boca Raton, CRC Press, pp. 357–68, 1991.

Pless, I. B. Concepts, terms, and methods. In *The Epidemiology of Childhood Disorders,* I. B Pless, ed. New York, Oxford, pp. 3–30, 1994.

Richardson, S. A., and H. Kuller. Mental retardation. In *The Epidemiology of Childhood Disorders,* I. B Pless, ed. New York, Oxford, pp. 227–303, 1994.

Sever, L. E. Occupational and environmental reproductive risks. In *Maternal and Child Health Practices,* 4th edn. H. M. Wallace, R. P. Nelson, and P. J. Sweeny eds. Oakland, CA, Third Party Publishing, pp. 309–20, 1994.

Sever, L. E. The state of the art and current issues regarding reproductive outcomes potentially associated with environmental exposures: reduced fertility, reproductive wastage, congenital malformations, and birth weight. Work Group on Reproductive and Developmental Epidemiology: Research Issues, Cincinnati, Ohio, October 24–26, 1988. US Environmental Protection Agency Report 600/8–89/103.

Sever, L. E., M. S. Lynberg, and L. D. Edmonds. The impact of congenital malformations on public health. *Teratology*, **48**, 547–9, 1993.

Sever, L. E., and M. L. Mortensen. Teratology and the epidemiology of birth defects: Occupational and environmental perspectives. In *Obstetrics: Normal and Problem Pregnancies*, 3rd edn, S. Gabbe, J. Niebyl and J. L. Simpson, eds. New York, Churchill Livingstone, pp. 185–6, 189–92, 1996.

Stanley, F. J., and E. Blair. Cerebral palsy. In *The Epidemiology of Childhood Disorders*, I. B Pless ed. New York, Oxford, pp. 473–97, 1994.

Stein, Z., M. Susser, D. Warburton, J. Wittes, and J. Kline. Spontaneous abortion as a screening device: the effect of fetal survival on the incidence of birth defects. *Am. J. Epidemiol.* **102**, 275–90, 1975.

US Public Health Service. Recommendations for the use of folic acid to reduce the number of cases of spina bifida and other neural tube defects. *MMWR* **41**, RR-14, 1992.

Wallace, H. M. Infant mortality. In *Maternal and Child Health Practices*, 4th edn. H M. Wallace, R. P. Nelson, and P. J. Sweeny eds. Oakland, CA, Third Party Publishing, pp. 429–52, 1994.

Watkins, M. L. Efficacy of folic acid prophylaxis for the prevention of neural tube defects. *Mental Retardation and Developmental Disabilities Research Reviews*, **4**, 282–90, 1998.

Weinberg, C. R., and A. J. Wilcox. Reproductive epidemiology. In *Modern Epidemiology*, 2nd edn., K. J Rothman and S. Greenland. Philadelphia, Lippincott–Raven. pp. 585–608, 1998.

Yeargin-Allsopp, M., C. C. Murphy, G. P. Oakley, R. K. Sikes, and the Metropolitan Atlanta Developmental Disabilities Study Staff. A multiple-source method for studying the prevalence of developmental disabilities in children: The Metropolitan Atlanta Developmental Disabilities Study. *Pediatrics*, **89**, 624–30, 1992.

Journals

American Journal of Epidemiology
American Journal of Public Health
Epidemiology
International Journal of Epidemiology
Paediatric and Perinatal Epidemiology
Teratology

Chapter 21

Dental epidemiology

Flemming Scheutz and Aubrey Sheiham

Introduction

Most dental students are introduced to their future profession through courses that reward reproduction of factual information such as anatomy, dental materials, and biochemistry. Later the dental students are also confronted with a heavy clinical workload. These facts form the dental students' views on dentistry and their future role as dentists. Given that epidemiology is different from the biologic sciences and has many logical elements, it is not surprising that many dental students often find epidemiology difficult and less relevant than clinical topics, in particular if they have not been exposed to problem-oriented learning earlier in their study.

We have chosen to use teaching and learning strategies that combine the best of traditional modes with more learner-centered methods seeking to provide a meaningful context, an approach that may best be described as guided discovery learning. The key feature is *learning how to learn through the process of discovery*. The long-term aim is deeply rooted in a belief that contemporary professionals need the skills of lifelong learning and the ability to deal with uncertainty and value conflicts. We do not therefore strive to cover every aspect of epidemiology, but aim to provide the students with the necessary theory and tools to become true professionals, i.e. critical and theoretically well grounded individuals within their particular field. Undergraduate dental students are primarily considered as *consumers of research* whereas postgraduate students are also potential or actual *producers of research*. This, and our teaching philosophy, guides us in the selection of teaching material on an undergraduate level. We would like to stress the importance of a comprehensive study guide that will assist students in their learning. A good study guide indicates what should be learned by specifying learning outcomes and helps students to set their own objectives and plan their learning. It should contain the answers to the questions: Where are we and how did we get here? Where are we going now and how will we get there? Thus, it provides guidance like a good tutor, but without the need for excessive staff–student contact.

Teaching objectives

The objective is to introduce dental students to the basic principles and methods of epidemiology in general and dental epidemiology in particular. And as we prefer to consider undergraduate dental students as *consumers of research*, we aim at producing *critical consumers* (Greenhalgh, 1998). Epidemiology is taught in combination with a basic course in biostatistics (Table 21.1) where the students are taught the most frequently used statistical methods in the dental literature (Jakobsen, 1999). The biostatistic part consists of lectures and exercises based on data from recent dental articles or textbooks and from the studies carried out by the department's staff. A short textbook in biostatistics covers the curriculum and the examination requirements (Swinscow and Campbell, 1996). A chapter in a book on community oral health (Scheutz, 1997) and an article about causation (Scheutz and Poulsen, 1999) cover the essentials of teaching in epidemiology, but there are several useful recommended introductory epidemiology textbooks (Greenberg *et al.*, 1993; Bhopal, 1997). During the course the students have access to computer programs that aid their learning and understanding of statistics (Stat-Aid, 1992; Statistix, 1998). The students are introduced to epidemiology as soon as they have understood and mastered the most elementary statistical methods. As the aim is to integrate statistics into the learning of epidemiology rather than teaching statistics separately, the teaching of the two disciplines is not delegated to particular teachers but given by teachers mutually responsible for the teaching and present during all lectures. The key issues of the teaching in epidemiology are presented in Table 21.2. Generally we focus on oral health as outlined below, but during the plenary teaching the students are also exposed to the key areas from medical epidemiology. Great emphasis is placed on validity and reliability when discussing study designs in epidemiology, bias, and confounding. Proficiency in epidemiology is considered to be just one element of *community oral health*, which comprises preventive dentistry, psychology, philosophy of science, health economics, sociology, health services research, planning of community oral health services, and information about private and public dental services.

A proper understanding of the basic theoretical aspects of biostatistics and epidemiology is of importance (Scheutz and Poulsen, 1999). For example, although the students learn to compute confidence intervals of point estimates this is usually a trivial exercise when the proper equation has been identified. The conceptual aspect of the formulas, proper understanding, and interpretation of a given confidence interval is far more important. Formulas, algebra, and calculations are thus merely looked upon as tools. All students are given a booklet that contains the formulas and tables they need for the exercises and for the assessment of their achievements.

Teaching contents

Dentistry has developed more or less independently of medicine. Because of this, undergraduate teaching in epidemiology has generally taken place separately, although the oral and dental field offers many illustrative and interesting studies. They comprise studies on the natural history and experiments of disease, problems of

Table 21.1 Student level of learning in different categories of statistic and epidemiologic measures

Category	Parameters and tests	Level of learning
Exploring, summarizing and presenting data (descriptive statistics)	Mean, median, mode, Gaussian distribution, standard deviation, percentiles, etc.	Understand, master, and interpret
	Graphs	Understand and interpret
Making inferences from data	Confidence intervals and hypothesis testing	Understand, master, and interpret
Parametric statistics	z-test, t-test, Pearson's correlation coefficient	Understand, master, and interpret
	ANOVA	Understand and interpret
Non-parametric statistics	Mann–Whitney rank sum test, Wilcoxon signed test, χ^2 test, Spearman's correlation coefficient	Understand, master, and interpret
Multivariable methods	Mantel–Haenszel's summary odds ratio and χ^2 test	Understand, master, and interpret
	Linear regression	Understand and interpret
	Logistic regression	Understand and interpret
Survival analysis	Life tables (actuarial analysis) and Kaplan–Meier product limit estimates	Understand and interpret
Measures of disease frequency	Prevalence, incidence rate, cumulative incidence	Understand, master, and interpret
Measures of association	Incidence rate ratio, relative risk, odds ratio	Understand, master, and interpret
Standardization	Direct and indirect standardization	Understand and interpret
The diagnostic matrix	Sensitivity, specificity, positive and negative predictive values	Understand, master, and interpret
Intra- and extra-examiner variability	Percent agreement, Pearson's correlation coefficient	Understand and interpret
	Kappa	Understand, master, and interpret

diagnosis and measurement, screening programs, intervention studies, and prevention, and are of particular interest to dental professionals, but they would also be instructive for medical students.

Table 21.2 Key issues in teaching undergraduates dental epidemiology in sequential order

Issue	Level of learning
Samples and sampling strategies	Understand and interpret
Validity and reliability	Understand and interpret
Bias and confounding	Understand and interpret
Misclassification	Understand and interpret
Diagnostic tests, screening, the diagnostic matrix	Understand, master, and interpret
Randomized controled trials	Understand and interpret

The four basic epidemiologic study types:
    Incidence studies
    Incidence case control studies
    Prevalence studies
    Prevalence case control studies
	Understand and interpret

Measures of disease frequency and measures of association	Understand, master, and interpret
Causation	Understand and interpret
Confounding	Understand and interpret
Control of confounding in design and analysis	Understand and interpret
Mantel–Haenszel's test Control of confounding, χ^2 test	Understand, master, and interpret

Multivariable analysis in epidemiology
    Linear regression
    Logistic regression
	Understand and interpret

Oral and dental epidemiology
    National and international figures
    and issues
	Learn

Descriptive and analytic issues particular to dental epidemiology	Understand
Interpretation of epidemiologic literature	Understand
How to read a paper	Master

Many diseases and conditions are seen in the facial region and the oral cavity, and should be dealt with during the teaching (Burt *et al.*, 1989). The two most common and also specific oral diseases are, however, dental caries and periodontal disease, and both exhibit particular epidemiologic features. They are therefore used as examples for teaching of dental epidemiology.

Dental caries

Diagnosing dental caries

Diagnosing dental caries illustrates a number of problems common to many diseases. These include definitions of lesions, the relationship between clinical, radiographic, and histologic diagnosis, measures of disease progress by estimating rates of progression of a lesion, the criteria for a good index, observer variation, and statistical methods of estimating examiner reproducibility and data analysis.

Quantification of dental caries

Dental caries can be quantified in several ways. Disease prevalence in populations with more than just a moderate prevalence is of limited usefulness. Under such circumstances the number of affected teeth or teeth surfaces per person provides more detailed information since it reflects differences in the amount of disease. In dental epidemiology it is therefore common to use different recording systems and disease indices, not only on an individual level but also at tooth and tooth site levels. Dental caries in the permanent dentition is assessed by the DMF index. The index can be used to measure teeth (DMF-T) or sites affected (DMF-S). It represents the sum of either decayed (D), missing (M), and filled (F) teeth (T) or surfaces (S) and expresses the total caries experience of the individual at the time of observation. The index takes into account present (D), eliminated (M) and treated (F) lesions. Whether they have been treated by extraction or filling is of little concern as the basic idea behind the DMF system is the principle of adding previous and present signs of caries. The chapter by Manji and Fejerskov in the *Textbook of Clinical Cariology* (Manji and Fejerskov, 1996) offers useful teaching background material for discussion on quantification of caries. The DMF index could also serve as a basis for a discussion of the problem of analysing dental data at a tooth site-to-site level and how disease frequency is influenced because the same individuals may contribute with up to 128 sites when the DMF-S index is used. A useful point for a discussion of the many requirements for indices measuring dental diseases is the fact that the recorded disease prevalence comprises treatment components, M and F in the index, which are both strongly dependent on the available dental services and treatment philosophy. Students may also be asked to carry out examinations on each other to illustrate problems such as definitions of lesions, measures of disease progression, observer variation, and the concepts of validity and reliability. Finally, the analytic opportunities that the mouth offers, such as split mouth trials, because caries occurs symmetrically on both sides of the jaw, or other types of paired design should also be mentioned (Væth and Poulsen, 1998).

Ecologic studies

Two classic ecologic studies contributed to our knowledge about dental decay (Murray and Naylor, 1996). The first was the finding that there was an association between fluoride level in water and low caries experience. The fluoride/caries studies started when the so-called *Colorado Brown Stain* of teeth was detected. It was hypothesized that the agent responsible for the mottling was in the water, but chemical analysis failed to discover anything common to all drinking water associated with mottling. It was shown that the children who used spring water were free of mottling whereas those using the usual supply were not. Children born subsequent to a change of drinking water did not have mottled teeth. Later, fluoride was identified as the element common to water supplies related to mottled enamel. Then it was noticed that there was less caries in the communities with mottling. It was postulated that the fluoride might be adjusted to balance the risk of mottling against the benefits of less dental caries. Some years later an inverse relationship between the prevalence of mottled teeth and caries was demonstrated. A low prevalence of caries and a very mild fluorosis were found among some children drinking water with fluoride content of 1 part per million (ppm). This finding led to studies of controlled fluoridation in which the fluoride concentration in water was increased to 1.0 and 1.2 ppm in the test, but not in the control communities. Dental caries was reduced by half in the test communities. Ninety-five controlled studies in 20 countries have confirmed the findings (Murray and Naylor, 1996), and this preventive effect has resulted in water fluoridation in many communities. These findings offer a good basis for a discussion on the dose–response relationship and the public health role that epidemiology can play, whilst taking into account possible negative outcomes on health, in this case mottling, equity, and health economic aspects of population preventive programs.

The second large scale ecologic study on dental caries was the effect of wartime food rationing on the decline of dental caries. The historic evidence of a strong association between refined sucrose and dental caries has been well documented (Rugg-Gunn, 1996). The prevalence of caries doubled between the eleventh and the seventeenth centuries, but the most dramatic increase occurred during the late nineteenth century, when sugar consumption increased because duties on sugar were removed. Thereafter, caries prevalence increased except during the First and Second World Wars. The increases and decreases in dental caries that coincided with sucrose consumption demonstrated a positive dose–response relationship between sucrose consumption and caries. Subsequent animal and laboratory studies have confirmed the sucrose/caries relationship (Rugg-Gunn, 1996). The association between the intake of refined sugars and dental caries may thus teach students the basic aspects of causal inference in epidemiology.

The natural history of dental caries

Dental caries does not progress in a linear pattern, but has periods of more rapid progression followed by periods of quiescence and regression. Standardized radiographs can be used in longitudinal studies to assess the pattern of progress. Students can be shown how to standardize and score radiographs and become familiar with statistical analysis in cohort studies; for example, survival analysis. Examples of differences in progression pattern can be used to illustrate the effects of preventive agents and other preventive measures (Ekanayake and Sheiham, 1988). The concept of the minimum induction period, defined as the period of time from causal action until disease initiation, and the latent period, defined as the time interval between disease occurrence and detection of disease, may be introduced within this context (Rothman and Greenland, 1998). Methodologic issues in cohort studies (Slade and Caplan, 1999), and advantages and disadvantages of this design could be compared to other types of epidemiologic studies such as cross-sectional and case control studies.

Confounding is common in epidemiologic studies and adjustment for this type bias may be achieved during data analysis through regression modeling. The theoretical foundation or underlying biologic model and the selection of variables may, however, often be questioned. Furthermore, the students' attention may also be drawn to the fact that many papers omit to describe that the necessary assumptions for carrying out a particular multivariable analysis were met.

Time trends: the rise and fall of dental caries

Most industrialized countries have experienced a dramatic decline in dental caries in children since the early 1970s (Petersson and Bratthall, 1996). The reason for the decline is a good basis for discussing the relative importance of fluoride in different forms, diet change, shifts in diagnostic criteria, and more speculative hypotheses such as herd immunity and increased use of antibiotics (Petersson and Bratthall, 1996; Burt and Fejerskov, 1996; Richards and Banting, 1996). It is interesting to observe that the preventive work carried out in the dental sector has a different status from that in the health and medical field at large. It is often stated that the successes in dental health promotion and preventive care could, in various ways, stimulate and enrich thinking in other sectors. On the other hand, general health promotion and changes in social factors and general patterns of eating and the availability of more sugar-free products may have contributed to the decline of caries (Nadanovsky and Sheiham, 1995).

Periodontal disease

Diagnosing periodontal disease

Periodontal conditions and diseases are routinely diagnosed by simple observation of the periodontal tissues, the gingiva and the periodontal pocket, with mouth mirrors and dental probes, often supplemented by intraoral radiographs. Diagnosing periodontal disease can be used to illustrate many of the same problems concerning diagnosis of caries (Papapanou and Lindhe, 1997).

Quantification of periodontal disease

The quantification of periodontal disease poses similar problems to that of dental caries: practically all persons have experienced the disease. Consequently, comparison of fractions of the population affected by the disease is of little value. As a result, oral epidemiologists have constructed indices where they have used teeth or tooth surfaces as the basic unit. Whereas the DMF caries index could be considered relatively simple and straightforward, this is not the case with many gingival and periodontal indices. Most are a mixture of inflammation of gingiva, presence of dental calculus, pocket formation, or attachment loss around the teeth. Nevertheless, periodontal indices have been used extensively in many surveys. The chapter by Papapanou and Lindhe (1997) and the WHO publication, *Oral Health Surveys* (World Health Organization, 1997), may serve as an introduction to a discussion of the concept of these indices, and how they may have influenced our interpretation of epidemiologic periodontal studies and dental health policy.

The natural history of periodontal disease

The widely accepted model of the life history of periodontal disease is a disease that starts as gingivitis and inevitably progresses to destructive periodontal disease if no intervention occurs has been challenged (Socransky et al., 1984; Papapanou and Lindhe, 1997). The main criticism of the old model is misinterpretation of epidemiologic information and methods. Adult forms of destructive periodontal disease appear to be characterized by relatively short periods of exacerbation (bursts) separated by periods of remission lasting from a few days to a few years. The cumulative loss of periodontal attachment from the bursts of destruction is the basis for the old idea that destructive periodontal disease is a continuous, slowly progressive disease. A feature of periodontal diseases is the distribution of lesions in affected people. All the periodontal tissues adjacent to the 128 surfaces of teeth at risk are not at equal risk. The disease does not affect sites at random. It is also common in epidemiologic studies of periodontal disease to measure disease only at selected sites on a few teeth, so-called index teeth, which may give incorrect estimates of the disease in the population surveyed. Finally, the interpretation of data from epidemiologic studies of periodontal disease can be used to indicate how misinterpretations and incorrect statistical analysis can lead to major health policy and treatment decisions (Imrey, 1986).

Screening for oral disease

Screening for disease is commonly used and studies from within dentistry could serve as useful examples when discussing the principles and methods of screening for disease. A well known form of screening is the half-yearly dental examination. The scientific basis, the WHO criteria for screening, and public health aspects of such screening programs should be discussed (Wilson and Jungner, 1968; McNeil et al., 1975). Furthermore, the reproducibility and the accuracy of a diagnostic method expressed in terms of sensitivity and specificity should be discussed, with particular attention directed to the poor sensitivity and specificity regarding the diagnosis of caries. Students should be trained in entering hypothetical data into a diagnostic decision matrix to calculate and understand the importance of positive and negative predictive values of a diagnostic test, and especially how these values depend on disease prevalence. Hypothetical or 'real' caries data may be used to construct a curve showing the positive predictive values at different possible prevalence values (Hausen, 1997). The consequences concerning treatment in general and dental caries treatment in particular should be discussed, especially in view of the decline in caries.

Causal inference in oral epidemiology

As the search for causes is one of the main aims of epidemiology, considerable emphasis should be given to this subject (Rothman and Greenland, 1998; Scheutz and Poulsen, 1999). Numerous studies on dental caries offer an excellent opportunity to illustrate and discuss models of causation and the concept of sufficient and component causes. Causation and prevention may be considered relative terms and viewed as two sides of the same coin. Saying that dental caries is a multifactorial disease just reflects the fact that bacteria, as well as sugar and other factors, are needed for the caries to develop. However, refined sugars are a necessary factor for the occurrence of the disease. The other factors, such as the amount and type of sugar, frequency of sugar intake, age of the dentition, and availability of fluorides, are additional to sugars, not alternatives to them (Scheutz and Poulsen, 1999). When looking for causes of pathologic states the main emphasis should be on identifying those factors that determine whether or not people actually develop the disease. Prevention of dental caries may thus be used to illustrate that there can be many ways to prevent disease. For example, to suffer from caries there must be certain types of bacteria present, and refined sugars must be eaten frequently. The first condition is satisfied, as far as we know, in most individuals. The second, however, varies and it is this variation that is responsible for a high or low caries incidence. Analytic studies can be used to illustrate their use in the search for determinants. The simplistic model of periodontal destructive disease that evolved from epidemiologic studies and clinical research argues that the main 'cause' of the disease is dirty teeth. It might be worthwhile looking at how the concept developed of dirty teeth alone being sufficient to produce disease, and how this coincides with Rothman's model causal inference (Rothman and Greenland, 1998). Finally, it could be worthwhile to examine Bradford Hill's criteria for causal inference (Hill, 1965) with regard to dental caries and periodontal disease.

Epidemiologic information as a tool for planning interventions

Epidemiologic methods are used for identifying causes of diseases and establishing priorities and health activities. It is a commonly held assumption in the provision and organization of health services, including dental health services, that the need for healthcare can be determined objectively by clinical assessment by professionals. However, it is increasingly recognized that healthcare needs may be defined in other ways because the definition of a given state of ill-health, including dental ill-health, is open to much wider interpretation than the narrow clinical definition. Reference should be made to the impact of dental diseases on individuals and on society, the degrees of disability and dysfunction created by the disease, the perceptions and the attitudes of patients towards ill-health, and the social origins of many common illnesses (Sheiham and Spencer, 1997).

Students can carry out small surveys on people to assess their oral health needs. The gap between normative and perceived needs can be demonstrated by interviewing respondents about their needs. Here medical sociology and health economics can be integrated by discussing the concepts of health and illness, and putting the professional and lay views in a broader context. Epidemiology should be used to assist in making decisions on priorities and strategies. The concepts of high risk and population strategies described by Rose (1993) are used to illustrate how epidemiology and policy are interrelated. That is done by applying Rose's concepts to the current policy debate in dentistry, namely, should the main emphasis be on detecting and treating those at higher risk of disease rather than directing resources at the whole community to lower disease levels (Sheiham and Joffe, 1991). The advantages and disadvantages of the two approaches can be outlined. The implication of the high-risk strategy is that one should reach those most in need of intervention. This approach invites the question 'How can we identify them?' Another question is the ability of any method of screening to separate high- and low-risk groups in terms of sensitivity, specificity, and predictive values. Just as the high-risk strategy requires a scientific basis, both in technical matters (methods of identifying those at high risk) and evaluation (validity, effectiveness), the same is true of the whole population strategy. It depends upon epidemiologic, sociologic, and other kinds of research to identify important determinants of the diseases in question, and acting to change their prevalence in the appropriate direction. Rose (1993) has eloquently discussed the scientific basis for the whole population strategy. He draws the distinction between two kinds of etiologic questions: the first seeks the causes of cases: 'Why do some people get caries at this time?' and the second, the causes of the incidence 'Why do some populations have much caries while in others it is uncommon?' The whole population strategy attempts to control the determinants of the incidence and is therefore a more radical strategy.

Teaching methods and format

The key concepts and items to be taught on an undergraduate level course are covered during a two week course (Tables 21.1 and 21.2). The course takes place in the dental students' third year and the teaching is problem-based. All the teaching material is distributed to the students one week before the course starts. The material comprises relevant scientific articles, questions focusing on important aspects of the articles, small independent exercises based on real datasets, and one larger exercise to be completed on an individual basis after completion of the course. The background material consists of two books covering the basics of biostatistics and epidemiology, copies of a few relevant publications, and a booklet of formulae in statistics and epidemiology. To facilitate the learning process, the core elements of the biostatistics and epidemiology are also available on the internet at the department's homepage (*www.odont.au.dk/s&p*). Most of the teaching takes place in the computer lab where the students have access to various statistical packages and spreadsheets to facilitate the computations. Only a few core lectures are given during the course, either at the beginning of the day or when needed during the day. The exercises are completed as group work and all groups' answers and solutions are put on the department's home page. After the completion of each exercise a student from one group discusses the answers with another group, with a student from this group in a plenary session.

Assessing students' achievements

All teachers monitor the students' achievements throughout the course by their ability to complete exercises, the solutions produced by the group, and their contribution in the discussions. We seek to give feedback on performance to each student throughout the course. The final evaluation of each student is based on the answers to the exercise that must be completed after the course has finished. It is our firm belief that the format and teaching methods we use during the course enhance our objective to teach dental students basic statistics and epidemiological methods and to transform dental students into *critical consumers* of scientific dental research.

References

Bhopal, R. (1997). Which book? A comparative review of 25 introductory epidemiology textbooks. *Journal of Epidemiology and Community Health*, **51**, 612–22.

Burt, B. A., Albino, J. E., Carlos, J. P. *et al.* (1989). Advances in the epidemiological study of oral-facial diseases. *Advances in Dental Research*, **3**, 30–41.

Burt, B. A. and Fejerskov, O. (1996). Water fluoridation. In *Fluoride in dentistry*. (eds. O. Fejerskov, J. Ekstrand and B. A. Burt), pp. 275–90. Munksgaard, Copenhagen.

Ekanayake, L. E. and Sheiham, A. (1988). A method for analysing caries progression data. *Community Dental Health*, **5**, 19–27.

Greenberg, R. S., Daniels, S. R., Flanders, D., Eley, J. W. and Boring, J. R. (1993). *Medical epidemiology*, Prentice Hall International Limited, London.

Greenhalgh, T. (1998). *How to read a paper. The basics of evidence based medicine*, BMJ Publishing Group, London.

Hausen, H. (1997). Caries prediction – state of the art. *Community Dentistry and Oral Epidemiology*, **25**, 87–96.

Hill, B. (1965). The environment and disease: Association or causation. *Proceedings of the Royal Society of Medicine*, **55**, 295–300.

Imrey, P. B. (1986). Considerations in the statistical analyses of clinical trial in periodontics. *Journal of Clinical Periodontology*, **13**, 517–28.

Jakobsen, J. R. (1999). A survey of statistical methods used in dental literature. *Journal of Dental Education*, **63**, 350–2.

Manji, F. and Fejerskov, O. (1996). An epidemiological approach to dental caries. In *Textbook of clinical cariology*. (eds. A. Thylstrup and O. Fejerskov), pp. 159–91. Munksgaard, Copenhagen.

McNeil, B. J., Keeler, E. and Adelstein, S. J. (1975). Primer on certain elements of medical decision making. *N Engl J Med*, **293**, 211–15.

Murray, J. J. and Naylor, M. N. (1996). Fluorides and dental caries. In *The prevention of dental disease*. (ed. J. J. Murray), pp. 32–67. Oxford University Press, Oxford.

Nadanovsky, P. and Sheiham, A. (1995). Relative contribution of dental services to the changes in caries levels of 12-year-old-children in 18 industrialized countries in the early 1970s and early 1980s. *Community Dentistry and Oral Epidemiology*, **23**, 331–9.

Papapanou, P. N. and Lindhe, J. (1997). Epidemiology of periodontal disease. In *Clinical periodontology and implant dentistry*.(eds. J. Lindhe, T. Karring and N. P. Lang), pp. 69–101. Munksgaard, Copenhagen.

Petersson, H. G. and Bratthall, D. (1996). The caries decline: a review of reviews. *European Journal Oral Sciences*, **104**, 436–43.

Richards, A. and Banting, D. W. (1996). Fluoride in dentistry. In *Fluoride in dentistry*. (eds. O. Fejerskov, J. Ekstrand and B. A. Burt), pp. 328–346. Munksgaard, Copenhagen.

Rose, G. (1993). *The strategy of preventive medicine*, Oxford University Press, Oxford.

Rothman, K. J. and Greenland, S. (1998). *Modern epidemiology*, Lippincott-Raven Publishers, Philadelphia, PA.

Rugg-Gunn, A. J. (1996). Diet and dental caries. In *The prevention of dental disease.* (ed. J. J. Murray), pp. 3–31. Oxford University Press, Oxford.

Scheutz, F. and Poulsen, S. (1999). Determining causation in epidemiology. *Community Dentistry and Oral Epidemiology,* **27**, 161–70.

Scheutz, F. (1997). Basic principles and methods of oral epidemiology. In *Community Oral Health.* (ed. C. M. Pine), pp. 55–74. Butterworth–Heinemann, Oxford.

Sheiham, A. and Spencer, J. (1997). Health needs assessment. In *Community Oral Health.* (ed. C. M. Pine), pp. 39–54. Butterworth–Heinemann, Oxford.

Sheiham, A. and Joffe, M. (1991). Public dental health strategies for identifying and controlling dental caries in high and low risk populations. In *Markers of high and low risk groups and individuals for dental caries.* (ed. N. W. Johnson), Cambridge University Press, Cambridge.

Slade, G. D. and Caplan, D. J. (1999). Methodological issues in longitudinal epidemiologic studies of dental caries. *Community Dentistry and Oral Epidemiology,* **27**, 236–48.

Socransky, S. S., Haffajee, A. D., Goodson, J. M. and Lindhe, J. (1984). New concepts of destructive periodontal disease. *Journal of Clinical Periodontology,* **11**, 21–32.

Stat-Aid. *Programmed Learning for Understanding Statistics* (1992). R. Riegelman, L. Riegelman and R. Hirsch. Blackwell Science, Cambridge, Massachusetts, USA.

Statistix version 4.1 (1998). Analytical Software, Tallahassee, FL, USA.

Swinscow, T. D. V. and Campbell, M. J. (1996). *Statistics at square one,* BMJ Publishing Group, London.

Væth, M. and Poulsen, S. (1998). Comments on a commentary: statistical evaluation of split mouth caries trials. *Community Dentistry and Oral Epidemiology,* **26**, 80–3.

Wilson, J. M. G. and Jungner, G. (1968). *Principles and practice for screening for disease,* Public Health Paper No. 34. World Health Organization, Geneva.

World Health Organization (1997). *Oral health surveys, basic methods,* World Health Organization, Geneva.

Chapter 22

Epidemiology of injuries

Eleni Petridou and Dimitrios Trichopoulos

Introduction

Because epidemiology is the basic science of public health, and injuries represent a major public health problem, injury epidemiology should dominate the corresponding field, whereas injury prevention and control should be a priority in allocation of public health resources. This is rarely the case, however, and the course instructor should try to explain to the students why injury epidemiology has received so little attention, and so few epidemiologists have chosen injury as the topic of their preference.

Epidemiology has been the principal discipline in preparing the grounds for the prevention of infectious diseases, several forms of cancer, and most cardiovascular diseases. It should be admitted, however, that it has contributed relatively little towards the understanding of causation and towards the prevention of injuries. The teacher should put forward three possible issues, not necessarily mutually exclusive, that could explain the limited success of injury epidemiology in the past:

1. Currently used epidemiologic methods are not as appropriate for the investigation of injury occurrence as for the study of other diseases and causes of death.

2. Injuries have not been recognized as a major public health problem until relatively recently.

3. Different disciplines (e.g. medicine, public health, sociology, psychology, engineering, product design and city planning, political sciences, standardization bodies, law enforcement agencies) and different sectors of the economy, each with different interests and research methodologies, compete for the leadership in the effort towards injury prevention, a fact which may be an important underlying cause for the fragmented research and evaluation efforts that characterize this field.

The first issue should not be casually dismissed. Many of the component causes of cardiovascular, neoplastic, or infectious diseases are identifiable biologic entities, whereas the factors contributing to injuries are frequently of behavioral origin, poorly defined, and inadequately operationalized. Moreover, there are distinct differences in the natural history of acute and chronic diseases, on the one hand, and accidents and their consequences on the other. In addition, cohort studies which represent the method of choice in traditional epidemiology are compromised in injury research by our inability to specify in advance the proximal behavioral or environmental exposures that may have triggered an accident – for example, how a driver reacted to the exciting news announced on the radio or how a sexy poster by the road affected the attention of a motorcyclist. Case control studies have also specific limitations in injury research because instantaneous death and post-traumatic shock or denial of responsibility on the part of those involved in an accident tend to create serious selection and information bias. These arguments, although legitimate, do not challenge the applicability of the discipline of epidemiology to injury research, because neither animal studies nor randomized experiments can be contemplated in this field of research.

The second issue is the lack of awareness about the magnitude of the public health impact of injuries. It is a source of frustration for both injury researchers and health and safety workers. Even now, there are people who are very concerned about dioxin levels in food but pay no attention to the speed at which they drive, despite that reducing average speed by one kilometer per hour will reduce crashes by 4%, whereas quadrupling the average concentration of dioxin in the food could probably have no discernible effects. In addition, the high proportion of injuries among the young has a disproportionally large impact on life expectancy, a fact which is not immediately recognized by lay people or even some health professionals.

Thirdly, prevention of injuries and particularly of those caused by road traffic accidents is frequently mixed with strong economic interests and power politics. Safety regulations and aspects of road construction, for instance, frequently overwhelm epidemiologic arguments supported by valid data and plain logic.

This introduction, although defensive, may be more effective in capturing the interest of the students compared to the traditional one that relies on description of the magnitude of the injury problem but fails to address the applicability of the epidemiologic methods to injury etiology and prevention.[1, 2]

Teaching objectives

A course of general injury epidemiology for health professionals is usually of rather short duration. This is mainly because injury epidemiology is much more time-, place-, culture-, technology- and activity-specific than other branches of epidemiology. Moreover, the epidemiologic process for accidents (events) and injuries (lesions) is generally deductive rather than inductive, because causation of accidents and consequent injuries in the abstract can be easily conceptualized in the context of the laws of physics and chemistry. Thus, to expand on factual information about when, where, and by which mechanism accidents have been caused in a particular place or at a particular time serves no general course objective.

The overall goal of a short course on the epidemiology of accidents and injuries is to document the importance of this field of epidemiology for the prevention of accidents and consequent injuries. More specifically, the course should aim:

1. To familiarize students with research on environmental or personal risk factors for injuries.

2. To enable students to assess the relative effectiveness of alternative intervention strategies for injury prevention.

3. To enable students to evaluate the quality of health provision services and the impact of therapeutic interventions and rehabilitative processes.

Prevention of accidents corresponds to primary prevention, whereas prevention of death or serious injuries following an accident corresponds to secondary prevention. The overall goals can be accomplished by setting specific objectives. Thus, at the end of the course, the student is expected to be able:

+ To identify the reasons for the limited success of injury epidemiology in comparison to other fields of epidemiology.

+ To use the terms 'accident' or 'injury' correctly in particular situations.

+ To provide an adequate description for the causation of accidents in terms of energy transfer.

+ To name the major classification systems for accidents and injuries.

+ To describe the sources of data for accidents and injuries as well as their strengths and limitations.

+ To apportion fatal injuries in major etiologic categories.

+ To delineate the contribution of descriptive data on the circumstances surrounding the accident to the prevention of injuries.

+ To appreciate the potential of sentinel injury data collection and early warning systems for identification of hazardous products and evaluation of injury prevention programs.

+ To make the right choice of the epidemiologic study design that better addresses the working hypothesis.

+ To point out the limitations of traditional study designs, either cohort and case control studies or randomized controlled trials, when applied to injury epidemiology, and recognize the need to take into account complex exposure patterns in the assessment of injury risks.

+ To comment on the strengths and weaknesses of new epidemiologic designs, such as the case-crossover design.

+ To rank injuries correctly among other causes of ill-health with respect to mortality, morbidity, and potential years of life lost.

+ To explain why human behavior is frequently implicated in the causation of accidents, although it may not represent a priority target for accident control.

+ To distinguish between active and passive safety measures.

+ To write down the two basic physical equations that allow the determination of injury severity in road traffic accidents, falls, and other injuries caused by transfer of physical energy.

+ To describe the ten stages that summarize the theory of accident prevention, as conceptualized by William Haddon.

- To identify the importance of age and gender, occupation, socioeconomic status, and nature of leisure or other activities as risk factors for accidents.

- To distinguish between idiosyncratic accident proneness and accident proneness because of use of alcohol or psychotropic drugs.

- To name five transient events that may trigger an accident and indicate the appropriate methodology for the investigation of the role of such events in accident causation.

- To provide examples of how the increase of the area of dispersion and the prolongation of time required for energy dispersion reduces the severity of injuries.

- To explain why the severity of injuries is not a linear function of the speed of a vehicle involved in a crash.

- To describe the simple equations of physics that underlie the role of seat belts and protective helmets in reducing the severity of injuries.

- To indicate the approximate fraction of corresponding fatality that could be reduced by use of seat belts, child car restraints, and helmets.

- To identify at least one major difficulty in conducting an epidemiologic study aiming to assess the role of alcohol drinking on accident causation.

- To explain why the incidence of home and leisure accidents is grossly underestimated.

- To indicate whether active or passive safety measures should be a priority in occupational settings.

- To define how study results can be used for injury prevention and control.

Teaching contents

Terminology, classification, and sources of data

Issues of terminology, classification, and data sources need to be presented, even though it takes an extraordinary teacher to make this presentation without boring the students. It is preferable to define injuries as the consequences of involuntary transfer of energy as suggested by Haddon.[3]

The term 'accident' is distinct from the term 'injury' since accident is generally a cause of injury. However, there is a tendency in the scientific community to use the term injury in every instance, because the term accident overestimates the role of chance and discourages efforts to identify risk factors for injuries.[4,5] Intentional injuries, namely those caused by violence as well as suicides or suicide attempts, are not included among accidents, which is a pity, because these subjects, usually covered by forensic medicine and psychiatry, are generally more exciting for the students.

Accidents as causes of morbidity and mortality are classified either in terms of the nature and location of injury or on the basis of the conditions of occurrence of the accident. The student should be guided to the more widely used classification systems that describe the conditions of accidents, including the supplementary classification of external causes of injuries and poisonings (E-codes) of the World Health

Organization (WHO) International Statistical Classification of Diseases, Injuries and Causes of Death (International Classification of Diseases, ICD) in its ninth and tenth revision (ICD-9, ICD-10).[6,7] Despite their widespread use, these E-codes have been criticized as being inadequate for prevention purposes.[8] In response to these concerns, additional codings, such as NOMESCO[9] and ICECI[10], have been developed.

In clinical settings, injuries as a consequence of accidents but also as a result of violence can be evaluated on the basis of their nature (e.g. burns, poisonings, fractures) and anatomic location, according to ICD-9 or ICD-10. Moreover, the severity of injuries can be assessed through the use of various scales; some of which focus on the extent of anatomic damage, such as the abbreviated injury scale (AIS), the injury severity score (ISS), the pediatric trauma score (PTS), whereas others focus on the functional severity of a trauma, e.g. revised trauma score (RTS) and Glasgow coma scale (GCS).[11–15]

Students should be reminded that correct classification is a prerequisite for:

♦ Comparability of data between and within countries
♦ Assessment of time trends
♦ Evaluation of preventive efforts.

Deaths from accidents are usually accurately recorded, although problems can be generated by misclassification of suicides as accidental deaths or when there is a long delay between an accident and the subsequent death. Even among the European Union member states there may be a variable time limit to assign a hospital death to an injury. Thus, when the death occured, for example, within a week after the accident, this accident was considered as the underlying cause of death, whereas another adverse condition was cited as the underlying cause when the death occurred after a longer time interval.

In contrast to mortality statistics, morbidity data, including those derived from hospital admissions, are generally of limited reliability, with the exception of hospital statistics from Scandinavian countries, in which the unique identifying number system allows data linkage. Even in these countries, however, accidents not requiring hospitalization are inadequately recorded. In many countries there is now a trend to establish large databases covering all types of injuries that require hospital contact, although not necessarily hospital admission. Such databases are invaluable when the total dimensions of the injury problem need to be evaluated and when hospital statistics are unreliable or of questionable validity. Because sources of injury data vary by time and place the teacher should be familiar with the conditions relevant to the students and the nationality of the audience.[16]

Descriptive epidemiology

Among the 17 major categories of diseases and causes of death in the classification that has been adopted by the World Health Organization, injuries represent in the developed countries the third most common cause of death, following diseases of the circulatory system, and malignant neoplasms. It is worth emphasizing that, in many countries, injuries are responsible for as many or more years of life lost than cardiovascular diseases and malignant neoplasms, because the latter two categories generally affect older people, whereas injuries are concentrated among younger population groups.

In most developed countries after the first year of life and until the age of about 45 years accidents cause more deaths than any other category of disease (Table 22.1). Mortality rates from accidents are twice as high among men as women, and mortality by age follows a more or less typical pattern.[17] It declines gradually until the age of 5 years, is very low during the decade from 5 to 14 years, jumps to a very high level between 15 and 25 years, particularly among men, declines slowly until the age of about 45 years and then it increases progressively with ageing without reaching the very high levels noted among young men. Long-term trends depicting mortality rates from accidents were increasing in most developed countries until the 1950s, mainly on account of the increasing frequency of road traffic accidents. Subsequently, the trends have been reversed and declining rates have been observed following implementation of specific policies for injury prevention. In proportional terms, more than 50% of fatal injuries are caused by road traffic accidents, about one-third from home and leisure accidents, whereas 10–15% are of an occupational nature. Fatal accidents represent the peak of the pyramid that depicts the magnitude of the injury problem. Every case of fatal injury corresponds to about 30 cases of serious injury that require hospitalization and may lead to permanent disability, and about 500 cases of injuries that require some form of medical attention.

Etiologic considerations

Injuries are caused when energy is transferred to the human body at a rate and density that exceeds the resistance of human tissues.[17–19] Human behavior, however, can be a critical determinant of the frequency and severity of injuries, by affecting the frequency and the duration of exposure to various sources of energy as well as the rate and the density of energy transfer in susceptible individuals. Thus, most accidents have multifactorial etiology and their prevention, or the reduction of severity of the resulting injuries, can be accomplished through intervention at either the medium by which energy is transferred or by changing the behavior of the susceptible individual, which can reduce the frequency or duration of exposure to the source of energy. For example, the serious consequences for car occupants following a crash can be avoided through change of the behavior of the driver, so that the probability of an accident is reduced, or through passive protection measures built into the car and aiming to ameliorate the consequences of the accident.

It should be obvious that the multifactorial etiology of accidents is not conceptually different from the multifactorial etiology of most diseases. It is instructive to point out the existing parallels, e.g. the etiologic sequence of an agent (be that *Plasmodium vivax* in the case of malaria or kinetic energy in the case of a fracture) that via a vector (be that a mosquito or a motor vehicle, respectively) and following an exposure event (be that a mosquito bite or a car crash) results in human damage (malaria or fracture). In all instances, prevention can be accomplished by focusing on the etiologically interacting factor that appears more amenable to some form of intervention. Thus, childhood poisoning with aspirin is the result of a number of factors acting in conjunction: the tendency of babies to taste everything they touch; the accessibility of

Table 22.1 Leading causes of death in high-income countries (both sexes) 1998

Rank	0–4 years	5–14 years	15–44 years	45–59 years	≥ 60 years	All ages
1	Perinatal conditions 53 198	Road traffic injuries 5 313	Road traffic injuries 76 249	Ischaemic heart disease 140 620	Ischaemic heart disease 1 719 015	Ischaemic heart disease 1 883 763
2	Congenital abnormalities 25 459	Congenital abnormalities 1 491	[???]	Trachea/bronchus/ lung cancers 67 308	Cerebrovascular disease 835 735	Cerebrovascular disease 893 182
3	Acute lower respiratory infections 5 744	Leukaemia 1 470	Interpersonal violence 26 196	Cerebrovascular disease 43 867	Trachea/bronchus/ lung cancers 346 568	Trachea/bronchus/ lung cancers 422 347
4	Measles 5 342	[???]	Ischaemic heart disease 24 128	Breast cancers 40 126	Acute lower respiratory infections 286 658	Acute lower respiratory infections 306 187
5	Diarrhoeal diseases 4 192	Interpersonal violence 926	HIV/AIDS 23 462	Cirroesis of the liver 38 948	Chronic obstructive pulmonary disease 264 968	Chronic obstructive pulmonary disease 280 168
6	Pertussis 3 475	Acute lower respiratory infections 821	Cirrhosis of the liver 13 285	Self-infected injuries 31 851	Colon/rectum cancers 207 234	Colon/rectum cancers 242 996
7	Road traffic injuries 2 328	Nutritional/ endocrine disorders 775	Cerebrovascular disease 12 680	Colon/rectum cancers 30 481	Diabetes mellitus 143 018	Diabetes mellitus 161 069
8	Nutritional/ endocrine disorders 1 853	Self-[???]infected injuries[???]	Breast cancers 12 137	Road traffic injuries 22 105	Stomach cancers 118 001	Breast cancers 160 139

Table 22.1 Leading causes of death in high-income countries (both sexes) 1998 *continued*

Rank	0–4 years	5–14 years	15–44 years	45–59 years	≥ 60 years	All ages
9	[???]	Fires 666	Trachea/bronchus/ lung cancers 8 433	Stomach cancers 20 447	Prostate cancers 111 173	Stomach cancers 143 310
10	Interpersonal violence 1 311	Cerebrovascular disease 407	[???]7 700	Pancreas cancers 13 814	Breast cancers 107 874	Road traffic injuries 141 656
11	Meningitis 1 144	Inflammatory cardiac disease 396	Leukaemia 6 753	Chronic obstructive pulmonary disease 13 759	Dementias 97 966	Self-infected injuries[???] 129 933
12	Fires 1 048	Lymphoma 337	Lymphoma 6 286	Diabetes mellitus 13 716	Pancreas cancers 83 422	Cirrhosis of the liver 121 816
13	Dementias 959	War injuries 301	Inflammatory cardiac disease 5 963	Lymphoma 13 412 81 798	Nephritis/nephrosis	Prostate cancers 114 807
14	Inflammatory cardiac disease 851	Dementias 297	Colon/rectum cancers 5 267	Mouth and oropharynx cancers 12 840	Lymphoma 70 824	Dementias 104 719
15	Tetanus 741	[???]	[???]	Oesophagus cancers 10 735	Cirrhosis of the liver 69 489	Pancreas cancers 99 126

Source: World Health Report 1999 Database.

pills when they are packaged in childproof containers, the appealing color of child-hood aspirin pills; the carelessness of the parents, who may leave medicines and other dangerous chemicals in easily accessible places; the lack of supervision; the large num-ber of pills in each package allowing poisoning with large doses. The constellation of these factors can be depicted by a triangle that is formed by the responsible factors; that is, the poisoning agent (aspirin), the host (child's developmental characteristics) and the environment (container, storage, supervision).

In this instance, it is difficult to allocate degrees of responsibility to individual fac-tors even when the other interactive causal factors remain intact. Therefore, the pri-mary objective of epidemiologic research towards the prevention of injuries relies on the recognition of the multifactorial origin of accidents and subsequent injuries, and the identification of the 'weak link' in the causal sequence. The use of safe packaging that precludes easy opening by toddlers can solve the problem to a very large extent, without attempting to change behavioral interacting factors that are known to be difficult to modify. This is why there is a general tendency to implement measures of passive prevention which are essentially technological, rather than measures of active prevention which focus on behavioral modification. Examples of passive prevention measures are: use of childproof packaging for medicines and chemicals; use of bal-cony fences that are sufficiently high and dense to restrict the toddlers from falling from a height; the institution of smoking detectors; and the regulation of thermostats so that hot water burns can be avoided. It should be emphasized, however, that most accidents involve manmade factors, whether in connection with motor vehicles, high-ways, poisonous chemicals, consumer products or swimming pools. In fact, the envi-ronment that causes injuries is the one that has been created by mankind; in this sense it can be redesigned by human beings to become safer.[16]

At this stage, it is worth repeating to the students that injuries are caused by the transfer of energy to susceptible individuals and to indicate that the transfer of mechanical energy is the most common mechanism of injuries. Indeed, road traffic accidents and falls are caused by the transfer of mechanical energy. Students are usu-ally eager to learn how to quantify the expected energy transfer and thus estimate the expected damage. They should be reminded of two basic equations in physics:

$$E = \tfrac{1}{2} mv^2 \qquad \text{(Equation 1)}$$

where E = energy, m = mass and v = velocity,

$$V = \sqrt{2gs} \qquad \text{(Equation 2)}$$

where v = velocity, g = acceleration or deceleration and s = the distance covered under the influence of acceleration or deceleration.

Thus, two cars crashing while moving in opposite directions with the relatively small speed of 25 km/h (~7 m/s) each, confer to their occupants consequences equal to those that would have been created if they were freefalling from a height of 10 m under the influence of gravity (the reference speed should be 25 km/h * 2 = 14 m/s).

Solving the second of the two equations for g indicates that the deceleration, which reduces the speed to zero, is inversely proportional to the distance covered by an individual during that crash. This is the principle underlying the widely used measure of passive safety that consists of the gradual (prolonged) collapse of the anterior or posterior part of the car as contrasted to the passenger cabin that should remain intact.

In a similar spirit, in explaining the risk factors for electrocution, the teacher should invoke the principles of physics regarding electricity. The consequences of electrocution are a function of the intensity of the electric current, which in turn is inversely related to the electric resistance of the body. The latter is substantially reduced (more than 10-fold) when the body is wet.

The theory of accident prevention

In presenting the theory of accident prevention the teacher should avoid trivializing the subject by invoking a collection of simple unrelated advisory statements, however useful the latter may be. Instead, the teacher should discuss the prevention of accidents in the context of the ten discrete countermeasure strategies, as conceptionalized by the late William Haddon, a pioneer in this field.[3,20] These are indicated below:

1. Preventing creation of an agent by creating conditions that control energy release without actually reducing it (e.g. by increasing the distance between the wheels of a car, by installation of thermostats that control water temperature in the household, or by building nuclear power plants far from inhabited areas).

2. Reducing the amount, and thus the density, of the agent, by controling the dispersion of the sources of energy (e.g. prescription of drugs in limited quantities, storage of toxic materials in much smaller quantities, establishment of nuclear power plants with smaller size reactors).

3. Preventing release of the agent, namely avoidance of the risk by preventing or reducing the release of energy (e.g. speed limits).

4. Modifying the rate or spatial distribution of the agent (e.g. use of seat belts, installing slow burning materials in airplane cabins).

5. Separating the host and the agent in space or time (e.g. exclusion of speed boats from swimming areas, or regulation of traffic through traffic lights).

6. Separating the agent (energy source) from the susceptible host by interposition of a material barrier facilitates the dispersion of energy over a greater area (e.g. helmets, airbags).

7. Modifying the relevant qualities of the agent, namely reducing the hazardous characteristics of the energy source (e.g. smoothing of angles or cutting endings of household utensils and furniture).

8. Strengthening the susceptible host by increasing the resistance of the human body (e.g. good nutrition and physical activity).

9. Countering the injury already caused by the agent, through timely postimpact care aiming to reduce the consequences of energy release (e.g. first aid system, intensive care units).

10. Stabilizing, repairing, and rehabilitating the injured host by means of specialized personnel and health care units.

It is clear that there are substantial overlappings between these ten countermeasures and also that the majority focus on primary prevention, whereas others focus on secondary prevention and on traditional care. In general, when the energy release is substantial, prevention should focus on one of the first described countermeasure strategies, whereas when the energy release is limited, control should be based on one or more of the latter ones.

Risk factors for accidents

There are no risk factors that are important for every type of accident in every population group. In general, however, the frequency and severity of accidents depend on a series of factors, such as:

- Age and gender (men are usually at higher risk and the risk is higher among the 15–24 year age group and towards the end of life).

- Occupational type (construction workers are generally at higher risk) or nature of leisure activity (the risk is very high among rock climbers).

- The safety coefficient of structures, processes, consumer products, etc. which is a function of legislation, regulations, and safety standards.

- The area of dispersion and the prolongation of the time required for energy dispersion are inversely associated with the risk and the severity of accidents. Helmets increase the dispersion of the energy from a crash, whereas seat belts increase both the time for deceleration as well as the spread of the energy over the various sites of the body.

- Accident proneness, which may be caused by neurologic diseases or created through use of psychotropic drugs or by some behavioral patterns.

- Transient high-risk behaviors (emotional stress, attention detraction by using a cellular phone or changing a radio program, etc.) dominate the etiology of about two-thirds of accidents.[21,22]

Although behavioral problems contribute to the majority of accidents it is not easy to identify individuals at high risk for such behaviors on the basis of a psychological profile. Instead, high-risk individuals should be identified through their tendency to drink or to use psychotropic drugs while driving, or among those who drive very long distances, like truck drivers. The teacher should treat this issue carefully, by avoiding stigmatization of a category of individuals as 'accident prone'. At the same time he/she should stress the fact that widespread behaviors can be instrumental in the causation of several accidents. This is the point to introduce the philosophy of legal measures that have a strict paternalistic dimension, an issue that has been controversial in libertarian circles: 'It is not the business of the state to force me to use a seat belt, so long as I do not endanger the life of anybody than myself' is a hollow but commonly used argument.

It has always been challenging for the investigators to develop formulas that would derive probabilities of accidents (risks) associated with various occupational or leisure activities taking into account exposure-related variables. This is also a request on the part of professional organizations such as sports associations as well as of insurance companies. As Sue Baker has stressed, however:

... the search for personal risk factors that would predict which members of a homogeneous group would be injured was doomed to failure and distracted the investigators from performing a descriptive study of the circumstances of injury that would have had far greater potential for injury reduction.[18]

Major accident categories

Road traffic accidents

Road traffic accidents (RTA) are responsible for about 50% of accidents in most developed countries, and a gradually increasing proportion in developing countries. Thus, they deserve special consideration. The teacher, however, should be careful to avoid sentimentalism and instead concentrate on issues that emerge from the examination of the basic issues related to the causation of injuries. In an RTA the severity of injuries depends on the deceleration which is imposed on the riders of the cars, or the pedestrians who are hit by vehicles during the so-called 'secondary' or 'human' stage of the crash. During this stage the speed of the riders on account of the inertia is suddenly reduced to zero as their bodies crash into the mechanical objects of the immobilized vehicle. Similarly, the speed acquired by the pedestrians after a vehicle hits them is suddenly reduced to zero, following their secondary crash on to the road or another immovable object.

The deceleration is a function of the ratio v^2/s, where v = velocity and s = the distance covered by the body during the time that the speed is reduced to zero, under the influence of deceleration during the secondary crash. The numerator demonstrates why high speeds have disproportionally large consequences, since a crash at 60 km/h has almost ten times more serious consequences than a crash with a speed of 20 km/h.

The examination of the role of the denominator in the ratio v^2/s demonstrates the importance of the seat belt. During the crash of the vehicle (primary crash) the anterior mechanical parts of most modern vehicles are squeezed in such a progressive way that the energy is gradually absorbed. As a consequence, the reduction of the speed of the vehicle to zero is accomplished in a distance of about 30–50 cm. The car cabin and the belted occupants follow the same trajectory. In contrast, a passenger who is not using a seat belt crashes (on account of the inertia) with the full original speed of the vehicle to the anterior mechanical part of the car. In this latter instance, the reduction of the original speed to zero takes place while a distance of only a few centimeters is covered. The consequences of the high deceleration of the body should be obvious. It is clear that seat belts are useful because they force the users to follow the movement of the vehicle, and allow them to exploit the much smaller deceleration of the primary crash, rather than the high deceleration that would have characterized the secondary crash. A seat belt has been estimated to reduce the probability of serious injury or death by about 40%.

The expansion of the airbag at the moment of crash also contributes to the prolongation of the distance covered while velocity declines to zero. Moreover, it conveys additional protection because the released energy is spread over a larger area. It should be obvious that seat belts, preferably three-point seat belts, and airbags (in passenger cars) should be available for as many car occupants as possible.

The teacher should also make sure that sufficient information is provided to the students about child car restraints, because children are frequently over-represented among car crash victims. The effectiveness of child car restraints in reducing serious injuries and deaths has been estimated to exceed 70%.

Case fatality ratio is particularly high among motorcycle riders but can be reduced by about 80% through the use of suitable and properly functioning helmets. It is worth stressing that the effectiveness of injury protection provided by helmets is a function of their quality and that quality helmets have a dated life, indicated by an expiry date.

The prevention of RTA can be substantially advanced by the investigation of place and time variables, namely place clustering, time periodicity and time–place clustering. It is unfortunate that deductive epidemiology studies are not more frequently used for road traffic injuries, because small 'outbreaks' of injuries may be as common as outbreaks of infectious diseases.

The emphasis on injury epidemiology in relation to behavioral factors should not lead the instructor to underestimate the critical importance of technical factors. These factors refer to vehicles or to the road system and may focus on secondary prevention, e.g. larger cars, seat belts or unyielding car cabins, as well as on primary prevention, e.g. increased visibility, antiblocking systems or elevated braking lights. Research and implementation of these developments by contemporary car industry as well as road auditing have a potentially high contribution to the reduction of the RTA toll.

A final but epidemiologically complicated issue is the role of ethanol and recreational drugs in the causation of road traffic injuries. None has the right to challenge the basic principle that drinking and driving should be separate activities. Nevertheless, one should also admit that the undertaking of proper analytic studies to evaluate the relation between drinking of alcoholic beverages or consumption of recreational drugs and driving, especially among the younger or relatively inexperienced drivers, is a methodologically extremely demanding task.

Home and leisure accidents

Home and leisure accidents (HLA) are extremely common but their low fatality reduces their importance in terms of mortality rates. A characteristic of HLA and of their associated injuries is that their epidemiologic study relies on very limited data in comparison to those available for the study of RTA. The teacher should lose no opportunity to stress the importance of HLA databases that have been relatively recently established in several countries and are providing the means for the documentation of the characteristics of HLA.[23]

Until recently, progress in the prevention of HLA has relied on descriptive information concerning case series or even case reports. Examples of preventive measures that were instituted on the basis of simple descriptive epidemiologic data are usually given by mechanism of injury; that is, falls and exposure to inanimate mechanical forces, burns, poisoning, drowning and submersion, and contact with heat or hot substances. Examples of such preventive measures can be found in textbooks concerning the epidemiology and prevention of injuries.[16–19]

Occupational injuries

Epidemiologic studies on occupational injuries, however imperfect, have converged in indicating that the prevention of these injuries should rely on passive measures and not require special attention or precautions on the part of the worker. The role of epidemiology, in this instance, is to document the existence of excess risk in various types of jobs or activities, and to provide risk profiles and attributable risks. The epidemiologic approach does not differ much from that commonly used in occupational medicine: calculation of standardized ratios or, at a minimum, proportional ratios.

Upgrading injury epidemiology

In developed countries injuries represent the most common cause of death during the first four decades of life and reduce life expectancy as much as malignant neoplasms and cardiovascular disease.[23] Likewise, RTAs account for more years of potential life lost than any other specific nosologic entity (Figs 22.1 and 22.2). Perhaps more importantly, deaths from injuries are at least 20 times more frequent than deaths from AIDS, environmental pollution, passive smoking, ozone depletion, and many other causes that have galvanized social reaction. It is generally accepted that advancements in epidemiology have preceded the curtailment of mortality rates from infectious and cardiovascular diseases and several forms of cancer. It is clear, however, that the epidemic of injuries in many populations remains unabated and there is an urgent need to expand the inductive and deductive epidemiologic investigation of injuries.

Injury epidemiology may not be as intriguing and intellectually stimulating as some other branches of epidemiology, but it has considerable potential to prepare the grounds for further reduction of premature mortality.[24] It is the duty of teachers of epidemiology to present these facts to all health professionals. In particular, epidemiologists need training to convey to the students that social responsibility is as important as intellectual satisfaction in the personal agendas of health professionals.

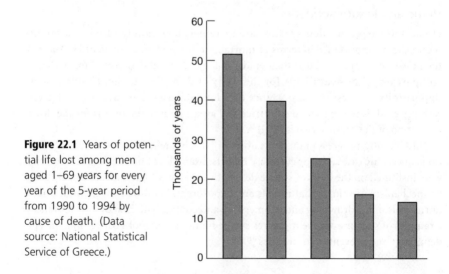

Figure 22.1 Years of potential life lost among men aged 1–69 years for every year of the 5-year period from 1990 to 1994 by cause of death. (Data source: National Statistical Service of Greece.)

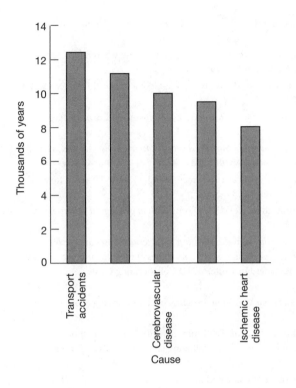

Figure 22.2 Years of potential life lost among women aged 1–69 years for every year of the 5-year period from 1990 to 1994 by cause of death. (Data source: National Statistical Service of Greece.)

Course evaluation and student's assessment

For lower level students, the ability to recall basic data of general applicability, especially to study design, and ability to link particular preventive measures to Haddon stages and basic laws of physics, should represent adequate evidence that they have met the course objectives. A series of multiple choice questions distributed to students for self-evaluation and subsequently discussed in the class provides an opportunity to refresh the recently acquired knowledge. Short essays or multiple choice questions could cover the evaluation component of the overall assessment of the students after the course.

Advanced level students in injury epidemiology can be evaluated by the development of a study design to investigate the role of a particular condition or activity in the causation of accidents. Alternatively, students can describe issues associated with assessment of an intervention project. The process is challenging for both the student and the instructor; in some cases the teacher may be challenged because injury epidemiology is full of subtle and complex issues.

References

1. **Petridou E.** Injury prevention: an uphill battle. *Injury Prevention* 1995;1:8.
2. **Petridou E.** Epidemiology and injury prevention. *Injury Prevention* 1998;3:75–6.

3. **Haddon W. Jr.** Energy damage and the ten countermeasure strategies. *Human Factors* 1973;15:355–66.

4. **Langley J. D.** The need to discontinue the use of the term 'accident' when referring to unintentional injury events. *Accid Anal Prev* 1988;20:1–8.

5. **Loimer H., Driur M., Guarnieri M.** Accidents and acts of God: a history of the terms. *Am J Public Health* 1996;86:101–7.

6. World Health Organization. *International Classification of Diseases*, 9th revision. Geneva, WHO, 1977.

7. World Health Organization. *International Statistical Classification of Diseases and related health problems*, 10th revision. Geneva, WHO, 1992.

8. **Langley J. D., Chalmers D. J.** Coding the circumstances of injury: ICD-10 a step forward or backwards? *Injury Prevention* 1999;5:247–53.

9. Nordic Medico-Statistical Committee. *NOMESCO classification of external causes of injuries.* Copenhagen, NOMESCO, 1996.

10. World Health Organization. *International classification for external causes of injuries (ICECI): guidelines for counting and classifying external causes of injuries for prevention and control.* Amsterdam, Consumer Safety Institute, WHO Collaborating Center on Injury Surveillance, 1998.

11. **Copes W. S., Champion H. R., Sacco W. J.** *et al.* Progress in characterizing anatomic injury. *J Trauma* 1990;30:1200–6.

12. **Baker S. P., O'Neill B., Haddon W. Jr.** *et al.* The Injury Severity Score. A method for describing patients with multiple injuries and evaluating emergency care. *J Trauma* 1974;14:187–96.

13. **Teasdale G., Jennett B.** Assessment of coma and impaired consciousness: a practical scale. *Lancet* 1974;ii:81–3.

14. **Champion H. R., Sacco W. J., Carnazzo A. J., Copes W., Fouty W. J.** Trauma Score. *Crit Care Med* 1981;9:672–6.

15. **Tepas J. J., Mollitt D. L., Talbert J. L., Bryant M.** The pediatric trauma score as a predictor of injury severity in the injured child. *J Pediat Surg* 1987;22:14–18.

16. **Christoffel T., Scavo Gallagher S.** *Injury prevention and public health: practical knowledge, skills and strategies.* Gaithersburg, Maryland, Aspen Publishers, Inc., 1999.

17. **Baker S. P., O'Neil B., Ginsburg M. J., Guohua L.** *The injury fact book*, 2nd edn. New York, Oxford University Press, 1992.

18. **Mohan D., Tiwari G.** *Injury prevention and control.* London, Taylor & Francis, 2000.

19. **Robertson L. S.** *Injury epidemiology.* New York, Oxford University Press, 1992.

20. **Haddon W. Jr.** On the escape of tigers: an ecological note. *Am J Public Health* 1970;60:2229–34.

21. **Redelmeier D. A., Tibshirani R. J.** Association between cellular telephone calls and motor vehicle collisions. *N Engl J Med* 1997;336:453–8.

22. **Petridou E., Trichopoulos D., Trohanis D., Dessypris N., Karpathios Th.** Transient exposures and the risk of childhood injury: a case-crossover study in Greece. *Epidemiology* 1998;9:622–5.

23. **Krug E.** *Injury: a leading cause of the global burden of disease.* Geneva, WHO, 1999.

24. **Petridou E.** Childhood injuries in the European Union: can epidemiology contribute to their control? *Acta Paediatr,* accepted for publication

Selected websites

- American Association of Poison Control Centers
  http://www.aapcc.org
- Association for the Advancement of Automotive Medicine
  http://www.carcrash.org
- Building Safe Communities
  http://www.edc.org/HHD/csn/bsc
- E-codes (workbook/spreadsheet-based listing of ICD-9-CM E-codes and their associated mechanisms and intent groups)
  http://www.pgh.auhs.edu/cvic/Ecode%20CDC%20matrix%20lookup.zip
- Harvard Injury Control Research Center
  http://www.hsph.harvard.edu/Organizations/hera/hicc.html
- Injury Control and Emergency Health Services Section of the American Public Health Association
  http://www.injurycontrol.com/ICEHS/
- Injury Prevention (journal)
  http://www.bmjpg.com/data/jip.htm
- Johns Hopkins Center for Injury Research and Policy
  http://jhsph.edu/Research/Centers/CIRP
- National Center for Injury Prevention and Control (CDC)
  http://www.cdc.gov/ncipc
- National Injury Surveillance Unit (Australia)
  http://www.nisu.flinders.edu.au/welcome.html

Chapter 23

Genetic epidemiology

Harry Campbell

Introduction

A major challenge for epidemiology in the future is understanding the role of genetic risk factors and how genetic factors interact with environmental factors in causing disease. There is a clear need for all epidemiologists to understand the potential for investigation of genetic risk opened up by the sequencing of the human genome and by the developments in genetic technology. Genetic epidemiology concerns itself with questions such as:

+ What is the prevalence of gene variants in different populations?
+ What is the risk (absolute and relative) of disease associated with these variants?
+ What is the contribution of gene variants to the occurrence of disease in different populations? (attributable risk)
+ What is the risk of disease associated with gene–gene and gene–environment interactions?
+ What is the validity of genetic tests?

To read relevant textbooks and follow leading articles published in the field of genetic epidemiology, it is important that students have or acquire a minimum literacy in the use of basic genetics terms and concepts, and have some knowledge of basic genetic laboratory techniques. A number of 'primers' have been published in textbooks or appear on the Internet. Teachers should recommend one they can make easily accessible to their students (see list of web resources below).

There are relatively few books that could serve as a course text in genetic epidemiology. A major problem is that, as genetic technology advances rapidly, new approaches to the study of genetic risk factors become possible and supersede previous approaches that become less favored or obsolete. It is more likely, therefore, that background reading to complement teaching will be based on selected recent journal articles or web resources than on one or two textbooks. It is important that students are directed towards and introduced to relevant journals and web sites in which the latest methods are described and discussed. This serves as an adjunct to coursework but also supports students' subsequent education in genetic epidemiology after they have completed the formal taught course. Journals that fit into this category (such as the *American Journal of Human Genetics*) can be found in the web resources noted below. In addition, general epidemiology journals such as *American Journal of Epidemiology*, *Epidemiology Reviews*, *Epidemiology*, and *International Journal of Epidemiology* are increasingly publishing articles of investigations of genetic risk factors and reviews of genetic epidemiology study designs. These are usually rather more comprehensible to the student than the more detailed discussion found in specialist journals such as *Genetic Epidemiology*.

Teaching objectives

An introductory course should concentrate on principles and important concepts together with a general introduction to specific methods or analytic procedures. More detailed exploration of specific methods is best targeted at students who are currently undertaking research which requires the application of these methods since, as noted above, the precise details of methods and analysis programs are regularly evolving and improving. A short course for undergraduate students could cover basic genetic concepts, define genetic epidemiology and the type of research questions it addresses, give a concise description of the main approaches, and note their uses, advantages, and disadvantages. A postgraduate course could follow the curricular outline given below. This could be presented as a module within a general MSc program in epidemiology, a stand-alone course, or as a complete MSc in genetic epidemiology. The length of the course would govern the depth of coverage and amount of 'hands-on' practical sessions working with computer programs. Longer courses would normally contain a supervised assignment or research project that requires students to apply the knowledge and skills acquired in the course.

All courses should equip students with a basic understanding of how to address the following hierarchy of research questions in genetic epidemiology:

♦ Does the disease cluster in families?

♦ Is the clustering caused by genetic or environmental factors?

♦ Is there evidence for a genetic factor? (Can a specific mode of inheritance be identified?)

♦ Can the genetic risk factor be localized?

♦ Do environmental factors modify the expression of the genetic factor? (Is there evidence of gene–environment interaction?)

Teaching contents

The exact content of the course will depend on the students' background, their particular interests, and the length of time available for the course. One suggestion for the structure of an introductory course in genetic epidemiology for those interested in understanding common complex disorders (rather than rare Mendelian disorders) is given in Table 23.1.

Table 23.1 Example of a course curriculum

1. Review of basic genetic concepts and principles of laboratory genetic techniques (optional)

2. Genotypes and phenotypes

    Hardy–Weinberg equilibrium

    Penetrance

    Heterogeneity

    Other concepts – anticipation, imprinting, genetic drift, founder effects, mutation, selection

3. How to study whether a disease has a 'genetic' component

    Twin studies

    Adoption studies

    Admixture studies

    Migration studies

    Segregation analysis

    Measurement of the risk ratio, lambda

4. How to identify whether specific genetic factors are related to disease

    Approaches to complex disease:

    Family-based and population-based approaches

    Candidate gene and whole genome screen (positional cloning) approaches

    Population characteristics favoring study of genetic factors

    Need for multidisciplinary collaboration

    Important epidemiologic considerations

    Ascertainment bias

    Sample size

    Multiple testing

    Confounding

    Causal inference

5. Major study designs

    Parametric linkage analysis

    Non-parametric linkage analysis

    Association studies based on linkage disequilibrium

    Comparison of strengths and weaknesses of linkage and association approaches

    Shared segment analysis

    Approaches to study of quantitative traits

Table 23.1 Example of a course curriculum   *continued*

6. How to study gene–environment interactions
Study designs
Sample size
Quantification of risk
7. Laboratory genetic analysis
Genotype misclassification
DNA collection and storage
8. Ethical and public health issues
The impact of genetic research on patients and their families
9. Computer programs for data analysis

Teaching method and format

Principles and concepts can be taught by didactic methods but are best illustrated with many examples from the literature and from the teacher's own experience. Many concepts may be difficult to grasp initially. The liberal use of examples reinforces the points made by approaching the concept from a different angle and may aid understanding. It can also help pace the teaching so that the course does not simply present a large number of new ideas without a break, risking students becoming lost or losing concentration. Examples can be presented in a way that invites active participation by the class and is therefore a useful way of checking whether or not students have understood new concepts.

It is essential that there is a strong 'hands-on' element, with computer practicals so that students can gain experience in handling data and can be introduced to computer programs used for analysis. At the very least this should be provided as a demonstration. Ideally, students should have the opportunity for guided practice. However, there are relatively few people using 'genetic epidemiology' programs and methods are constantly being updated. This has resulted in there being much less investment in making user-friendly interfaces to these programs than in other areas of epidemiology. This presents a problem for teaching computer practical sessions. In an introductory course much time can be wasted instructing students in the mechanics of how to operate command-driven programs with user-unfriendly interfaces. Teachers should avoid devoting any significant time to this unless the course specifically aims to teach skills in a particular technique or with specific programs. When the computer programs are complicated to operate it is better either to give a demonstration or to give each student a detailed set of instructions of the steps required so time is not wasted. Teachers should end each session by summarizing the aims of the session and reviewing what was done. They should also highlight general principles that can be taken from the example. This helps to offset the tendency for students to become so involved in details of the operation of the program that they lose sight of the relevance of what they are doing. These sessions should also give details of where these programs can be obtained. An outstanding example of a web resource giving these details is the Rockefeller website (see references).

Where calculations can be performed easily by hand tabulation or by use of a simple spreadsheet then opportunities should be given in the course for students to tackle the analysis of illustrative datasets. Examples of where this may be appropriate include the analysis of data from transmission disequilibrium test (TDT) studies or using data to illustrate the effect of population stratification on risk estimates in association studies.

Once the principles of a particular method have been taught and an example given in a computer demonstration or guided worked example, then it may be helpful to give students a reprint of a recent publication which uses this approach and ask them to read this critically overnight. This can then be discussed as a class exercise the following day. This is a useful way of reinforcing understanding of the method by setting it in context. It can also be used to check that students have grasped the key issues and for introducing further refinements or more advanced issues for individual follow-up by students.

In some courses the teacher may wish to consider setting aside time to demonstrate a few basic techniques in a genetics laboratory. This investment of time is, depending on the background of students, worthwhile as part of the introductory section of a longer course which is run over several weeks or months. An appreciation of the complexity and validity of laboratory methods can help students read published reports critically and interpret results appropriately.

Teaching notes

This section will follow the curricular outline described above, will draw attention to some key issues to cover, and will identify teaching resources which could be used to develop teaching materials on these topics. There are many textbooks and web resources which can be used to explain basic genetic concepts (see examples in the list of web resources below). It is essential that the teacher check understanding of concepts as they occur in the course or, if necessary, at the outset of the course.

It is worth spending time ensuring that students understand the Hardy–Weinberg equilibrium. Students should be shown how to count allele frequencies and how to calculate genotype frequencies in the next generation given known allele frequencies. They should be aware of some of the applications of measuring or comparing allele frequencies; for example, in comparing two populations or in association studies.

How to study whether a disease has a 'genetic' component

The role of more traditional epidemiologic study designs such as adoption studies, admixture studies, and migration studies has been reviewed in the textbook by Khoury (Khoury *et al.* 1993). The teacher may decide to focus the teaching on the more recent DNA-based study approaches described below or may wish to review briefly the role of the more traditional approaches in estimating the relative contribution of genetic and environmental components of disease risk.

Twin studies can measure the contribution of a genetic component to total variation: this is based on measuring concordance between twins. Students should understand that concordance can be quoted in two different ways (pair-wise and proband-wise). They should be familiar with the correct interpretation of the main comparisons between monozygous and dizygous twins (reared together or apart) and their other siblings. They should understand that the calculated heritability estimates are not absolute but may vary in different environmental settings. A published example of estimating heritability by means of a twin study should be discussed with students.

The risk ratio, lambda, is based on the measurement of the (increased) risk of disease for relatives of cases compared to the population risk. This can be calculated for all types of relative but is most often quoted for siblings of cases (lambda sib). This serves as a measure of familial clustering. Since this clustering could be in whole or in part caused by environmental factors, an adoption study would be required to determine the relative importance of genetic and environmental sharing. Lambda is often estimated in studies that recruit cases retrospectively from clinic records and then study disease in relatives. It should be highlighted that this tends to lead to overestimation of lambda since families with multiple cases tend to be selected. There are also problems with determining affective status of unaffected relatives of young age in adult onset disease and with diseases that influence reproduction. Comparison of values of lambda for different sets of relatives can give clues as to the nature of the underlying genetic model (as has been done for schizophrenia) but is highly dependent on the precision of estimates published in the literature.

Estimating a parameter such as lambda sib or carrying out segregation analysis can be an important first step in studying the role of genetic factors in a disease. It can provide direction concerning whether or not further investment of resources into trying to identify specific alleles is justified and, if so, which approach may be more appropriate. It is a critical determinant of the power of affected sib pair studies.

Segregation analysis investigates whether familial clustering is consistent with Mendelian transmission patterns by estimating the proportion of affected offspring and comparing this to the expected proportion based on Mendelian inheritance. An introduction to segregation analysis should begin with an explanation of types of ascertainment (complete, single incomplete, and multiple incomplete), ascertainment bias, and the methods of correction for this bias in the different types of ascertainment. Students should be made aware of the general principles of segregation analysis and where to obtain computer programs for this analysis. However, computer practicals on this approach should be left to more advanced courses for those who intend to use this approach in their work.

How to identify whether specific genetic factors are related to disease: qualitative traits

(Parametric) linkage analysis

This approach is particularly suited to studying genes with major effects on disease risk. It is one method of mapping disease susceptibility genes and involves analysing segregation patterns in families with multiple affected members. Introductory teaching should start by covering concepts of recombination, recombination fraction, genetic distance, and, if necessary, likelihood theory (maximum likelihood estimates and likelihood ratio test). Properties of the LOD (logarithm of the likelihood ratio in favour of linkage) score should be outlined: that LOD scores greater than 0 generally favor linkage, that LOD scores can be added across families, and that the maximum LOD score over all recombination fractions less than 0.5 provides a good test statistic for the presence of linkage. The interpretation of maximum LOD scores should be discussed by outlining the theoretical and empirical basis for the traditional position of taking a maximum LOD score of greater than 3 as evidence of linkage. The influence of multiple tests such as that which occurs in genome-wide screening should also be discussed. Students should understand that, since the LOD score is a 'conditional likelihood of the markers given the disease', then linkage analysis is robust to ascertainment bias and hence it is valid to select high-risk families for study. Similarly, although linkage analysis is based on an underlying model, the type 1 error rate (significance level) is valid even when the model parameters are misspecified. However, misspecification of marker allele frequencies (and in particular assuming an allele is rarer than it actually is) can invalidate LOD score results and lead to false-positive findings. The relative advantages of two contrasting approaches to specifying allele frequencies, using published frequencies from large samples from the same ethnic group and of using maximum likelihood estimates from observed allele counts over all study pedigrees with the ILINK genetic analysis program (see list of web resources), can be compared.

Since linkage analysis uses DNA markers which are polymorphic, students should know about the advantages and disadvantages of the two major types: repeat polymorphisms based on length difference and single nucleotide polymorphisms (SNPs) based on point changes in single nucleotides.

Simple example pedigrees (assuming that the Mendelian inheritance pattern is known, that the marker and disease status of everyone is known, single genes and no phenocopies) can be used to hand-count the number of recombinant and non-recombinant offspring in increasingly more complex situations. The concept of phase should be illustrated through these examples. Example tables of LOD scores at various recombination fractions and LOD score curves should be given to the class for group discussion of their interpretation. The use of computer simulation methods (for example, using the SLINK genetic analysis program (see list of web resources) to determine expected LOD scores) to assess the power of a family or set of families to detect linkage should be described.

Once basic principles have been covered, concepts such as incomplete penetrance (penetrance functions and liability classes), inbreeding loops, and genetic heterogeneity (heterogeneity LOD score) can be introduced. The importance of considering genetic heterogeneity in circumstances in which more than one gene may be involved in the etiology of the disease under study should be emphasized. The teacher should describe the strategy of calculating posterior probabilities of linkage for each family (once linkage to the first locus is established) to identify families from which to search for linkage with another marker. Finally, the principles of multipoint analysis can be presented. Fine mapping is dependent on correct model specification, and the results of multipoint analysis are therefore very sensitive to misspecification (quantitative trait locus, QTL; methods which are discussed below tend to be more stable).

Examples of the successful use of this approach (for example, in breast cancer) should be used as a way of reviewing and summarizing this approach. Students should be introduced to linkage programs by means of a demonstration or closely guided worked example. Details should be given of how to access available linkage analysis programs (see Rockefeller site in list of web resources) and related textbooks (see, for example, Terwilliger and Ott, 1994). If students are to be taken beyond this point to gain competence in handling the individual programs, then there are a number of computer-based courses run regularly which are designed for this purpose (see list of web resources).

(Non-parametric) linkage analysis

This approach restricts attention to those affected only and assesses whether there is more sharing of alleles which are identical by descent (IBD) in groups of affected relatives than you would expect if there were no linkage. An introduction to this method should cover the limitations of parametric linkage analysis when studying complex disease. The teacher should check that students understand the concepts of IBD and identity by state (IBS) and familial relative risk. Teachers should point out that advantages of studying affected relatives include: increased probability that a genetic cause is present and that affected relatives have the same genetic cause, and that large shared segments among relatives should be identifiable. The theoretical basis of the affected sib pair test should be laid out and then the principles for dealing with multiple affected individuals described. Formulas for calculating the power of a sib pair study should be given. The relationship between power and the familial relative risk in sibs (lambda sib) should be highlighted and ways of increasing this value (for example, by defining the phenotype in another way such as by selecting cases with early age of onset or more extreme clinical findings) discussed. Students should appreciate that empirically derived values of lambda sib may reflect the effect of many genes and the value for the gene under study may be lower than this. Examples of the successful use of this approach (for example, in diabetes) should be used as a way of reviewing and summarizing this approach.

More general non-parametric tests aimed at detecting linkage by testing for increased marker similarity between the affected members of a pedigree can be explained in outline. The problem of distinguishing between IBD and IBS in adult onset disease (when parents may not be available for study), and the use of other siblings in an attempt to reconstruct parental genotypes or of adjacent markers to provide additional information to help distinguish IBD and IBS should be discussed.

Students should be asked to calculate means tests or chi-squared values for various patterns of observed sharing and then to derive values of lambda as a way of reinforcing their understanding of underlying principles. They should then be introduced to programs such as MAPMAKER SIBS or GENEHUNTER by means of a demonstration or closely worked example (see details in Rockefeller website in list of web resources).

Once both this approach and association analysis have been covered in the course the advantages and disadvantages of these two approaches for the study of complex disease should be compared. One dimension of this should be to discuss their relative power to detect genetic risk factors of modest effect.

A number of issues pertinent to both parametric and non-parametric linkage analysis should be reviewed at this stage. A review of linkage statistics is helpful: LOD scores, location scores (in multipoint linkage programs), and non-parametric linkage scores (from the GENEHUNTER program), since these have different interpretations, with a LOD score of 3 being roughly equivalent to a location score of 13.8 or a non-parametric linkage score of 3.7. The calculation of 95% confidence limits or 1 or 3 LOD limits should be described, highlighting that stringent LOD score criteria are particularly important for genome searches.

Association studies (allelic association)

The principles of this approach are similar to that of a traditional case control study with their inherent strengths and weaknesses. The approach is based on showing a higher or lower allele frequency among cases than controls. In most studies the (marker) allele under investigation is a marker which was very close to the disease-causing allele at the time in history when this mutation arose and has remained in linkage disequilibrium with the disease-causing allele since that time. However, this approach can also be used to study candidate genes presumed to include the disease-causing alleles. It should be pointed out that this approach studies association of alleles (not genetic loci) in contrast to linkage analysis which studies linkage of genetic loci (not alleles).

Since there are some differences in approach to traditional case control studies, it is important that students are taken through the steps in an association study starting with checking that both the control and case alleles are in Hardy–Weinberg equilibrium. Only if this is the case can allele counts be assumed to be independent and thus the comparison between them be considered valid. If either set of alleles are not found to be in Hardy–Weinberg equilibrium then a comparison of genotype counts (combining genotypes with small numbers, if necessary) is more valid but has considerably less power. This may be due to chance, laboratory typing errors, or population stratification and can be explored by checking laboratory results and studying other markers. The teacher should check for understanding of the concept of linkage disequilibrium and revise this, if necessary.

Students should appreciate the problem of interpretation of positive results in association tests and be aware of the many examples in the literature of reported positive associations which have not been repeated by subsequent studies. Strategies for distinguishing between the various explanations for observed positive associations – chance, population stratification, linkage disequilibrium, and causal association – should be presented. These include repeating the study in a different population with the same or different study design (for example, with a TDT study after a positive reported association in a study with external controls), investigating evidence of association with several markers in different areas of the genome (to detect stratification effects), and studying markers close to that reported to show association (since association to these markers might be expected if linkage disequilibrium were the likely explanation). The latter should be checked in the control and the case chromosomes since background linkage disequilibrium can be fairly extensive in some isolate populations.

Students should understand the distinction between external and internal controls and the reasons for developing the latter study designs to overcome problems of population stratification. The underlying principles and methods of analysis of the TDT and the haplotype relative risk method should be explained. The use of other markers to check for population stratification should be noted. The TDT design is currently favored in the literature and students should understand how to conduct and analyze data from a TDT study. Students should understand that different types of family structure can be studied and analyzed together. The reasons for the need for high marker heterozygosity should be explained. A major disadvantage is missing data from one of the parents in the study of adult onset complex disease. More recent extensions to the TDT method involving inference of parental genotype from unaffected sibs and S-TDT and 1-TDT methods when direct parental genotyping is not possible but can be mentioned.

Sample size considerations should be described and a comparison made between the power of this approach compared to non-parametric linkage analysis of complex diseases, as mentioned above. In outbred populations the TDT approach may be particularly suitable for the candidate gene approach. Current marker maps are not sufficiently dense to permit a genome wide screen (because of the small degree of linkage disequilibrium detectable by association studies). However, in the near future the use of clusters of intragenic polymorphisms (SNPs) in identified human genes should be feasible. This approach would be particularly powerful if functional polymorphisms were to be studied since the amount of linkage disequilibrium would be irrelevant if the hypothesis is that the disease-causing allele is being studied.

Simple datasets from TDT studies can be given to students to hand-tally results and so gain experience in the analysis of TDT data. Computer programs for the analysis of TDT data should be introduced (see details in list of web resources).

Analysis of shared segments

There is an increasing interest in the potential of the analysis of shared segments in isolate populations. This is based on the identification of shared IBD segments which have come from a common ancestor. The larger the number of generations since the common ancestor, the smaller the size of the shared segment. Approaches such as homozygosity mapping and ancestral haplotype reconstruction work best in populations in which there is a high probability that patients share a common ancestor. The principles underlying these methods should be outlined. A discussion of the favorable characteristics of populations to support these studies can serve as a useful session to introduce or review understanding of concepts from population genetics such as founder effects, genetic drift, and genetic heterogeneity.

How to identify whether specific genetic factors are related to disease: quantitative traits

Genetic epidemiologic approaches for the study of continuous traits should be described. Students should understand why looking at a population distribution is not a good way of identifying major genetic effects. The potential gain of information from this approach compared to analysis of qualitative traits should be noted but with the recognition that there have been few examples of successful mapping of quantitative trait loci (QTL) in humans. In part, this may be because of insufficient power. Just as the value of lambda is a critical determinant of the power in non-parametric linkage analysis so the value of rho (the proportion of variance caused by the gene under study) is critical for the power of QTL analysis. To have sufficient power, 10–15% of the variance observed should be caused by the genetic locus under study. Limiting the variance from environmental factors (for example, by studying smaller family structures such as twins) might be one way of increasing this value.

A number of different strategies can be employed, including affected sib pair analysis, analysis of large multiplex pedigrees, or association studies. References can also be given to other approaches such as the maximum likelihood binomial approach which is a model free method for linkage analysis on nuclear families. Published examples have most commonly adopted the sib pair approach. The gain in power by studying extreme concordant or discordant sib pairs should be considered, together with the need to sample from across the whole range of values of the trait to aid interpretation of results. Students should be shown how to handle families with more than two sibs.

Students should be asked to give examples of how similarity/dissimilarity can be measured. The basis of QTL analysis is that IBD status is negatively correlated with some measure of dissimilarity. The classic Haseman Elston, the rank-based statistic (found in MAPMAKER SIBS program) and variance component analysis approaches should be introduced. The requirement of Haseman Elston for the difference measure to be normally distributed should be pointed out and strategies for dealing with violation of this requirement (variable transformation, use of non-parametric tests, or use of permutation test) noted.

Students should be given a closely guided worked example of QTL analysis (for example, using GENEHUNTER) that uses different methods of analysis so that results can be compared.

Gene–environment interactions

A major challenge in the study of the role of genetic factors in complex disease is that causal pathways may involve a number of genetic variants interacting with each other and with environmental factors. It is likely that individual genetic variants will have a small effect at an individual level (although at a population level they may be important – as measured by population attributable risk). It is helpful to review the various possible mechanisms of gene–environment interaction and how these can be identified. The power of various study designs for detecting gene–environment interaction should be discussed with students. Ways of adapting the various approaches already covered in the course to study gene–environment interaction should be described.

Support after the course

After an initial course students can be informed about specific courses that focus solely on practical instruction in specific techniques. These are run by a number of different agencies, including those listed in the web resources. Students should also be encouraged to read the journals noted above regularly as new methods are usually published first in these journals (see, for example, current issues of relevant journals at http://www.hum-molgen.de/journals/index.html).

Assessing students' achievements

Short courses of undergraduate teaching in genetic epidemiology should check students' understanding of important concepts and principles. A variety of methods, including short essay or multiple choice questions, can be adopted depending on the overall assessment strategy for the course. At the postgraduate level the summative assessment should, in addition, address application of these principles and handling and analysis of simple datasets. This is probably best achieved by a supervised research project. This can be supplemented by assessments requiring critical appraisal of published studies and analysis of simple datasets (using either spreadsheet or specialist genetic epidemiology computer programs which were used in the course). Teachers may also choose to include assessment of the students' understanding of the public health, ethical, social, or legal implications of advances in the understanding of the role of genetic factors in common diseases. Examples of opportunities for checking understanding and giving feedback through formative (in course) assessment have been given throughout this chapter.

Conclusion

This chapter has focused on some of the key principles of genetic epidemiology which underpin study design approaches currently employed in the investigation of the role of genetic risk factors in diseases of public health significance. Although study methods are evolving rapidly, most of these principles will remain relevant and valid in the future. Nevertheless, it is particularly important in genetic epidemiology that teachers should keep up to date with current literature or attend courses which present latest developments in genetic epidemiology.

Acknowledgements

The author would like to acknowledge with thanks those that have taught him in the Erasmus Summer School in Rotterdam in the Netherlands, the European School of Genetic Epidemiology in Pavia in Italy, and in the Human Genome Mapping courses in the UK. What is presented in this chapter is based to a large extent on reflections on experience of being a student on these courses over a number of years as well as of teaching genetic epidemiology.

Further reading

Textbooks

Haynes, J. L., Vance, P. *Design of genetic mapping studies for complex diseases.* J Wiley, 1998.

Khuory, M. H. Genetic epidemiology. In: Rothman, K. J. and Greenland, S. (eds) *Modern Epidemiology* 2nd edition, pp. 609–22. Lippincott-Raven: Philadelphia USA, 1998.

Schulte, P. A., Perera, F. P. *Molecular epidemiology: principles and practices.* Academic Press, San Diego, USA, 1993.

Terwilliger, J., Ott, J. *Handbook of human genetic linkage.* Johns Hopkins University Press, London, 1994.

Original articles

General

Lander, E. S., Schork, N. J. Genetic dissection of complex traits. *Science* 1994; **265**, 2037–48.

Risch, N., Merikangas, K. The future of genetic studies of complex human diseases [see comments]. *Science* 1996; **273**, 1516–17.

Parametric linkage analysis

Lander, E., Kruglyak, L. Genetic dissection of complex traits: guidelines for interpreting and reporting linkage results. *Nature Genetics* 1995; **11**, 241–7.

Kruglyak, L. What is significant in whole-genome linkage disequilibrium studies? *American Journal of Human Genetics* 1997; **61**, 810–12.

Non-parametric linkage analysis

Risch, N., Zhang, H. Extreme discordant sib pairs for mapping quantitative trait loci in humans. *Science* 1995; **268**, 1584–9.

Risch, N. Linkage strategies for genetically complex traits. II. The power of affected relative pairs. *American Journal of Human Genetics* 1990; **46**, 229–41.

Association analysis

Spielman, R. S., Ewens, W. J. The TDT and other family-based tests for linkage disequilibrium and association. *American Journal of Human Genetics* 1996; 9:983–9.

Shared segments

Houwen, R. H., Baharloo, S., Blankenship, K., Raeymaekers, P., Juyn, J., Sandkuijl, L. A., Freimer, N. B. Genome screening by searching for shared segments: mapping a gene for benign recurrent intrahepatic cholestasis. *Nature Genetics* 1994; 8:380–6.

Lander, E. S., Botstein, D. Homozygosity mapping: a way to map human recessive traits with the DNA of inbred children. *Science* 1987; **236**, 1567–70.

Service, S. K., Lang, D. W., Freimer, N. B., Sandkuijl, L. A. Linkage-disequilibrium mapping of disease genes by reconstruction of ancestral haplotypes in founder populations. *American Journal of Human Genetics* 1999; **64**, 1728–38.

Gene–environment interaction

Hwang, S. J., Beaty, T. H., Liang, K. Y., Coresh, J., Khoury, M. J. Minimum sample size estimation to detect gene-environment interaction in case-control designs. *American Journal of Epidemiology* 1994; **140**, 1029–37.

Khoury, M. J., Flanders, W. D. Nontraditional epidemiologic approaches in the analysis of gene-environment interaction: case-control studies with no controls. *American Journal of Epidemiology* 1996; **144**, 207–13.

Yang, Q., Khoury, M. J., Flanders, W. D. Sample size requirements in case-only designs to detect gene-environment interaction. *American Journal of Epidemiology* 1997; **146**, 713–20.

Yang, Q., Khoury, M. J. Evolving methods in genetic epidemiology. III. Gene-environment interaction in epidemiologic research. *Epidemiologic Reviews* 1997; **19**, 33–43.

Quantitative traits

Zhang, H., Risch, N. Mapping quantitative-trait loci in humans by use of extreme concordant sib pairs: selected sampling by parental phenotypes. *American Journal of Human Genetics* 1996; **59**, 951–7.

Selected web resources

Human Genetic Epidemiology Network
http://www.cdc.gov/genetics/hugenet/
(HuGE Net is a global collaboration of individuals and organizations committed to the development and dissemination of population-based information on the human genome; the web site acts as an information exchange network on genetic epidemiology.)

Web Resources of Genetic Linkage Analysis at Rockefeller University
http://linkage.rockefeller.edu/
(This contains access to a wide variety of statistical programs for the analysis of genetic epidemiologic studies, updated bibliographies on selected study design approaches in genetic epidemiology, links to relevant online genetics journals, details of training courses in genetic epidemiology, and details of other relevant web resources.)

Forum in Human Genetics (HUM-MOLGEN)
http://linkage.rockefeller.edu/hum-molgen/index.html
(HUM-MOLGEN is a moderated, interactive communication and information list-server in Human Genetics. It is available over the Internet. It covers news in human genetics, calls for collaboration, announcements, literature reviews, ethical and social issues, diagnostics, computational genetics, special topics in genetics and biotechnology.)

UK Public Health Genetics Network.
http://www.medinfo.cam.ac.uk/phgu/links/links.asp
(This web site contains a regular newsletter with commentary on recently published important articles on genetic epidemiology or genetics and public health, and details of a wide range of relevant web resources, including those in genetic epidemiology, genetics education and training, genetics dictionaries and glossaries, links to relevant online journals, and ethical, legal, and social implications of human genetics.)

Human Genome Project Information
http://www.ornl.gov/TechResources/Human_Genome/links.html
(This contains an enormous variety of genetics resources, including a primer on molecular genetics at http://ornl.gov/hgmis/publicat/primer/intro.html, a directory of education resources in genetics, a glossary of genetic terms, and links to relevant online genetics journals.)

Links to relevant online genetics journals can be found at:
http://linkage.rockefeller.edu/hum-molgen/journals.html
Link to ongoing MEDLINE literature search on genetic epidemiology and details of
selected recent special issues of journals on genetic epidemiology can be found at:
http://www.cdc.gov/genetics/resources/medical/htm

Chapter 24

Study of clustering and outbreaks

Paul Elliott

Introduction

This chapter is concerned with understanding the principles underlying the detection and investigation of possible clusters of disease, and the extent to which they might contribute to knowledge on potential environmental causes. The focus is almost exclusively on the investigation of outbreaks of chronic disease, or at least outbreaks potentially related to chronic environmental 'exposures'. The investigation of acute outbreaks, including infectious diseases (such as food poisoning) in general requires a different approach, not least rapid identification of the causative organism, and often a questionnaire survey using the case control approach to identify common predisposing factors. These issues are discussed elsewhere in this volume.

The issues covered in this chapter would usually be considered part of postgraduate training in epidemiology or public health, especially branches of those disciplines concerned with the effects of the physical environment on health. However, the topic has general interest, and would be suitable for teaching to an undergraduate audience with a quantitative background and an interest in health and the environment.

Teaching objectives

These are summarized as follows:

♦ Describe the context within which claims of disease clusters arise.

♦ Explain what is meant by a disease 'cluster' so that the students are able to define it in statistical or causal terms.

♦ Explain the distinction between a single disease cluster and a tendency for disease 'clustering'.

♦ Explain the importance of random variability in helping to determine spatial and temporal patterns of disease, especially involving small populations and small numbers of cases.

♦ Ensure that the students are aware of the data issues that affect interpretation of possible disease clusters, including those associated with the cases themselves (numerator), the population at risk (denominator), and geographic linkages between the two.

♦ Explain the concept of the standardized mortality or morbidity ratio (SMR) and describe how this is often used in the initial assessment of a possible disease cluster.

- Stress the importance of potential confounding, especially that caused by socio-economic factors.
- Describe the nature of, and potential for, bias in disease cluster studies.
- Describe what steps are required in a cluster investigation and when further investigation may be appropriate.

Teaching content

In line with the above objectives, the course should cover the following topics:

1. Context of the reporting of disease clusters.
2. Definitions of a disease cluster.
3. Random variability.
4. Initial investigation and statistical appraisal.
5. Interpretation and bias.

Each of these is now discussed in turn.

Context of the reporting of disease clusters

It is important that the students are aware of the key trends in disease occurrence over the past century so that they can put the reporting of disease clusters in proper context. The declines in the major infectious diseases, and increases (and later declines) in coronary heart disease and lung cancer in the UK, United States, and other developed countries, were largely related to improvements in hygiene and standards of living, and more recently to lifestyle, diet, and smoking patterns. These might be characterized as the internal environment, while public attention has focused increasingly on the possible health impact of the external or physical environment. This includes ionizing or non-ionizing radiation, emissions from local industry, or perceived threats from contaminated land, the water supply, or waste disposal.

These issues can usefully be discussed with reference to Doll and Peto's (1981) famous review on *The Causes of Cancer*. In Table 20 of that volume, they estimate that 4% of cancer mortality has occupational causes, 2% are due to pollution, 3% to geophysical factors (including ultraviolet light), while less than 1% are caused by industrial products. In contrast, some 30% of cancer deaths were estimated to be due to tobacco, and a further 35% to diet. The students should be invited to make their own ranking before comparison is made with Doll and Peto. Often (in common with public perception) the students will rank 'environment' much higher than do Doll and Peto.

Public concern is often accompanied by suspicions of disease excess in the local community, so-called cluster reports. These are often picked up by the media; examples can readily be found to illustrate the point. A case study on anophthalmia in England and Wales is given later in this chapter.

Definitions of a disease cluster

Clearly it is important to discuss with the students what is meant by the term 'disease cluster'. Knox (1989) suggested three alternative definitions, which should provide a useful springboard for discussion (Table 24.1).

Table 24.1 Definitions of a disease cluster according to Knox

A cluster is/is not:
a geographically and/or temporally bounded group of occurrences –
of a disease already known to occur characteristically in clusters
of sufficient size and concentration to be unlikely to have occurred by chance
related to each other through some social or biologic mechanism, or having a common relationship with some other event or circumstance

From: Knox, E.G. (1989). Detection of disease clusters. In: *Methodology of Enquiries into Disease Clustering* (ed. P. Elliott), p. 20. London: Small Area Health Statistics Unit (with permission).

With the first of these, little weight can be placed on any particular local excess; rather there is a general tendency for the disease itself to clump over space. Such a pattern has been seen, for example, with Hodgkin's disease (Alexander *et al.*, 1989), implicating a possible infectious etiology for that condition.

The second of Knox's definitions is purely statistical and does not deal with the question of possible etiology. None the less, it can be useful to screen for apparent clusters potentially worthy of further investigation among the many thousands of such investigations that could be done. The problem, though, of how to set the boundaries that determine 'sufficient size and concentration' needs to be discussed with and appreciated by the students: if the threshold is set too low (i.e. high sensitivity but low specificity) large numbers of 'false-positive' clusters are bound to occur. Neutra (1990) addresses these issues (see below).

Knox himself preferred the third definition, relying as it does on some notion of causation. He also posed the fundamental question underlying any cluster investigation: 'Is it real?'.

Random variability

A key issue for the students to understand is the nature of random variability. First there is a vast (often unacknowledged) problem of multiple testing in cluster studies, since to arrive at a single apparent 'cluster' in a given area and time period, a large number of observations ('tests') are potentially made – over thousands of small areas, different time periods, disease categories, over age and gender groups, and so on. Secondly, for rare diseases in small geographic areas or over short time periods, the expected number of cases is low, leading to large random variability. Elliott and Wakefield (1999, Fig. 1.12) give an example of apparent 'clusters' that were generated by a Poisson (random) process.

Clearly, the combination of multiple testing in one direction only (high values of the relative risk) and small expected numbers will lead to the reporting of many false-positive clusters. Students need to appreciate that distinguishing between false-positives and any true increase in risk ('Is it real?' in Knox's terminology) is at the heart of cluster detection and investigation.

Initial investigation and statistical appraisal

The UK Leukaemia Research Fund (1997) and US Centers for Disease Control (1990) give good accounts of the approach to a cluster investigation, which are useful as a basis for group discussion. It is important that the students are aware of the steps in a cluster investigation, and have an understanding of the key issues. The steps (see Elliott and Wakefield, 2001) include the following:

1. Form a hypothesis.
2. Select geographic region(s) and time period(s) for study.
3. Assemble and check the data.
4. Obtain an estimate of risk.
5. Write a report and feed back.
6. End study or further investigation as indicated.

Key points for discussion include:

♦ Differentiating between *a priori* and *post hoc* observations (the latter are notoriously difficult to evaluate as statistical testing is formally invalidated).

♦ The importance of data checking, as many apparent clusters may simply reflect anomalies in the data. For example, a case study is included below where census estimates in an area of rapid growth (Dalgety Bay in Scotland) gave biased risk estimates. The data issues affecting studies of this type are reviewed in Staines and Jarup (2000).

♦ The problem of 'boundary shrinkage' which may accentuate estimates of disease risk. According to Olsen *et al.* (1996): 'The more narrowly the underlying population is defined, the less will be the number of expected cases, the greater will be the estimate of the excess rate, and often the more pronounced will be the statistical significance.'

♦ Calculation of a risk estimate (for example, the SMR, which is often obtained by comparing the observed numbers of cases in areas near and more distant from a point source (or in high and low pollution areas) with the numbers expected based on the age and gender distribution of the population, using indirect standardization). Aylin *et al.* (1999) give details of the calculation of the SMR in the context of disease clusters and small area disease mapping. Breslow and Day (1987) discuss the properties of the SMR more generally. A worked example is included below.

♦ The importance of potential socioeconomic confounding, which can distort estimates of disease risk (Jolley *et al.*, 1992).

♦ The need to manage the hopes and expectations among the local community (which may be unrealistically high).

♦ How to terminate an investigation. According to the Leukaemia Research Fund (1997): 'There are no easy ways to conclude a cluster investigation. The vast majority of cluster investigations fail to achieve any firm or acceptable conclusions … If a clear and logical report is written and explained it can usually be accepted even by those who are most emotionally involved.'

Interpretation and bias

The students need to be aware of the difficult issues of interpretation if an apparent disease excess in a particular area is found. In particular, there are many sources of potential bias: Elliott and Wakefield (2000) provide discussion. These include:

+ Bias in the identification of areas for study, since an informal and poorly defined selection process is undertaken (areas at apparently low risk are never selected!).

+ The 'boundary shrinkage' problem, leading to accentuated estimates of risk.

+ Low population numbers and small numbers of cases, giving imprecise estimates.

+ Ill-defined hypotheses, or in some cases, lack of hypothesis.

+ Poorly defined or absent exposure data.

+ Incomplete or inaccurate health and population data, and migration between areas, especially where latency periods are prolonged (most cancers).

+ Confounding.

+ Reporting bias in areas where symptom surveys have been undertaken.

Teaching method and format

This should be a combination of lecture/seminar format, small group teaching, case studies and worked examples, and private study. Suggested breakdown of time would be lecture/seminar 30%; case studies and worked examples (small group teaching) 30%; reading and preparation time, and private study 40%. Seminars would typically include 20–30 students; small groups (for the case studies) might include three or four students working together and reporting back to the main group.

Typically, the course will be held over 2 or 3 days (four to six sessions, depending on the number of case studies), although it may be longer if computing sessions are included.

Some worked examples and case studies are given below. These could be set as class exercises, used as the basis for discussion, or modified for use in assessment. They do not require computing facilities, although the calculation of the SMR example requires calculators. Similar exercises using computer programs could be added, particularly for more advanced courses. Examples include CLUSTER software, SMRFIT (Hanrahan et al., 1990) and the GeoBUGS software for disease mapping (Thomas et al., 2000). The latter, in particular, is public domain software. A couple of worked examples are included in the on-line manual that comes with GeoBUGS; further practicals are to be added to the GeoBUGS web site in the near future.

Worked examples and case studies

Cluster report: anophthalmia in England and Wales

This case study illustrates the media reporting of alleged clusters of a rare disease and the steps that were required to investigate them. In *The Observer* newspaper of 17 January 1993 it was claimed under the headline 'Mystery of babies with no eyes' that there were localized clusters of anophthalmia across England and Wales. This is a serious birth defect where the infant is born without eye tissue (either unilateral or bilateral); it is closely related to microphthalmia, where some eye tissue is present. The newspaper linked the 'clusters' to the use of the pesticide Benomyl.

The article was accompanied by a map (Fig. 24.1) which illustrates well many of the problems and pitfalls in the reporting of alleged clusters. First, it is unclear from the map and accompanying article (and subsequent enquiry) what was the source of the cases, whether or not they were truly anophthalmia, whether or not there was duplicate reporting, and so forth. Secondly, no time scale was given for the occurrence of the cases, and only in Louth in the north-east of England was any clear geographic boundary given (40-mile radius), so that it would have been impossible to determine a denominator for the alleged clusters and hence obtain an estimate of the risk. Without such basic information, it was not possible to make any judgement as to whether or not there was any true excess of this condition, nor of course whether there was any geographic association with pesticide use (Dolk and Elliott, 1993).

Two weeks later, the newspaper again reported on the alleged cluster, this time under the alliterative headline 'Pesticide fears grow as numbers of babies born blind doubles'. As a result of the concerns raised by the newspaper reports, a birth prevalence study of anophthalmia and microphthalmia was set up, specifically to examine

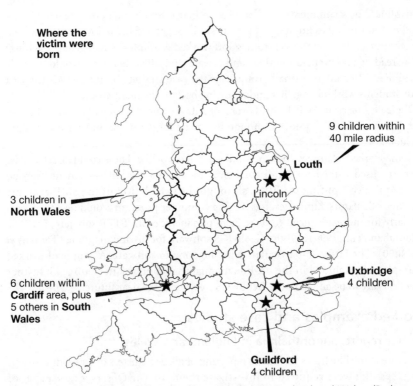

Figure 24.1 Map of alleged clusters of anophthalmia in England and Wales. (Redrawn from The Observer, 17 January 1993, with permission.)

for evidence of disease clusters or clustering of this condition. The study took 5 years to report; no evidence of specific clusters was found, although there did appear to be an unexplained excess in rural compared with urban areas (Dolk *et al.*, 1998).

Estimation of the SMR

The Leukaemia Research Fund (1997, pp. 60–8) includes a worked example of the SMR which can readily be adapted as a group exercise by preparing blank tables for the students to complete. It is based on data for the town of Antigo in Wisconsin, USA, together with reference data for the State of Wisconsin (Hanrahan *et al.*, 1990). In the Leukaemia Research Fund worked example, three cases of bladder cancer were included for Antigo from 1960 to 1969, and this is then compared to the expected number using disease rates for Wisconsin after standardization for age. One-sided significance testing for the SMR is also obtained based on the Poisson distribution (and found not to differ significantly from unity). The worked example includes detailed instruction on the calculations, which can readily be done on a calculator.

Denominator issues: Dalgety Bay in Scotland

This is an example of a small area investigation of cancer incidence in a small town in east-central Scotland following the discovery of small amounts of radium-226 on the foreshore (Black *et al.*, 1994). This was thought to emanate from radium-based luminous paint that was used in military aircraft that were disposed of by burning during the 1940s. Because of recent in-migration, the demography of Dalgety Bay had changed during the study period, so that careful attention to the denominator was needed in the calculation of SMRs. The paper also demonstrates, in its Table 2, the effect of allowing for socioeconomic deprivation in the calculation of SMRs (observed:expected ratios); since Dalgety Bay is an affluent area, some risk estimates were higher following adjustment for deprivation (e.g. lung cancer, stomach cancer), whilst others were lower (especially skin cancer where the observed:expected ratio was 1.50, 95% confidence interval (CI) 1.05–2.08, with age and sex adjustment, and 1.38, 95% CI 0.97–1.91, with adjustment also for deprivation). The students should be invited to discuss these issues, and also to give their views on the conduct and interpretation of the study.

A point source enquiry using routine data

This illustrates the typical course of an enquiry where routine data are used; it also shows the possibilities for largely automating an enquiry where the necessary data systems are in place, as is the case for the UK Small Area Health Statistics Unit (SAHSU). A Rapid Inquiry Facility within SAHSU can collate, analyse, and report on the health statistics around any point in the country within a few days. This facility offers the means to facilitate and speed up greatly the first steps of a cluster investigation (Aylin *et al.*, 1999).

A member of the public had complained to their Member of Parliament concerning possible health effects of chemical air pollution near two factories on the same site in a deprived area. No changes in illness patterns had been noted by local general practitioners. A detailed report had been compiled by local environmental health officers who had inspected the site. Respiratory mortality rates were generally high in that part of the district, and the local Department of Public Health focused the investigation on respiratory admissions and mortality rates near the two factories. The coordinates for the two factories were passed to the SAHSU Rapid Inquiry Facility.

After standardization for age, sex, and deprivation, mortality rate from respiratory disease appeared to be raised, although the excess was seen both within 2 km (RR 1.07, 95%CI 1.01–1.13) and more distant from the two factories (2–7.5 km; RR 1.09, 95% CI 1.08–1.11), suggesting that this might reflect generally higher rates than those of the standard region used for calculating expected values, rather than an excess associated specifically with the source. There was no excess of hospital admissions for respiratory illness <2 km from the source (RR 0.99, 95% CI 0.95–1.03) although there was an apparent small excess at 2–7.5 km (RR 1.05, 95% CI 1.04–1.07). The excesses observed were all less than 10%.

A report was provided to the referring department giving details of the request, data used, time period and geographic extent of the investigation, age and International Classification of Disease groups studied, maps of the area, including deprivation profile, results, and brief commentary, and an outline of limitations of the analysis. This was used to inform the local Department of Public Health's report and provide feedback. No further action was deemed necessary.

Follow-up study using routine data. Leukemia incidence near radio and TV transmitters in Great Britain

This study illustrates how an initial cluster report led to a national investigation using routine cancer data. Newspaper reports claimed that there was an excess of leukemia near the Sutton Coldfield radio and TV transmitter in England. An 83% excess incidence of leukemia was found within 2 km, apparently confirming the local reports of a disease excess (Dolk et al., 1997a). On its own, this result was difficult to interpret, however, especially since it was unclear whether the hypothesis of increased leukemia incidence arose a priori or as a post hoc observation. A follow-up study examined incidence of leukemia and selected cancers near all other transmitters in Great Britain (Dolk et al., 1997b). Although a shallow decline of leukemia risk with distance from the transmitters was observed, the report concluded that the magnitude and pattern of risk found near Sutton Coldfield did not appear to be replicated, and that the results gave, at most, only very weak support to the Sutton Coldfield findings (Dolk et al., 1997b).

Group discussion and debate: Rothman versus Neutra

In a landmark paper, Rothman (1990) argued that cluster investigation was hardly ever indicated; he advocated instead traditional hypothesis-led investigation, and (as required) the remediation of environmental concerns per se without reference to the health statistics. Neutra (1990), in his reply, largely agreed with Rothman's analysis. Although he found some justification for cluster investigation, this was only for rare diseases, with large relative risks (>20) associated with high specificity exposures, and where case aggregation met the criterion for minimum size (>5). These two papers together give an excellent background to the issues surrounding cluster investigation, and are compelling reading to the interested student.

Assessing students' achievements

Assessment will need to be based on the requirements of the course. Possibilities include short answer questions to interpret findings of apparent disease 'excess' in a particular locality/time period, and/or to delineate steps in the investigation. Students might be asked to carry out a paper critique of a cluster investigation or to present in small groups to the rest of the class. Another possibility is to carry out a computational exercise (e.g. calculation of the SMR and its assessment) using either a computer- or calculator-based practical. In all cases, it will be essential to determine that the students have gained critical appraisal and understanding to allow them to evaluate the cluster literature properly.

References

Alexander, F. E., Williams, J., McKinney, P. A., Cartwright, R. A. and Ricketts, T. J. (1989). A specialist leukaemia/lymphoma registry in the UK. Part 2: clustering of Hodgkin's disease. *Br. J. Cancer*, **60**, 948–952.

Aylin, P., Maheswaran, R., Wakefield, J. *et al.* (1999). A national facility for small area disease mapping and rapid initial assessment of apparent disease clusters around a point source: the UK Small Area Health Statistics Unit. *J. Publ. Health Med.*, **21**, 289–298.

Black, R. J., Sharp, L., Finlayson, A. R. and Harkness, E. F. (1994). Cancer incidence in a population potentially exposed to radium-226 at Dalgety Bay, Scotland. *Br. J. Cancer*, **69**, 140–143.

Breslow, N. E. and Day, N. E. (1987). Statistical methods in cancer research, Vol. II—*The design and analysis of cohort studies*. Lyon: IARC, pp. 61–79.

CDC (1990). Guidelines for investigating clusters of health events. *M. M. W. R.*, 39 (No. RR-11),1–23.

Dolk, H., Busby, A., Armstrong, B. G. and Walls, P. H. (1998). Geographical variation in anophthalmia and microphthalmia in England, 1988–94. *Br. Med. J.*, **317**, 905–910.

Dolk, H. and Elliott, P. (1993). Evidence for 'clusters of anophthalmia' is thin. *Br. Med. J.*, 307, 203 (letter to the editor).

Dolk, H., Shaddick, G., Walls, P., Grundy, C. and Elliott, P. (1997a). Cancer incidence near high power radio and TV transmitters in Great Britain: I. Sutton Coldfield transmitter. *Am. J. Epidemiol.*, **145**, 1–9.

Dolk, H., Elliott, P., Shaddick, G., Walls, P. and Grundy, C. (1997b). Cancer incidence near high power radio and TV transmitters in Great Britain: II. All transmitter sites. *Am. J. Epidemiol.*, **145**, 10–17.

Doll, R. and Peto, R. (1981). *The Causes of Cancer*. Oxford: Oxford University Press.

Elliott, P. and Wakefield, J. C. (1999). Small-area studies of environment and health. In: *Statistics for the Environment 4: Pollution Assessment and Control.* (eds V. Barnett, A. Stein, and K. Feridun Turkman). London: Wiley, pp. 3–27.

Elliott, P. and Wakefield, J. C. (2000). Bias and confounding in spatial epidemiology. In: *Spatial Epidemiology: Methods and Applications* (eds P. Elliott, J. C. Wakefield, N. G. Best and D. J. Briggs). Oxford: Oxford University Press, pp. 68–84.

Elliott, P. and Wakefield, J. C. (2001). Disease clusters: should they be investigated, and if so, when and how? *J. R. Statist. Soc. A*, 164, pp. 3–12.

Hanrahan, L. P., Mirkin, I., Olson, J., Anderson, H. A. and Fiore, B. J. (1990). SMRFIT: a Statistical Analysis System (SAS) program for Standardized Mortality Ratio analyses and Poisson regression model fits in community cluster investigations. *Am. J. Epidemiol.*, 132, S116-S122.

Jolley, D., Jarman, B. and Elliott, P. (1992). Socio-economic confounding. In: *Geographical and Environmental Epidemiology: Methods for Small-Area Studies* (eds P. Elliott, J. Cuzick, D. English, R. Stern), pp. 115–124. Oxford: Oxford University Press.

Knox, E. G. (1989). Detection of disease clusters. In: *Methodology of Enquiries into Disease Clustering* (ed. P. Elliott), pp. 17–20. London: Small Area Health Statistics Unit.

Leukaemia Research Fund (1997). *Handbook and Guide to the Investigation of Disease Clusters.* Leeds: Leukaemia Research Fund Centre for Clinical Epidemiology.

Neutra, R. (1990). Counterpoint from a cluster buster. *Am. J. Epidemiol*, **132**, 1–8.

Olsen, S. F., Martuzzi, M. and Elliott, P. (1996). Cluster analysis and disease mapping – why, when and how? *Br. Med. J.*, **313**, 863–866.

Rothman, K. J. (1990). A sobering start for the cluster busters' conference. *Am. J. Epidemiol*, **132**, S6–13.

Staines, A. and Jarup, L. (2000). Health event data. In: *Spatial Epidemiology: Methods and Applications* (eds P. Elliott, J. C. Wakefield, N. G. Best and D. J. Briggs). Oxford: Oxford University Press, pp. 15–29.

Thomas, A., Best, N. G., Arnold, R. A., and Spiegelhalter, D. J. (2000). *GeoBUGS User Manual, Demonstration Version 1.0,* Imperial College and MRC Biostatistics Unit, http://www.mrc-bsu.cam.ac.uk/bugs/winbugs/geobugs.shtml.

Chapter 25

Field studies in developing countries

Japhet Killewo and Anita Sandström

Introduction

Field studies in developing countries encompass a number of research activities geared at answering questions about a particular health problem using a variety of methods and population groups. In developing country settings, field studies obtain information from the study subjects directly through interviews and possibly through examinations and taking of specimens that are subsequently tested for a variety of ill-health conditions. Most field studies in developing countries involve investigation and control of communicable diseases. Accordingly, researchers in those countries must be equipped with the necessary tools to address such problems. From their nature, field studies should generate information from population samples that are so select-ed as to enable researchers to draw appropriate conclusions regarding the target pop-ulation. For this reason, researchers wishing to conduct field studies should pay attention to appropriate selection and sampling processes of the target population before attempting to study individuals. Although there are various ways of collecting survey data in the field, only a few are practical for developing country situations. For example, the use of telephones and the application of self-administered question-naires are not feasible options for developing countries because of the low telephone coverage and the high rates of illiteracy, respectively, in these countries. Instead, inter-views using prepared schedules provide a more practical and acceptable method of collecting data. Under the latter conditions, direct contact with the study subject by the researcher or research assistants is essential.

Training for field studies

The approach to be adopted in training those aspiring to do field research in develop-ing countries is to provide them with a set of guidelines that will help them to design appropriately and implement studies which can increase research skills and yet help to influence policy and improve health. However, before any field studies are under-taken, students must have a theoretical background of research methodology and related subjects. This background can be obtained either through a short course last-ing several weeks or through a staggered series of lectures and practicals on research methodology and related subjects. Such training can be carried out in the course of a specified training period for other purposes such as may be applicable for students of medicine, dentistry, pharmacy nursing, and the social sciences. This set of guidelines does not, however, assume prior knowledge of the subject among undergraduate students. It expects some basic skills and knowledge among postgraduate students to whom most of the guidelines may constitute a repetition of the subject but perhaps provide more practical skills.

The teaching approach in this chapter is targeted at both undergraduates and postgraduates in public health-related fields or clinical epidemiology in which part of their training involves field research. The content to be covered will range from skills to develop research plans, through fieldwork-related activities and data processing, to report writing and dissemination of results to the scientific community, policy makers, and the studied community. This content assumes knowledge of other general aspects of epidemiology such as principles and methods as well as research methodology that may have been covered separately. Knowledge of how to develop a research plan will provide skills on how to negotiate with funding agencies and how to justify research on the proposed topic. It will also provide skills on how to plan for field activities, how to document research ideas and how to work systematically following a specified protocol. Undergraduates will develop their research plans and implement studies in groups, while postgraduates will do the same but work more independently as a reflection of their expected level of scientific maturity.

Teaching objectives

The teaching objectives of a course focusing on field studies in developing countries should enable students to do the following at the successful completion of the course:

♦ Develop a study protocol on a research topic for which the student will do a field study. This will include skills in problem identification and justification for research, literature search and review, formulation of objectives, developing the methodology, developing the budget, and making a justification.

♦ Acquire skills in field procedures involving the study population such as defining and selecting a study sample, matching, randomization, making the required measurements, and follow-up.

♦ Acquire skills on the logistics of preparing for fieldwork, including carrying out a pilot study, pre-visits, arranging for transport, and accommodation for field workers.

♦ Acquire skills on how to approach study communities and individuals for successful enlisting of their cooperation to the study.

♦ Acquire skills in data collection procedures, including performing interviews in field situations and ensuring confidentiality and trust.

♦ Acquire skills in data analysis, presentation, and interpretation.

♦ Acquire skills in report writing and dissemination of results to the various stakeholders.

Teaching content

Development of a research protocol

Before students can embark on a field study they must be taken through the process of developing a research plan. This is the 'architectural' phase of a study. The research protocol will normally consist of a document that carries the relevant details of the various stages in a study. It contains, among others, the important sections of problem identification and definition, literature review, study objectives, study methodology, and budget. Each of the sections requires that the student has thorough knowledge of the theory behind the subject matter and must be able to translate concepts into practical realities. Many students have problems in conceptualizing a research problem, prioritizing problems for research, and formulating the specific objectives of a study. Groupwork on problem formulation and priority setting should be encouraged to give students the needed experience in this crucial task and to stress the importance of a well formulated problem for the success of the study. These initial areas require the instructors to spend more time in ensuring that the students grasp the subject matter before proceeding to the next sections. Regarding the methodology section, it is important to specify the study population and selection strategy, study design, and study instruments. Students should be made to understand that it is the nature of the research problem that determines the study design. Whether quantitative or qualitative, all study designs must be detailed enough to facilitate data collection. Specific quantitative study designs such as cross-sectional, descriptive, case control, cohort, experimental, and specific qualitative study designs like Focus group discussions and key informant interviews should be understood where relevant.

Field procedures involving the study population

Students should understand how and why to select a study area and population. The concepts of sampling and sample size determination, study methods, and the situations in which they are best used and how the field activities are related to the study objectives should be clearly explained. Before the final questionnaire or record form is produced in large numbers students should make sure that the questions or information being sought respond to the study objectives. They should also ensure that all the steps in the methodology are clear to each one of them. Undergraduate students should always perform role plays in asking the questions, followed by a pre-test of the questionnaire in a small population with characteristics similar to those of the actual study population. Any problems experienced during the pre-test are discussed and the necessary modifications made before actual fieldwork starts.

Concepts of measurements and determinants of their variation and validity should be clearly understood, and standardized procedures of measurement should be adopted to reduce interobserver variation where many data collectors are involved. Students should also learn the skills of designing questionnaires or data collection forms and how to record the responses in such a way as to facilitate computer data entry and analysis. The importance of a clear definition of a study population should be stressed. For example, students wishing to study a population by household should be able to define a household and who among those living in the household on a particular day should constitute the study population, irrespective if they are present at the time of the interview. For longitudinal studies the study base should be clearly defined.

Preparation for field work

Students should play a key role in the preparation for fieldwork. This requires first and foremost a clear understanding of what is going to be done in the field by each one of them. For undergraduate students who are expected to work in groups, all concerned should be familiar with the objectives of the study and what the expected outcome should be. Students are often a source of confusion and conflict for communities in the field, especially when they are placed in large numbers in one place. To reduce such problems, it is important that all students on a particular course attend the preparatory sessions so that they are familiar with what is to be done. It is also important that they are split into small and manageable groups, each with a supervisor, to be placed in different parts of the study area. However, postgraduates should make the necessary preparations on their own. Because they have a vested interest in the study in terms of fulfilment for a Masters' or PhD thesis they are often motivated to make good preparations.

Ethical clearance and permission to do the study in the selected area are important aspects that must be addressed when preparing for fieldwork. This skill will also include the ability to refine the protocol by addressing comments from either the supervisor or any relevant internal reviewer. Students should understand that research and ethical review processes are essential for any scientific work.

For large field surveys, a pre-visit to the study site by two or three students and one supervisor is always advisable because this is the time that the researcher can assess potential problems and plan for their solution before the actual study begins. A pre-visit allows the researcher to become familiar with the climatic conditions, socioeconomic situation, and the administrative structure of the study area, including who among the leaders is likely to be cooperative and therefore helpful and what type of support can be obtained from them. Transport and accommodation are common problems in field studies and these should be resolved well in advance. Students must make sure that all field requirements are prepared in advance. For example, if they are using questionnaires or data collection forms for a survey they must make sure that enough are produced in advance. Even if the study area may have facilities for producing questionnaires or data forms, researchers should not rely on them, as they may be committed or out of order when they are needed. Students should be prepared for bad weather conditions like rain, floods, and cold weather. They should also be prepared with first aid kits for most common local health problems. Students should learn the basic rules of camping, including those of tent pitching, construction of pit or other forms of latrines suitable for the area, and boiling of drinking water, all geared at maintaining good sanitation in the field to prevent diarrhea and other communicable diseases. In malaria-endemic areas they should be prepared and able to prevent mosquito bites. The whole study team should be prepared to assist those community members who happen to require healthcare or advice during the study period while those found to be sick in the course of medical examination as part of a study must be treated.

Undergraduate students should allocate tasks to each other and must choose one leader among them to be their spokesperson for the group in making communications with the community leadership. Group approach to community leaders should be avoided. Typical tasks for group sharing in an interview survey include typing of the questionnaire, making enough copies of the questionnaire, packaging the questionnaires, and making one individual responsible for their transportation to the field and distribution to individual interviewers. Food and accommodation should be the responsibility of another group, first aid and medications should be the responsibility of another, study instruments such as microscopes, blood pressure machines, test reagents, etc. should be the responsibility of another and so on and so forth. A supervisor or instructor advises the group and oversees the quality of the research and ensures social integrity in the group. For postgraduates the role of a supervisor is important, but postgraduates should be allowed to work more independently than undergraduates.

Approach to communities and individuals

Lack of sampling frames and proper addresses in developing country situations make it necessary to adopt study designs that are less than ideal. For example, the use of simple random sampling methodologies for rural and scattered populations may be impossible and, even when possible, it may be difficult to trace the study subjects. Only the very rare populations with well established health and demographic surveillance systems or regular census can allow simple random sampling procedures to be applied because such systems will have the necessary sampling frames and proper addresses for identifying and following up selected individuals. A case in point is the Bangladesh site for health and demographic surveillance system at Matlab, which was developed by the International Centre for Diarrhoeal Disease Research, Bangladesh (ICDDR,B) in the 1960s to collect data routinely from a population of about 210 000. The system therefore provides accurate, reliable longitudinal data which can be used by health planners, policy makers, and scientists. If proper addresses are lacking, a follow-up study is planned and routines for returning to the household/interviewee have to be developed.

During interviews, students should be able to explain what the objectives of the study are and why they are carrying out the study in the selected area. They should also be able to explain why a particular study subject has been selected for the study and not the others. This should be done in a simple language that can be understood by the ordinary person. Students should recite a common text to be used by each one of them to avoid different messages going around the communities as, for example, when obtaining informed consent. Students should be instructed to prepare interview settings that ensure confidentiality and trust, and allow free and open conversation. For overcrowded urban or periurban populations it may be necessary to divert the interest of an excited public by providing some form of entertainment while interviews are taking place. Community leadership should always be used but cautiously.

Students should learn to be independent of any kind of political, religious, or activist movement pressure in addressing research questions. Some community leaders are so popular or even unpopular that they will try to lead you to study certain people or to avoid studying certain people just to gain more popularity depending on how beneficial they perceive the study to be. They may also misunderstand the purpose of the study altogether and do the opposite of what was earlier agreed upon. In general, community leaders can be very useful for studies if approached properly. Some of the useful hints include the following:

1. Making them understand the purpose of the study and how the community may benefit from the study itself or its findings.

2. Making them participate in the study in ways that facilitate the study, including selection of study population using appropriate methods or giving needed guidance in locating people and places.

3. Asking them to play hosts to the study team by helping to identify suitable accommodation and food.

Researchers should be prepared with the necessary official permits to do research in the area. Sometimes nobody will ask about the permits, but it is worthwhile having them handy all the time just in case someone does ask. It is extremely embarrassing when one has to stop the study to return to base to find the permit which will probably have been misplaced and taking the trouble of going for a copy of the permit which may take several days. Such lack of preparedness leads to loss of time and confidence, making research work difficult.

Data collection procedures

Depending on the size and complexity of a study, a pilot study may be necessary for large and complex studies to test field methods and instruments to enable their refinement before a large scale study is undertaken. Data collection should be organized in a systematic way to avoid sampling houses or individuals that have already been sampled by another group. Students should be well versed with the appropriate research methods before embarking on data collection. Population sampling and data collection techniques differ between quantitative and qualitative studies, and these must be well studied to enable the researcher to answer the research questions at hand. If cluster sampling is used in a quantitative survey then all that will be needed is to make sure that the whole cluster is covered in data collection. All members of a cluster, regardless of their being at home or not, are eligible for inclusion in the study and any member left out will constitute a non-response to the study. Non-response is a serious bias to any study and must be avoided as much as possible. In follow-up studies, attrition or loss to follow-up should be minimized to increase the validity of the findings. At the end of each day students should sit down to review the day's work. Some information may not have been correctly recorded. Some responses may not have been recorded and yet some respondents may not have completed their responses. This is the time to correct such errors or to plan how to return to the respondents for missed responses. The supervisors should at this point check the questionnaires or data forms of each student and provide guidance in the right direction. Researchers should define criteria for inclusion or exclusion of a subject in a study. If age is the criteria for inclusion, a list of individuals with their corresponding ages should be made before selection to obtain the eligible population. Students should be informed that most quantitative studies require age or past time variables from each study member. In illiterate populations it may be difficult to remember the date of birth or when an event important for the study took place in the past. For such populations it may be advisable to construct local calendars that may facilitate the recall of such events by the study population. Local calendars may be in the form of the time when events of local importance (wars, earthquakes, death of an important person etc.) took place.

Data analysis, presentation, and interpretation

Before students attempt to collect their own data they should be instructed on how to perform data entry and analysis as well as how to make appropriate interpretations of the findings. This can best be done using a different dataset or a set of questionnaires or data forms used for a different purpose. This option provides the students with the necessary skills before they collect their own data. In this way they feel motivated to collect reliable information. Where computers are not available, traditional methods of data processing and analysis are adopted. However, in the 21st century it is expected that students undertaking research will have access to a computer with simple and public domain data entry and analysis packages such as EPIINFO. For undergraduates it may be difficult for each student to have access to a computer but for postgraduates it is a necessity for them to have hands-on experience in using computers. Undergraduate students may share computers to practise data entry, cleaning, and analysis. To facilitate this process, one computer with good projection equipment may be necessary so that the instructor can demonstrate how to enter, clean, and analyze data to a large group of students.

Students must also be given the skills of interpreting their results, particularly tables and figures. The correct row or column percentages must be well interpreted. Students often confuse the two. They must know the correct numerators and denominators. Students must be able to differentiate between incidence and prevalence, and know how to interpret results of odds ratios, risk ratios, risk rates, confidence limits, and P values. Students must learn how to translate results from computer printouts to easily digestible and understandable tables. They should know that a good table in a report or published paper could be a result of a combination of several tables produced by a computer. In presenting the results of the study, students must be prepared to explain the results of data analysis to others who were not part of their study. This can be done either by oral or poster presentations, as is common in scientific forums. For such presentations to be useful there must be a sizable audience available to the students to ask questions and to make comments on the presentations. The situation must mimic a scientific conference since this is to prepare students to be confident in making scientific presentations and addressing scientific communities. For this reason they should be made familiar with the different projection facilities, poster making, and use of flip charts. They should learn to develop presentation materials with short text, tables, and figures that are not crowded and are legible from a distance. They should learn to use large font size text and avoid projecting ordinary size text for the audience to read. They should also avoid making speeches and reading large amounts of text to the audience. For undergraduates, all the students should participate in the preparation of the presentation. However, only one student is selected by the group to make the presentation if it is brief, otherwise several of them are selected to present different aspects of the study depending on the time available. For postgraduates, however, the responsible student will make the presentation with little or no assistance. If the report is in the form of a dissertation or thesis it is necessary to prepare it in the prescribed format of the institution with the required number of copies so that appropriate dissemination, including sending copies to libraries, can be facilitated. Defending a thesis or dissertation should be in the form of a scientific presentation using appropriate equipment and materials such as overhead transparencies, flip charts, slides, etc.

Report writing and dissemination of results

Report writing is an important aspect of research. It provides materials for feedback to the studied communities, the policy makers, and the wider scientific community. In addition, it provides a constant reminder of the author's contribution to knowledge and the support provided by the funding agency. For the requirement of undergraduate students whose field study is expected to be brief, a formal study report should be prepared for assessment of students' performance and a copy must be kept in the library for records. From this type of report, materials for presentation at the end of the study and for feedback to the studied communities are extracted. Students should be aware that study communities are always curious to know how they will benefit from the study findings. For this reason, researchers should always try to provide feedback to studied communities to reciprocate their cooperation for the study. In some communities it may not be adequate to provide feedback through common channels such as the radio or newspapers but by direct means involving revisits to the population and taking advantage of public meetings to give the feedback. For postgraduates, however, who may have received funding for a field study of several months, there may be the additional need for a progress report as well as the final technical and financial reports. The students must therefore learn the techniques of reporting that must be timely and tally with the time and activity schedule as indicated in the study plan. If students are planning to publish the report in scientific journals they must learn the techniques of scientific writing. In addition, students must learn how to extract information from technical reports for the consumption of policy makers. Information for policy recommendation must be simple, brief, and to the point. Most importantly, recommendations must be seen to emanate from the study and must be practical and reflective of local realities.

Teaching method and format

Lectures should be given where a subject is being introduced for the first time and where theoretical knowledge about the subject matter is necessary. This should then be followed by a demonstration or a practical session during which students undertake a task themselves to gain practical skills. For the topic on development of a research plan, a 1-hour lecture should be given, followed by separate practical sessions on problem identification and justification, literature search and review, formulation of objectives, methodology, and budgeting, including budget justification. For each component, a brief practical should be prepared for groups of students to spend approximately half an hour discussion for which they should prepare one or two overheads to make a presentation to class members at the end.

The other topics should be prepared in the same way except that the time to be allocated for the lecture session will be shorter. For example, Table 25.1 shows the suggested topics, method of teaching, and the approximate time to be spent on each topic.

Assessing students' achievements

Objective assessment of students' performance is a difficult task for many instructors and an unwelcome event for many students. Some of the key questions that arise in the course of deciding to assess students' achievement are:

- When is it appropriate to make an assessment?
- What kind of assessment should be made?
- What style of questions should be asked?
- How many times should students be assessed?
- What scores should contribute most to reflect objective assessment of an individual student?

Generally, learning is reinforced when some form of reward is given by placing individual students in categories of performance as indicated by their scores. To assess students' performance in field studies and related subjects, performance levels should be assessed for each student by topic or subject, and regular assessment tests should be organized at the end of the training session, subject or topic. This is especially so for the staggered type of courses. For short non-staggered courses one test at the end of the course covering all the topics will be sufficient. Grading the quality of the study protocol, quality of the report, and quality of presentations for postgraduates is easy because individual performance is being assessed. However, for undergraduates who largely work in groups, difficulties may arise in making fair assessments for individual performance. For example, assessment of groupwork that indicates high quality performance may in reality be a reflection of a few bright or hardworking individuals in the group. For this reason, groupwork assessment grade should constitute a small fraction (e.g. 20%) of the overall assessment grade. For example if, in a given semester, students do five written tests and six group tasks, each marked out of 100, then the overall average grade should reflect true individual performance by giving less weight to group tasks (i.e. multiplying the group tasks average by 20% and the test average by 80%).

Conclusion

Training in field studies and related subjects is the key to providing practical skills for undergraduate and postgraduate students of medicine, dentistry, pharmacy, nursing,

Table 25.1

Suggested topic and subtopic	Teaching method and time required	
	Teaching method	Time in hours
Development of a research plan	Lecture	1
Problem identification	Practical	2
Literature search and review	Practical	2
Objectives	Practical	1
Methodology, including questionnaire design	Practical	4
Budgeting and budget justification	Practical	2
Preparation for fieldwork		
Understanding study objectives	Presentations and discussion	1
Sampling methods and sample size determination	Lecture	2
Concepts of measurement and validity	Lecture	1
Concepts of measurement and validity	Practical	1
Pre-visit of study area	Fieldwork	48
Preparation of questionnaires and other field materials	Groupwork	36
Approach to communities and individuals		
Logistics of seeking ethical clearance and permission	Lecture	1
Interview techniques	Lecture	2
Interview techniques	Practical	2
Living with the community during actual study	Fieldwork	All time
Data collection procedures		
Quantitative *versus* qualitative data collection techniques	Lecture	2
Questionnaire/data form design and pre-coding	Lecture	1
Questionnaire/data form design and pre-coding	Practical	2

Table 25.1 continued

Suggested topic and subtopic	Teaching method and time required	
	Teaching method	**Time in hours**
Actual fieldwork	Fieldwork	All time
Review of day's work in the field	Fieldwork	All time
Data processing, analysis, and interpretation		
Data entry and data cleaning	Lecture	2
Data entry and data cleaning	Practical	4
Data analysis	Lecture	1
Data analysis	Practical	4
Data presentation and interpretation	Lecture	2
Data presentation and interpretation	Practical	2
Report writing and dissemination of results		
Concepts of report writing	Lecture	1
Writing a paper for publication	Lecture	1
Critique of a published article	Lecture	1
Critique of a published article	Practical	2
Facilities and materials for aiding presentations	Lecture	1
Facilities and materials for aiding presentations	Practical	2
Feedback reporting	Fieldwork	48

and the social sciences in conducting health research in developing countries. While instructors providing guidance to students in this field should emphasize the need for doing good research, they should themselves be exemplary in so doing. They should provide the necessary guidance and contribute to students' research endeavors whenever possible so that new knowledge can also emanate from students' work. This chapter has attempted to provide instructors with the kind of steps needed to guide students, both undergraduates and postgraduates, to perform systematic field studies in the medical and social science disciplines.

Further reading

Abramson, J. H. *Survey methods in community medicine: Epidemiological studies, programme evaluation* (Fourth edition). Churchill Livingstone. Edinburgh, 1990.

Abramson, J. H. *Making sense of data. A self-instruction manual on the interpretation of epidemiologic data* (Second edition). Oxford University Press. Oxford, 1994.

Beaglehole, R., Bonita, R., Kjellstrom, T. *Basic epidemiology.* WHO, Geneva, 1993.

Fauveau, V. Data collection system and datasets available in Matlab. In Matlab: *Women, children and health.* Fauveau, V. (ed). International Centre for Diarrhoeal Disease Research, Bangladesh (ICDDR,B) special publication No. 35. 1994 Dhaka.

Hall, G. M. (Ed). *How to write a paper.* BMJ Publishing Group, London, 1994.

Huth, E. J. *How to write and publish papers in the medical sciences.* Second edition. Williams and Wilkins, London, 1990.

Kirkwood, B. *Essentials of Medical Statistics.* Blackwell Scientific Publications. Oxford, 1988.

Morris, L. L., Fitz-Gibbon, C. T., Freeman, M. E. *How to communicate evaluation findings.* SAGE Publications. London, 1987.

Polgar, S., Thomas, S. A. *Introduction to research in the health sciences* (Third edition). Churchill Livingstone. Melbourne, 1995.

Ross, D. A. and Vaughan, J. P. Health Interview Surveys in Developing Countries: A methodological Review. *Studies in Family Planning,* 1986 **17**, 78–94

Smith, P. G., Morrow, R. H. *Methods for field trials of interventions against tropical diseases: A toolbox.* Eds. P. G. Smith and Richard, H. Morrow. Oxford Medical Publications. Oxford University Press, Oxford 1991, Reprinted 1992 and 1993.

van Ginneken, J., Bairagi, R., de Francisco, A., Sarder, A. M., Vaugha, P. *Health and demographic surveillance in Matlab: Past, present and future.* International Centre for Diarrhoeal Disease Research, Bangladesh (ICDDR,B) special publication No. 72. 1998 Dhaka.

Pedagogies

Chapter 26

Epidemiology inside and outside the classroom

J. H. Abramson

Introduction

There is no single ideal way of teaching epidemiology. Teaching can take place in different situations, and its techniques and content may differ. A good teaching program is one that is geared to its students' needs, capacity, interests, and preferences, and exploits available teaching situations and techniques to provide learning opportunities that will achieve the educational objectives.

This chapter reviews some features of the teaching of epidemiology inside and outside the classroom. It starts with a discussion of the main factors that affect the choice of methods and then deals in turn with conventional classroom methods, laboratory teaching (problem-solving and other exercises), self-instruction, problem-oriented projects, and distance learning. Separate consideration is then given to teaching in the hospital and in the field (with special attention to teaching in a community health center).

Teaching objectives

Decisions about teaching methods

Many factors influence the choice of teaching methods. Prominent among these are the educational objectives of the teaching program, the students' interests and preferences, and practical considerations.

Educational objectives

The educational objectives, i.e. what it is hoped the students will learn to do, require careful specification (Mager, 1997). They may be categorized broadly as follows:

1. *Knowing* epidemiology: the ability to state specified facts about epidemiologic terms, principles and methods, and specified findings of epidemiologic studies, e.g. facts about the epidemiology of selected diseases.

2. *Using* epidemiology: the capacity to interpret and appraise epidemiologic findings, and to apply such knowledge when performing activities that are not primarily epidemiologic. Medical students may be expected to acquire skill in making clinical decisions founded on facts about the prevalence and incidence of diseases, the variability of biologic findings, the prognostic significance of risk

factors, the reliability and validity of test results, and the results of clinical trials. Students who are or will be involved in public health practice or policy formulation may similarly be expected to acquire skill in the use of epidemiologic findings when making decisions. For many teachers, the main goal is that students should be able to 'think logically' when appraising causal relationships. The capacity to read articles critically may be specified as an objective.

3. *Practising* ('doing') epidemiology: the capacity to perform specified epidemiologic activities. These may range from simple tasks such as tabulating data and calculating rates, through more complex activities, such as questionnaire design, the maintenance of disease registers, and data processing and analysis, to the comprehensive planning and performance of studies. Emphasis may be put on the ability to perform research designed to yield generalizable conclusions, or on more pragmatic studies aimed at the improvement of health or healthcare in specific communities or populations.

4. An ability to *teach* epidemiology, especially to other members of the health team, is often specified as an additional objective. A related but usually neglected objective is the ability to *communicate* epidemiologic findings – especially to decision-makers and the media – in such a way as to maximize their use and minimize their misuse.

The choice of situations and methods for teaching depends on the educational objectives. Students will learn to 'use' and 'practise' epidemiology best if they are taught in a context in which epidemiology is 'used' and 'practised', and if they are given practical experience (with suitable supervision) in 'using' and 'practising' it.

In general, educational objectives should be adapted to the needs of the students and the requirements of the population in which the students will work. Objectives may vary for medical students, physicians in clinical practice, clinicians who wish to undertake research, nursing students, nurses and other professionals engaged in patient care, medical assistants and other auxiliaries, aspiring professional epidemiologists, public health students and practitioners, community physicians, health administrators, health service researchers, statisticians, and auxiliary personnel engaged in epidemiologic and health service research, students who are not committed to a career in a health profession (Lilienfeld *et al.*, 1978; Fraser, 1987), and so on.

There is no consensus about educational objectives for specific categories of students, even in a single country. Some medical schools are satisfied if students learn the epidemiology of common diseases; others focus on the capacity for clinical decision-making or critical reading; and others expect students to learn how to make a community diagnosis and evaluate the outcome of a community health program. Although most teachers of epidemiology would probably regard all these aims as important, educational objectives are often limited by the restrictive views of curriculum committees or other constraints. Moreover, specific objectives will differ in communities with different health problems. The importance of training in the 'practice' of epidemiology may depend on the local availability of epidemiologic skills and personnel, and may vary in different healthcare systems.

The variation in objectives means that no teaching program can be regarded as the single best one for universal application to a given category of student.

Teaching contents

Students' interests and preferences

Some students have little interest in epidemiology, notably many medical students who see little relevance to their central concern, the care of individual patients. Apparently only after graduation is there a tendency towards a greater appreciation by physicians of the value of epidemiology (Krall *et al.*, 1983).

For such students, particularly in medical schools where teachers of other disciplines disparage epidemiology, it is important to concentrate on epidemiologic topics of obvious clinical relevance, especially for the treatment of hospital patients. 'Packaging' too may be important – the term 'epidemiology' may be a handicap; when asked to rate seminars, medical residents in New York gave lower ratings to those on epidemiology than to those on the sensitivity, specificity, and predictive value of laboratory tests, or on literature interpretation (Kantor and Griner, 1981).

The current interest in evidence-based medicine can motivate students to learn basic epidemiologic principles and methods, and increasing use is being made of evidence-based medicine as a vehicle for the teaching of epidemiology. In Boston, a controlled study indicated that exposure to four sessions on evidence-based medicine was enough to have a significant positive impact on critical appraisal skills (Ghali *et al.*, 2000). In a specimen classroom session on epidemiology and biostatistics in Oxford, a clinical scenario is presented and the students are asked to suggest likely explanations and the evidence needed to reach a diagnosis, and then discuss the validity and interpretation of this evidence; a journal article describing a clinical trial is circulated, and (first in small groups and then as a whole class) the students appraise the validity of the findings and their applicability to the case in question (Sackett *et al.*, 1997). A session might also center not on a specific case but on a recommended treatment protocol for a specific condition, and the evidence supporting this protocol. To break out of a narrow therapeutic context, the focus might also be placed on a preventive recommendation, such as avoiding coffee or eating more fruit and vegetables, or on broader aspects of healthcare, such as the role of community involvement.

Some teachers of epidemiology regard a clinical context as being as important as a clinical content, and prefer to teach in a hospital setting, or try to link their teaching with other courses, e.g. by teaching the epidemiology of infectious diseases in the framework of courses on microbiology or the clinical aspects of these diseases. In schools with an integrated 'problem-based' curriculum, epidemiology can be incorporated in the solution of the defined problems, which may relate to biomedical questions or to health economics, general practice, health education, etc. (Leeder and Sackett, 1976; Pemberton, 1986).

Even when the climate for the teaching of epidemiology is unfavorable, efforts should be made to broaden the interests of students beyond the care of the single patient. It needs only a few students to become interested in community healthcare or epidemiologic research to make these efforts worthwhile, or at least to seem so, to a teacher who may otherwise find his work frustrating.

Students whose central interest is in healthcare at a group or community level, such as graduate students of public health or health administration, generally recognize the importance of epidemiology. But here, too, the teaching should be brought as close as possible to the students' interests, in terms of specific situations (e.g. hospital or community health services), applications (research *versus* pragmatic epidemiology), and subject matter (heart disease, child health, etc.). A flexible program that permits choices by students is of especial value. This may be achieved by giving students a choice of assignments or projects, and (particularly in graduate courses) by providing a range of elective courses.

Students' preferences concerning methods of teaching should also be considered. Those who have had little experience, during or since their school days, of heuristic teaching aimed at helping them to discover for themselves rather than learning what they are told, may not take kindly to teaching based on a problem-solving approach. The capacity to solve problems is of central importance in 'practising' and 'using' epidemiology, and problem-solving exercises cannot easily be dispensed with; however, they may be more acceptable and effective in some student groups than in others, and in every group there will be some students who require more 'hand-holding' than others.

The effectiveness of all teaching methods varies for different students. Self-instruction, for example, may work well with some students and not with others. Some students enjoy working with computers, others are computer-shy. A flexible program that caters for different needs has obvious advantages. Students may be given a choice between attendance at lectures and reading, or between computerized and printed problem-solving exercises, and may be permitted to do the exercises in groups or alone, and in class or at home. Periodic surveillance of students' progress is especially important when such options are offered, as students may not always make the best choices. Not only the kind of teaching, but also the amount of teaching may vary for different students; special tutorials, summer projects, and elective courses have been advocated for those medical students who are interested in epidemiology: 'efforts should be concentrated where the interest is greatest' (Grufferman *et al.*, 1984).

Practical considerations

It is hardly necessary to stress the importance of practical constraints that may affect teaching methods, such as the availability of time, teachers, and other resources, and the capacity and interests of teachers. A community health center, for example, is likely to be a useful context for the teaching of epidemiology only if there is a sufficiency of tutors or preceptors, if the personnel are interested in the use of epidemiology, and if there are ongoing programs that demonstrate the utility of epidemiology in the provision of healthcare. Epidemiologic activities that appear to be conducted solely for teaching purposes may have a negative impact on students.

If medical students are to be given hands-on experience of the use of epidemiology in clinical work, an obvious basic requirement is allotment of time for this during the clinical years.

Teaching method and format

Classroom teaching

Lectures

An exceptional lecture or series of lectures by an exceptional lecturer can be an inspiring experience. However, by and large, lecturing is not the most effective way of teaching, although there may be little choice if teachers are scarce. In the UK, the proportion of public health teaching time allocated to lectures has decreased in recent years, whereas teaching by small group methods has increased (Edwards *et al.*, 1999). In a controlled trial of methods of teaching clinical epidemiology to medical students in Wales, lectures received the lowest evaluations and self-learning packages the highest (Gehlbach *et al.*, 1985). In Pennsylvania, 89% of medical students randomly allocated to small discussion groups rated the course as important in their medical education, as compared with 65% of those allotted to a large lecture group; there was no difference in examination performance (Romm *et al.*, 1989).

Good lectures can, of course, serve useful purposes. Apart from imparting facts, they can provide students with frameworks and models for use in their own explorations of the topic, and they can sometimes communicate enthusiasm and a motivation to learn. The value of a lecture is enhanced by careful preparation, preparatory reading assignments for students, an interesting, audible, systematic, and not overlong presentation, appropriate use of aids such as the blackboard, slides, transparencies, computer presentations, and handout material, sensitivity to the students' reactions, provision of opportunities to ask questions or discuss the content, and assignments based on the lecture.

Lectures alone cannot easily be used to teach skills but, in conjunction with practical exercises, they can serve a valuable function by presenting systematic frameworks for the performance of activities (how to appraise a screening test, how to plan a survey, how to investigate an outbreak, how to control for confounding, how to do a meta-analysis, etc.).

Group discussions

Group discussions with active student participation, i.e. with interaction among students as well as with teachers, are more effective than lectures, particularly if the group is small. If there are more than about 20 students, the same few students generally participate actively each time.

The discussion may center on topics presented by teachers or students; some or all of the students may have been given reading assignments in advance. The teacher's roles include:

♦ Preventing the session from degenerating into a bad lecture by an unskilled student lecturer.

♦ Drawing students into the discussion.

♦ Guiding the discussion to ensure that the teaching potential of the topic is adequately exploited.

♦ Ensuring that students come away feeling they have learnt something, and knowing what it is that they have learnt.

Discussions of articles presented by students (and preferably that all students have been asked to read) provide an opportunity not only to learn about the topic, but also to learn how to evaluate study methods and appraise the validity of findings and conclusions. They constitute a useful teaching method in programs where the ability to read critically is a defined objective. Some teachers recommend 'classical' papers (Buck *et al.*, 1988) that illustrate important epidemiologic concepts or methods; others prefer recent papers of current interest.

Discussions of recent articles may be organized in a 'journal club' framework, generally in the context of continuing education for physicians or other professionals.

Other methods

Role playing may be a useful technique, for example, in teaching the use of interviews in surveys. Students interview one another in front of the class, using schedules they have prepared themselves, and this provides a basis for discussions of the effects of the wording or sequencing of questions, interview technique, and so on.

Other classroom methods include panel discussions, in which experts discuss a topic among themselves and answer students' questions, and symposia, in which presentations are made by a number of experts.

Laboratory teaching

'Laboratory' teaching is a convenient term for a variety of activities that aim to teach epidemiologic skills in a systematic way.

Problem-solving exercises

Problem-solving exercises generally present facts derived from actual or imaginary studies, and require students to analyse and appraise the facts, draw inferences, and reach decisions concerning the need for further investigations and/or intervention. The role of such exercises in the teaching of epidemiology is similar to that of the examination of patients in the teaching of clinical medicine (Lowe and Kostrzewski, 1973). The exercises provide practical experience, under laboratory conditions, in the use of epidemiologic tools: methods of investigation, analysis, and data interpretation. Students may be required to gather data (generally from documentary sources), prepare tabulations and charts, perform statistical analyses, and formulate and test hypotheses. Library research may be needed. The exercises are often constructed serially; at each step students are asked what additional information they need, and then given new facts and new tasks. The exercises may center on epidemiologic methods, the epidemiology of selected conditions, or specified epidemiologic concepts. They are probably most effective if they deal with problems and techniques of obvious relevance to the students' interests.

The exercises may be carried out by students working alone or in small groups (of, say, four or five), inside or outside the classroom. Students are usually advised to summarize their answers in writing, for their own later use; some teachers require the submission of written answers. When the exercises are done in a classroom, instructors generally circulate among the groups to guide the students and review their answers, and the class may be brought together from time to time for a more general discussion.

Serially constructed exercises that provide printed solutions and comments (for example see Abramson and Abramson, 2001) can be used either for self-instruction or in group situations, and have the advantage that students or groups can work at their own pace.

Problem-solving exercises may also be used primarily as a basis for group discussions (in groups of, say, up to 20). 'Seminar exercises' of this kind were first popularized by Terris (1966). A set of facts and questions is distributed, and some time later a group discussion is conducted, dealing with the answers, the methods of reaching them, and relevant concepts and subject matter. It is helpful for the instructors to decide in advance what topics they wish the discussion to cover.

These two methods of using exercises may be combined. For example, students may be given an exercise to do, and then provided with additional facts and questions as a basis for a subsequent group discussion.

Exercises in specific techniques

Exercises in specific techniques, performed in the classroom or as 'homework', are commonly used to provide experience in performing epidemiologic procedures and to reinforce or extend the student's knowledge of epidemiologic principles or facts. Such exercises, which do not necessarily present the intellectual challenge of problem-solving, may be used as adjuncts to lecture or reading courses, or may be the chief element of a course. A course on survey methods, for example, may include exercises on the choice of a study design, the formulation of study objectives, the choice of controls, the selection of a sampling method, the use of random numbers, the choice and definition of variables, the measurement of validity and reliability, the design of questions and questionnaires, data processing, and so on. These may be more than pencil-and-paper exercises: an unforgettable demonstration of observer variation, for example, can be staged by asking all the students in a group to measure a volunteer's height and weight, or to determine blood pressures based on a film of sphygmomanometer readings. Some topics, for example the use of statistical methods in epidemiology, can hardly be taught without the practical drill that systematic exercises provide.

Computer exercises

Exercises involving the use of a computer are especially important in graduate courses in which students are required to conduct projects involving the use of computer databases or computer analysis. While the use of commercial software packages may be unavoidable for some purposes, it is advisable to give students experience in the use of readily available public-domain programs, such as EpiInfo (Dean *et al.*, 1994), which streamlines data entry, does analyses, and can convert data to formats suitable for use with various statistical packages, and PEPI, a collection of statistical programs for epidemiologists (Abramson and Gahlinger, 2001).

Self-instruction

Self-instruction (Atkinson and Wilson, 1969) is practicable in instances where suitable materials are available, i.e. a parcel of reading material, exercises and other printed aids, a self-instructional computer program or access to one on the Internet, or a package using audiotapes, videotapes, slides, or other components.

Many students find self-instruction attractive because they can choose their own pace and sequencing, working alone or with friends. Some students need only be 'pointed in the right direction' and can then be largely left to their own devices; others require considerable ongoing guidance. An important advantage of self-instruction is that it nurtures the capacity to learn in a self-directed way. Unless students have this skill they will cease to learn when they complete their formal tuition and are exposed to 'the "future shock" they could encounter after graduation ... their world will be characterized by rapid change, and by many facts and skills which have [a] half-life of ten years or less' (Higgs, 1982). A major goal of an epidemiology course, it has been said, is 'to provide you with some perspectives and tools that will prevent you from becoming obsolete after you leave medical school' (Ernster, 1979).

In theory, self-instruction saves teachers' time. In practice it may not do so because of the need to prepare appropriate learning guides and other material, and to provide supplementary individual tutoring. But if suitable self-teaching aids are already available, the technique may be a valuable one where teachers of epidemiology are scarce (Acheson, 1973; Lobo and Jouval, 1973).

Published 'do-it-yourself' books include study guides (Morton *et al.*, 1996; Unwin *et al.*, 1997) and a manual on the interpretation of epidemiologic data (Abramson and Abramson, 2001).

Computer-assisted learning programs

Increasing use of computer-assisted learning programs is to be expected. DoEpi, for example, a set of interactive exercises built around the EpiInfo software, with modules concerned with outbreak investigation, public health surveillance, and a research study, provides experience in computing as well as in epidemiologic methods (Dean *et al.*, 1998). For many students, the main attraction of computer-assisted instruction is that it provides a non-threatening private learning environment in which they can work at their own pace and make errors without fear of ridicule from peers or teachers (Larson, 1984).

If the required facilities are available, computer-assisted instruction can be cost-effective. Tests of its use in the education of health professionals have shown that students learn as well as with more traditional teaching strategies, but in one-third to one-half the time (Larson, 1984). However, teachers who propose to write their own computer programs should be ready to devote considerable time to this; estimates of the time required to develop 1 hour of computer-based instruction range from 20 hours (Veloski, 1986) (with more time needed for pilot testing, evaluation, and revision) to 228 hours (Reinhardt, 1995) or more. The DoEpi package includes a 'Wizard' facility that can permit the construction of a new exercise in a few days, given the necessary computer skills (Dean *et al.*, 1998).

A teacher wishing to use a computer-assisted learning program (or other ready-made self-instruction package) should ensure that its content meets the requirements of the epidemiology course, and that the presentation is appropriate. A computer program should not be just an 'electronic page turner' that has few advantages over printed material, but should exploit the computer's capacity to interact with the user; it should permit the learner to choose topics and their sequence and (where appropriate) to control the level of difficulty, and should carry on a dialog by providing immediate feedback appropriate to the user's responses (correct or incorrect). Well designed programs provide specific feedback, enabling the student to assess his or her own knowledge and progress and, where necessary, reinforce learning. Some programs can promote creative problem-solving by allowing the student to manipulate variables: they 'open up the world of "what if's"' to the learner (Larson, 1984). The program should be user-friendly – easy to operate, with lucid and unambiguous text, uncluttered displays, clear and simple instructions, and readily available on-screen help; it should permit the correction of mistakes and the changing of answers, allow for easy transition to previous screens, provide an easy way of quitting the program, and so on (Johnson, 1985; Skiba, 1985; Kearsley, 1989).

Reading

Self-instruction by reading is, of course, an ancillary method in all epidemiology courses. Students are generally given lists of required and recommended reading. This may be regarded as background learning, or it may be given more prominence by requiring its use in class presentations or discussions or in written assignments. Some lecturers expect students to read designated material before the lecture, which they confine to topics that emerge from this reading; however, students often ignore these assignments, especially if they are extensive.

Many teachers of epidemiology find that there is no single textbook they can recommend, if only because the objectives of courses vary, as do the contents, emphases, and approaches of textbooks. Some books deal only with specific aspects of epidemiology, and those that claim to be comprehensive generally have gaps. A book written for a defined audience may meet its purpose well but be of restricted value for other readers. Students are often advised to read specified parts of different textbooks, as well as selected journal articles. Some teachers prepare compilations of chosen materials.

Students should be encouraged to seek relevant material on the Internet. If library facilities are lacking, the rapidly growing collection of lectures of the 'Epidemiology Supercourse' may be useful (http://www.pitt.edu/~super1/main/epi.htm); but it should be noted that lectures provided in written format have most of the disadvantages and none of the advantages of oral lectures.

Projects

Problem-oriented projects

Problem-oriented projects pose students with tasks that require employment of epidemiologic knowledge and methods. They provide valuable hands-on experience in addressing real life or simulated problems. Students may evaluate such projects more favorably than formal teaching, and with no detriment to their examination results (Marantz et al., 1991).

Projects may be assigned to individuals or (more usually) to groups. Group projects have the ancillary advantage of providing experience in teamwork. Most students perform well in group projects, even if there are some who leave the work to their more interested and conscientious colleagues. Whole-class projects may be undertaken in which tasks are divided among different groups. Ongoing tutoring is usually provided. For graduate students particularly, projects may have an appreciable element of self-instruction; students may be required to crystallize their own objectives and reach their own decisions about methods of investigation. Classroom sessions may be organized to review the planning and progress of the projects, so that learning experiences can be shared. Final reports are generally presented orally to the whole class, as well as in writing. A project may form the basis for a thesis; this is a requirement in some courses, especially those that aim to produce researchers or teachers (Zvarova et al., 1997).

The nature and scope of projects vary, depending on students' and teachers' specific interests, the time available, and other considerations of feasibility. Some projects are restricted to library research, particularly for undergraduate students, who may be asked to find, read and critically appraise articles with a bearing on a decision required in clinical or community healthcare. Most projects involve systematic data gathering, in the field or from clinical records (which may be particularly attractive to medical students). Field projects may enhance students' awareness of the role of the community in health development (Persson and Wall, 1993). The project may be concerned with the health status of a group or community, the determinants of health, or the provision of healthcare, and may be descriptive or analytical; it is often evaluative in nature.

Students are generally asked to make recommendations based on their findings to provide experience in the interpretation and use of epidemiologic findings. Students of public health (Gofin et al., 1985) and health management (Mercenier and van Balen, 1973) may be required to make practical use of the findings for planning or evaluating healthcare. The use of findings in the development of student-organized action programs, and the controlled evaluation of a program originated by a previous group of students, have been found to be strong incentives (Schofield and Muller, 1973).

Projects sometimes take the form of research aimed at the acquisition of generalizable new knowledge. This kind of experience is a requirement for some graduate students. It has also been advocated as an important and productive contribution to the teaching of epidemiology to undergraduates, sometimes leading to publications; but even with grant support for an adequate infrastructure of personnel and equipment, several generations of students may have to work on each study, and faculty members may have to complete student-initiated projects (Grufferman et al., 1984). Requiring medical students to write a research protocol has been advocated as a method of teaching research design, even if there is no intention of performing the study (Linskey et al., 1987); projects in research design have also been included in undergraduate nursing courses (Laschinger et al., 1990). In West Virginia, a course that focused on the writing of a research proposal was found to be more effective and acceptable to medical students than previous approaches to the teaching of epidemiology, and led in some instances to actual research (Garland and Pearson, 1989).

Distance learning

As communication technologies advance, distance learning (which is characterized by the physical separation between instructor and learner) is growing in popularity, and numerous academic programs are in existence. Traditional correspondence courses are being replaced by methods that range from the placing of 'lectures' on the Internet, and electronic mail, to more elaborate methods of transmission and mechanisms that allow real-time interaction between teachers and students or among students. The curriculum may include self-instruction components, problem-solving and other exercises, and even group projects.

Emphasis has been given to the role of distance learning in epidemiology for students and professionals in developing countries, where teachers are scarce, and to its potential for enhancing practical and research collaboration between public health workers in developing and developed countries. One program, which defines its aim as 'to provide health workers with solutions to problems which they face in their everyday work', has modules on nutritional surveillance, the role of epidemiology in the care of refugees, nutritional surveillance, and rapid epidemiologic appraisal (MacFarlane et al., 1996).

The preparation of material (if not already available) may of course be very time-consuming, and teachers have reported that 'providing effective feedback for students required nearly as much time as in an ordinary course with the same number of students'. They also commented that about 25% of the messages were devoted to technical problems of computer communication (Ostbye, 1989).

Teachers interested in distance learning should be prepared to learn new skills or to collaborate with experts on technical aspects. A useful primer on distance learning in public health (Segal, 1999) has been prepared by the US Center for Disease Control and Prevention. It reports that practical experience indicates that the best distance learning programs combine a variety of media, selected for different purposes, and that success is enhanced if students are organized into groups under a local facilitator, especially if the groups meet periodically. Evaluations have shown that learners prefer well designed instruction using a distance learning strategy to other approaches. The primer includes a handbook describing the concepts and strategies of distance learning (Yoakam and Chute, 1999); among the methods listed are audio conferences, computer conferences, audiographics, and one-way and two-way video.

Teaching in the hospital

Teaching epidemiology in the hospital is of special importance for medical students and others whose main concern is the clinical care of patients, and for students with a special interest in hospital services.

For the former category, where the challenge is to bring the students to realize the relevance of epidemiology to their clinical interests, emphasis may be placed on topics that are closely related to the clinical problems they encounter. Students may be required to perform 'literature critiques' on problems that interest them, or to undertake surveys based on samples of hospital patients and dealing with clinical problems.

In some medical schools epidemiologists participate in ward rounds and case discussions, or run ward rounds themselves (Stone, 1998) to ensure coverage of the epidemiologic features of common diseases and the principles of clinical epidemiology or evidence-based medicine, i.e. the use of epidemiologic knowledge and methods in diagnosis, in prognosis, and in decisions about care (Sackett *et al.*, 1991; 1997). This 'bedside' approach probably depends for its success on the attitude of key clinicians to epidemiology and on the availability of teachers who are versed in clinical medicine as well as in epidemiology; clinical epidemiology is possibly best taught by clinicians who know and use epidemiology (Lobo and Jouval, 1973; Jenicek and Fletcher, 1977). The bedside approach is not necessarily effective, even for teaching its limited epidemiologic agenda. In a London medical school where bedside teaching by epidemiologists was replaced by a seminar course based on small group sessions and practical exercises, the new course was positively evaluated by students and led to a greater appreciation of the importance of epidemiology for clinical practice (Heller and Peach, 1984).

For students with a special interest in hospital services, the hospital situation offers a wide variety of opportunities for experience in the application of epidemiologic methods. Projects may be concerned with such topics as nosocomial infections, physical hazards in the hospital environment, sickness absences of personnel, factors influencing the use of services and compliance with care, the effectiveness and safety of various diagnostic and therapeutic services, and the impact of the hospital on community health.

Teaching in the field

Field projects

Field projects provide valuable learning experiences. The projects may be undertaken by individual students or by small or large groups. They generally involve surveys of diseases or health status in selected samples or population groups, surveys of environmental and other determinants of health, and/or studies of healthcare. Use may be made of available data as well as, or instead of, data gathered by the students. As published examples show, the topics of field projects range over the whole field of public health (Lowe and Kostrzewski, 1973; Pemberton, 1973; Bennett, 1979). For most students, the experience is most interesting if the project has the aim of solving or alleviating a known health problem.

Tutoring is generally a combined responsibility of teachers of epidemiology (and other subjects) and personnel of the services or agencies with whose help the projects are conducted. The latter act as preceptors, and the feasibility of projects often depends on the availability of suitable preceptors.

Field projects have been used for teaching epidemiology to health workers of different kinds, ranging from graduate specialists to practical nurses (Kurtzman and Block, 1983) and community health workers (WHO, 1981), and also as opportunities for bringing together groups of students of different disciplines, e.g. medical students and health inspector students (Bennett, 1981), to assist them to learn to function in teams concerned with common tasks.

Field projects based on local community services can serve useful educational purposes for all students, but students with a specific interest in public health services at a regional or national level may require projects that go beyond a local community. 'Learning while doing' may be the central feature of the training of health professionals for careers in applied epidemiology and preventive medicine, as in the Epidemiologic Intelligence Service program of the US Public Health Service (which provides 2 years of practical experience in field investigations and epidemiologic research of local, state, national, or international importance) (Goodman *et al.*, 1990; Thacker *et al.*, 1990) and similar field epidemiology training programs in other countries (Brachman and Music, 1989; Cardenas *et al.*, 1998).

Teaching in a community health center

A community health center (or any other primary care service that serves a defined population) offers special opportunities for a wide variety of epidemiologic projects of interest to various categories of students. Possible topics include common diseases and disabilities; familial, social, environmental and behavioural factors, and their effects on health and disease; processes of growth, development, and aging; and various aspects of the care of people living in their own homes.

A health center or service that practises community-oriented primary care (COPC) can be a particularly useful teaching context. COPC, which denotes the combination of the care of individuals and the care of the community as a whole in a single integrated practice, is characterized by the development of defined community programs to deal with the health needs of the community and its subgroups (Abramson and Kark, 1983; Kark *et al.*, 1994; Rhyne *et al.*, 1998). Epidemiology is built in as the basis for the appraisal and elucidation of these needs and for the planning and ongoing monitoring and evaluation of the programs – epidemiology in practice, incarnate. Attractive features for medical students are the emphasis on a real community problem (a 'community case') and the similarity of the COPC cycle (examination and community diagnosis, consideration of different interventions and their probable effectiveness, intervention, surveillance, evaluation, and modification of intervention) to the approach they have learnt to apply in clinical work.

The opportunities that a COPC practice provides for teaching epidemiology (Kark *et al.*, 1973; Gofin *et al.*, 1985; Boufford and Shonubi, 1986; Osborne *et al.*, 1986) may be used in at least four ways. First, students can be exposed to the COPC programs, and observe how epidemiology can contribute to community healthcare. They will see what methods are used: how community diagnosis and health surveillance are conducted, how the findings are used in the planning of community programs, how the programs are monitored and evaluated, and how new findings are used as a basis for program modifications (Abramson and Abramson, 1999). Second, students can be given 'laboratory' exercises based on data collected in the practice. Third, they can undertake projects related to the center's activities. These may be directed at collecting information that may help in modifying existing programs or developing new ones, or they may be less pragmatic 'research'-oriented studies that make use of the center's accumulated data and other resources. Fourth, students may be asked to apply what they have learnt by planning COPC programs for the communities in which they work or will work, using available information about these communities and their health services; problem-solving projects of this kind are best performed by small groups of students, at least one of whom knows the community well.

Integrated workshops on COPC, incorporating most or all of these approaches, together with teaching concerned with basic management skills, community health education, community organization, and other topics, have been provided for public health students, residents in family medicine, pediatricians, and others (Kark *et al.*, 1973; Gofin *et al.*, 1985). In general they have been favorably received, and most participants subsequently reported that they were applying what they had learnt. In a number of instances the students' plans for health programs in other communities were put into operation.

Field demonstrations

Field demonstrations based on visits to agencies concerned with the collection, analysis, or use of epidemiologic data are useful only if they are well prepared and organized, and clearly concerned with topics of interest to the students. Otherwise they can easily deteriorate into casual sightseeing trips.

Combined methods of teaching

The most effective teaching programs are probably those that use a variety of different approaches, exploiting the special advantages of each. They may include courses dealing with different topics and using different teaching methods; with good sequencing and coordination, these can reinforce each other. Even in a single short course the use of varied methods may be beneficial and receive a positive evaluation from students (Clarke *et al.*, 1980; Fowkes *et al.*, 1984).

References

Abramson, J. H. and Abramson, Z. H. (2001). *Making sense of data: A self-instruction manual on the interpretation of epidemiological data*, 3rd edn. New York: Oxford University Press.

Abramson, J. H. and Abramson, Z. H. (1999). *Survey methods in community medicine: epidemiological research, programme evaluation, clinical trials*, 5th edn. Churchill Livingstone, Edinburgh, pp. 387–405.

Abramson, J. H. and Gahlinger, P. M. (2001). *Computer programs for epidemiologists: PEPI version 4.00*. Sagebrush Press, Salt Lake City, Utah.

Abramson, J. H. and Kark, S. L. (1983). Community oriented primary care: meaning and scope. In: Connor, E. and Mullan, F. (eds) *Community oriented primary care: New directions for health services delivery*. National Academy Press, Washington DC, pp. 21–59.

Acheson, R. M. (1973). Epidemiology in medical education: introduction to the symposium. *International Journal of Epidemiology* 2, 355–7.

Atkinson, R. C. and Wilson, H. E. (1969). *Computer-assisted instruction: a book of readings*. Academic Press, New York.

Bennett, F. J. (ed.) (1979). *Community diagnosis and health action: a manual for tropical and rural areas*. Macmillan, London.

Bennett, F. J. (1981). Community diagnosis: its uses in the training of community health workers and in primary health care in East Africa. *Israel Journal of Medical Sciences* **17**, 129–37.

Boufford, J. I. and Shonubi, P. A. (1986). *Community oriented primary care. Training for urban practice.* Praeger, New York.

Brachman, P. S, and Music, S. I. (1989). Epidemiology training and public health practice. *Epidemiology and Infection,* **102**, 199–204.

Buck, C., Llopis, A., Najera, E. and Terris, M. (eds) (1988). *The challenge of epidemiology— issues and selected readings.* Pan American Health Organization, Washington DC.

Cardenas, V., Sanchez, C., De la Hoz *et al.* (1998). Colombian field epidemiology training program. *American Journal of Public Health* **88**, 1404–5.

Clarke, M., Clayton, D. G. and Donaldson, L. J. (1980). Teaching epidemiology and statistics to medical students – the Leicester experience. *International Journal of Epidemiology* **9**, 179–85.

Dean, A. G., Shah, S. P. and Churchill, J. E. (1998). DoEpi: computer-assisted instruction in epidemiology and computing and a framework for creating new exercises. *American Journal of Preventive Medicine* **14**, 367–71.

Dean, A. G., Dean, J. A., Coulombier, D. *et al.* (1994). *Epi Info, version 6: a word processing, database, and statistics program for public health on IBM-compatible microcomputers.* Centers for Disease Control and Prevention, Atlanta, GA.

Edwards, R., White, M., Chappel, D. and Gray, J. (1999). Teaching public health to medical students in the United Kingdom – are the General Medical Council's recommendations being implemented? *Journal of Public Health Medicine* **21**, 150–7.

Ernster, V. L. (1979). On the teaching of epidemiology to medical students. *American Journal of Epidemiology* **109**, 617–18.

Fowkes, F. G. R., Gehlbach, S. H., Farrow, S. C., West, R. R. and Roberts, C. J. (1984). Epidemiology for medical students: a course relevant to clinical practice. *International Journal of Epidemiology* **13**, 538–41.

Fraser, D. W. (1987). Epidemiology as a liberal art. *New England Journal of Medicine* **316**, 309–14.

Garland, B. K. and Pearson, R. J. C. (1989). Epidemiology course for medical students focuses on proposal writing. *American Journal of Preventive Medicine* **5**, 240–3.

Gehlbach, S. H., Farrow, S. C., Fowkes, F. G. R., West, R. R. and Roberts, C. J. (1985). Epidemiology for medical students: a controlled trial of three teaching methods. *International Journal of Epidemiology* **14**, 178–81.

Ghali, W. A., Saitz, R., Eskew, A. H., Gupta, M., Quam, H. and Hershman, W. Y. (2000). Successful teaching in evidence-based medicine. *Medical Education* **34**, 18–22.

Gofin, J., Mainemer, N. and Kark, S. L. (1985). Community health in primary care – a workshop on community-oriented primary care. In: Laaser, U., Senault, R. and Viefhus, H. (eds) *Primary health care in the making.* Springer-Verlag, Berlin, pp. 17–21.

Goodman, R. A., Bauman, C. F., Gregg, M. B., Videtto, J. F., Stroup, D. F. and Chalmers, N. P. (1990). Epidemiologic field investigations by the Centers for Disease Control and Epidemic Intelligence Service, 1946–87. *Public Health Reports* **105**, 604–10.

Grufferman, S., Kimm, S. Y. S. and Maile, M. C. (1984). Teaching epidemiology in medical schools: a workable model. *American Journal of Epidemiology* **120**, 203–9.

Heller, R. F. and Peach, H. (1984). Evaluation of a new course to teach the principles and clinical applications of epidemiology to medical students. *International Journal of Epidemiology* **13**, 533–7.

Higgs, J. (1982). Self-instructional materials as components of courses. In: Ewan, C. E. (ed.) *Self-instruction: a strategy for education of health personnel*. Kensington, NSW, Australia: University of New South Wales Center for Medical Education Research and Development, WHO Regional Teacher Training Centre for Health Personnel; Review Paper No. 1, pp. 2–22.

Jenicek, M. and Fletcher, R. H. (1977). Epidemiology for Canadian medical students – desirable attitudes, knowledge and skills. *International Journal of Epidemiology* **6**, 69–72.

Johnson, A. T. (1985). User friendliness in microcomputer programs. *Comput Programs Biomed* **19**, 127–30.

Kantor, S. M. and Griner, P. F. (1981). Educational needs in general internal medicine as perceived by prior residents. *Journal of Medical Education* **56**, 748–56.

Kark, S. L., Kark, E., Abramson, J. H. and Gofin, J. (eds.) (1994). *Atencion primaria orientada a la comunidad (APOC)*, Ediciones Doyma S. A., Barcelona.

Kark, S. L., Mainemer, N., Abramson, J. H., Levav, I. and Kurtzman, C. (1973). Community medicine and primary health care: a field workshop on the use of epidemiology in practice. *International Journal of Epidemiology* **2**, 419–26.

Kearsley, G. (1989) Good versus bad software: what makes the difference? *Computers in Life Science Education* **6**, 1–3.

Krall, J. M., Hall, D. S., Garland, B. K. and Pearson, R. J. C. (1983). Physicians' views on the teaching and utility of courses in epidemiology and biostatistics. *Journal of Medical Education* **58**, 815–17.

Kurtzman, C. and Block, D. (1983). Preparation of nurses for community orientation in primary health care in Israel. *Israel Journal of Medical Sciences* **19**, 768–70.

Larson, D. E. (1984). Using computer-assisted instruction in the education of health care professionals: what the dean needs to know. *Computers in Life Science Education* **1**, 65–7.

Laschinger, H. S., Johnson, G. and Kohr, R. (1990). Building undergraduate nursing students' knowledge of the research process in nursing. *Journal of Nursing Education* **29**, 114–17.

Leeder, S. R. and Sackett, D. L. (1976). The medical undergraduate programme at McMaster University: learning epidemiology and biostatistics in an integrated curriculum. *Medical Journal of Australia* **2**, 875–81.

Lilienfeld, A. M., Garagliano, F. and Lilienfeld, D. E. (1978). Epidemiology 101: the new frontier. *International Journal of Epidemiology* **7**, 377–80.

Linskey, M. E., Neugut, A. I., Hall, E. and Cox, J. D. (1987). A course in medical research study design and analysis. *Journal of Medical Education* **62**, 143–5.

Lobo, L. C. G. and Jouval, H. E. Jr (1973). The use of new educational technology in the development of health manpower in Latin America: its implications in the teaching of epidemiology. *International Journal of Epidemiology* **2**, 359–66.

Lowe, C. R. and Kostrzewski, J. (eds.) (1973). *Epidemiology: a guide to teaching methods*. Churchill Livingstone, Edinburgh.

MacFarlane, S. B., Cuevas, L. E., Moody, J. B., Russell, W. B., and Schlecht, B. J. (1996). Epidemiology training for primary health care: the use of computer-assisted distance learning. *Journal of the Royal Society of Health* **116**, 317–21.

Mager, R. F. (1997). *Preparing instructional objectives*, 3rd edn. Center for Effective Performance, Atlanta, GA.

Marantz, P. R., Wassertheil-Soller, S., Croen, L. and Lukashok, H. (1991). Teaching clinical epidemiology to medical studets using a collaborative learning model. *American Journal of Preventive Medicine* 7, 121–3.

Mercenier, P. and van Balen, H. (1973). The experience, development and evaluation of the International Course in Health Management. *International Journal of Epidemiology* 2, 129–35.

Morton, R. F., Hebel, J. R., McCarter, R. J. (1996). *A study guide to epidemiology and biostatistics*, 4th edn. Aspen Publishers, Gaithersburg, Md.

Osborne, E. H. S., Hearst, N., Lashof, J. C. and Smith, W. M. (1986). Teaching community-oriented primary care (COPC): a practical approach. *Journal of Community Health* 11, 165–71.

Ostbye, T. (1989). An 'electronic' extramural course in epidemiology and medical statistics. *International Journal of Epidemiology* 18, 275–9.

Pemberton, J. (1973). Practical work in epidemiology and community medicine for medical undergraduates. *International Journal of Epidemiology* 2, 399–405.

Pemberton, J. (1986). Strengthening the practice of epidemiology in the European community. *International Journal of Epidemiology* 15, 449–53.

Persson, L. A. and Wall, S. (1993). Epidemiology teaching and the community perspective. *World Health Forum* 14, 36–41.

Reinhardt, A. (1995). New ways to learn. *Byte Magazine* 20(3), 50.

Rhyne, R., Bogue, R., Kukulka, G. and Fulmer, H. (1998). *Community-oriented primary care: health care for the 21st century.* American Public Health Association, Washington DC.

Romm, F. J., Dignan, M. and Herman, J. M. (1989). Teaching clinical epidemiology: a controlled trial of two methods. *American Journal or Preventive Medicine* 5, 50–1.

Sackett, D. L., Haynes, R. B. and Tugwell, P. (1991). *Clinical epidemiology: a basic science for clinical medicine*, 2nd edn. Lippincott, Williams and Wilkins.

Sackett, D. L., Richardson, W. S., Rosenberg, W. and Haynes, R. B. (1997). *Evidence-based medicine: how to practice and teach EBM.* Churchill-Livingstone, New York.

Schofield, F. D. and Muller, A. S. (1973). Epidemiology in the undergraduate curriculum of an African medical school. *International Journal of Epidemiology* 2, 407–13.

Segal, B. S. (1999). Distance learning primer. Currently available on Internet: www.cdc.gov/phtn/primer.htm

Skiba, D. J. (1985). Evaluation of computer-assisted instruction courseware. *Computers in Life Science Education* 2, 11–14.

Stone, D. H. (1998). The clinical epidemiology ward round: can we teach public health medicine at the bedside? *Journal of Public Health Medicine* 20, 377–81.

Terris, M. (1966). The teaching of epidemiology to medical students. *Archives of Environmental Health* 12, 801–13.

Thacker, S. B., Goodman, R. A. and Dicker, R. C. (1990). Teaching and service in public health practice, 1951–90—CDC's Epidemic Intelligence Service. *Public Health Reports* 105, 599–604.

Unwin, N., Carr. S. M., Leeson, L. and Pless-Mulloli, T. (1997). *An introductory study guide to public health and epidemiology.* Open University Press.

Veloski, J. J. (1986). The integration of the computer into medical education. In: Javitt, J. (ed.) *Computers in medicine: applications and possibilities.* W. B. Saunders Co., Philadelphia, pp. 134–53.

WHO (1981). *The use of epidemiology by front-line health workers in developing countries.* Geneva: WHO publ. SHS/SPM/B1.3.

Yoakam, M. and Chute, A. (1999). Overview of distance learning concepts and strategies. Currently available on Internet: www.cdc.gov/phtn/primer.htm

Zvarova, J., Engelbrecht, R., van Bernmel, J. H. (1997). Education and training in medical informatics, statistics and epidemiology in EuroMISE. *International Journal of Medical Informatics* 45, 3–8.

Chapter 27

Computer-assisted learning – principles and practice

Charles du V. Florey

Introduction

Computers linked to the Internet and to local intranets have revolutionized communication with students. The change from conventional paper-based communication to the use of computers has taken place so recently that students tend to be more aware of the medium's potential than teachers. The resistance of staff to learning about computer methods of instruction is probably founded on the belief that the investment in learning a totally new skill is too great to make it worthwhile. Others may wish to try their hand at developing computer-based material but do not know what skills they require.

In this chapter some of the principles for the use of computers to aid teaching and the skills required for writing interesting material are described. I have assumed that anyone reading this chapter already has basic keyboard skills and is familiar with the Windows or Mac interfaces.

Teaching objectives and contents

The writing of quality computer-assisted learning (CAL) should be guided by a number of principles. I have listed those by which our own work[1] was guided.

A teaching or learning aid

CAL means exactly what it says. Students need several ways of approaching their subject to help them overcome blocks to understanding. CAL is only one approach. It is best to consider it as one of many learning resources and to write it only for those aspects of a subject where the computer enhances the presentation. CAL may be planned within the context of a taught course so that its place within the overall syllabus can be understood. It is essential to provide back-up to the CAL with human tutors.

Not a book

The most convenient way in which to read conventional material is from a book or set of paper-based notes. It can be carried and read in almost any circumstances and does not require any technology for reading it. Material committed to the computer should not be a book on a screen because it will either not be read or will be printed by the student, thus removing the point of the computer.

This is the most important principle of all.

High level of interaction

Students need something to do most of the time they are in front of the screen. If they are expected to read a lot of text without other interaction they are likely to lose concentration and abandon the effort. Interaction means answering questions (this can also become boring if too many are asked or it is the only form of interaction), using simulations, and carrying out analyses. Interactive exercises should dominate the material.

Different results each time

In real life, each new study presents new problems and a different set of data. Interactive exercises should as far as possible mimic life by changing the data each time the program is run. This allows students to test themselves in changing situations rather than learning by heart the solution to a single expression of a problem. Obviously this is not possible for all problems, but when there are opportunities to introduce variation in successive attempts to solve a problem they should be taken. Examples include simulation of data to show a particular distribution or the taking of random samples from a larger body of data.

Immediate feedback

Students should be able to test their understanding by interaction with the computer and receive immediate feedback on their performance. The test might be a multiple choice question. It should be impossible to see the answer before answering, but once the student's answer has been irrevocably entered into the computer, the correct answer should be displayed immediately. This approach ensures that the student attempts the question before looking at the answer, but spares the student the irritation of having to write down the answers to be compared with the correct answers at a later time.

'Not invented here' syndrome

One of the barriers to the greater use of other authors' CAL is the feeling that the approach used is incompatible with your own way of teaching and neither covers the subjects adequately nor uses data relevant to your own locality. If the CAL is to be used by others beyond your own institution it must be written in a way that allows adaptation. For example, a module on death certification should allow the user to insert the certificate of the country where the CAL is to be used. The program should allow the use of population data relevant to the students' own country or region. If you are prepared to take the extra trouble required to generalize your programs, your efforts are likely to be much more acceptable in the marketplace. Areas suitable for allowing changes to suit local conditions include:

- 'Expert' commentaries
- Glossary
- Multiple choice questions
- Text in general (this allows, among other things, translation into other languages)
- Tutor's notes
- Links to other programs and the Internet .

Sparing use of generic programs

If you are writing CAL to sell or for use by others working away from your institution, you must consider carefully whether the users will have access to the generic programs (e.g. spreadsheets) available to you during programming. If you use word-processed files, they must be in a form that can be read by all or most modern word processors (e.g. rich text format: rtf). If you use a spreadsheet it must be available to all the potential users of your program. Some programs come with the operating system of the computer so that it will be available to all or most users. For the PC these include Notepad, WordPad, Paint, and programs designed for displaying Help files. Web browsers can be downloaded free from the Internet. Other programs for which a licence fee must be paid should be avoided if possible.

Developments in computing

Computers, peripherals, and software are changing so quickly that some of what I write here will be out of date by the time you read it. For example, within the last few years there have been three changes to the way in which Help files are displayed on PCs, the last taking a radically different approach based on browser techniques. The introduction of rewritable CDs and digital video disks (DVD) will change the way non-professional programs can be distributed and what can be shown. The increasing speed of Internet connections will facilitate what is currently not worthwhile, such as transmission of video clips. Planning CAL now requires some appreciation of what is likely to take place in computing over the next 5 years. New software should be flexible enough so that it can be easily altered to take advantage of advances in hardware.

Maintenance

When you have written your CAL you will need to have a plan for maintaining it. You may have to revise the factual content every year and make suitable changes. You may be asked to add new modules to give greater depth to the student's experience. You may need to update the way in which the software operates, using new computing software and hardware. This aspect of writing CAL material should not be overlooked unless you are happy to see your work become outdated within 12–24 months.

Assessing students' achievements

Assessing computer-assisted learning material

Before assessing any material, you should decide what you want for your students. If you are uncertain about what CAL can offer, it may be best to look at what is available to you before deciding where you feel CAL may contribute to your course. Initially, particularly if you have no wish to make changes to the program, you might apply the following basic criteria to the software:

+ Speed: does it run fast enough to avoid irritation using the computing facilities available to you?

+ Navigation: is it easy to find your way around the material? Are there search facilities in the program?

+ Presentation: does the choice of font make for easy reading? Is the general layout attractive, or does it deter you from exploring the material? Is there attractive use of colour? Does it use joke graphics that deter use?

+ Content: are educational objectives stated? Does the content cover the areas of your subject clearly and in a way you will be happy to support when teaching your students face-to-face?

This may be sufficient for you to decide whether you want to investigate the software further. Your next step is to ask students to assess the program. Student assessment should use at least three approaches. The first should cover the students' own assessments under the above four criteria. The second should be an observational assessment of how the students use the material. For example, do they read the text or skip to the interactive parts? Do they read the instructions or attempt to use the program intuitively? Do they perform any of the exercises? Do they get lost? The third assessment should be to determine how much the students have learned using CAL compared to conventional material and the stated educational objectives. This assessment should also measure the amount of face-to-face time spent with students under the two types of presentation.

Teaching method and format

CAL material may be used in any course. We have found that it is unwise to run a course that depends solely on CAL, as most students require further explanation from a member of staff. We have run a variety of epidemiologic courses originally designed for conventional delivery to undergraduate and graduate students, and have subsequently introduced the CAL as a further learning resource. The taught part of a course is structured to take advantage of the subjects of the CAL, but it has been our policy to discuss the subjects in class before asking the students to do the CAL. For medical undergraduates, whose motivation to understand epidemiology tends to be less than that of graduates, it is essential to indicate at which points in a course the various CAL programs should be run. Asking students to do the CAL in their own time results in a poor response.

One of the aims of CAL is to reduce the time spent in face-to-face teaching. Integration of the CAL into an otherwise conventionally delivered course should take this into account by reducing the length of lectures on subjects covered by the CAL and by omitting some of the classroom exercises which the CAL may present in a more challenging way. We have used this in a 4-week course on the elements of systematic review in which we gave a series of 20-minute talks on methodologic issues and then asked the students to revise the subjects using all means at their disposal, including CAL. At the end of the course, the students' knowledge and ability to use it in practice was markedly greater than when we had taught the same subjects by lecture and classroom practical.

Writing computer-aided learning material

The principles for desiging CAL described above may be so daunting that you would rather not read the rest of this chapter. You may believe that you cannot muster the resources to get started. You may feel you will never acquire the skills to get even your paper-based notes into a respectable format for presentation on a computer screen. In this section three levels at which you might operate are described. I believe that most teachers working in higher education institutions should be able to acquire the skills for level 1 within a very short time. For those who become excited by the medium, raising one's skill to level 2 may take up to 2 weeks of on-the-job experience with help from people who are already experienced. Level 3 requires a team of people with a range of expertise, dedication and, not least, funding.

Level 1: moving text from paper handouts to the computer

The most basic use of computers and the Internet is for making instructions and timetables readily available to students without having to ensure complete paper-based coverage. It allows access from any computer that can be connected to the institutional intranet or the Internet. The text can be updated as frequently as the author desires.

Skills required

The creation of the material requires a sound knowledge of a word processing package to produce text, a spreadsheet or similar program for the creation of graphs and a paint program for manipulating clip art (ready made drawings or paintings for inclusion in your own files) or photographs. If you are able to scan photographs and other printed material into your computer (an extremely simple process), the range of illustration you can add to the basic text is enormous.

At this level you will need the help of someone skilled in putting material onto a web site. Alternatively, you should be able to save the file(s) containing your electronic handout in a form which software available to the student can process and to locate it in a place where students can gain access to it.

At this level the skills required are simply those for transferring existing material from a paper version to a computer-readable version. In principle this is not a sound use of the computer as it tends be boring for the student and, unless printed out, only accessible by computer. If printed out, the only gains from computerization are the ability of the teacher to update the material easily and for students at a distance to gain access to it. Such a situation exists for distance learning courses for which this level of computerization may be valuable or indispensable.

Level 2: creating hypertext links

At level 2, the author begins to use the computer in a way that no longer completely mimics the printed page. The computer allows words or diagrams or even parts of diagrams to be linked to other parts of the computer file, to other programs or, for example, to the Internet. This means it is possible to give instantaneous access to definitions and explanations of technical terms in the main text by simply clicking the mouse button when the mouse cursor is over the unknown word. Paper-based notes cannot replicate this attribute of the computer nor can they offer immediate direct or teacher-controlled access to the enormous amount of information on the Internet. These techniques are illustrated in the files displayed on web sites and in help files that come with almost every modern software application.

The strength of hypertext is that you can include different tracks in the same structure so that the presentation of the material can be varied according to level of student, type of illustrative materials, and level of complexity of an exercise, and so on. The advantage of hypertext for epidemiology is that the principles and techniques of the subject are the same for all students, regardless of background, but the detail and applications can be varied according to the level of the course.

To write instructional material with hyperlinks requires planning before the material is written. A map of the pages should be drawn up so that links between them can be defined. Diagrams for use in the material should be prepared in computer-readable form (preferably in colour) and hyperlinks from them defined. A list should be made of words that require definitions and Internet sites that the student should visit.

Once the plan has been written and agreed among the teachers the material must be assembled in a suitable way for using with the program used to display it. There are authoring programs specially designed for use by people inexperienced with programming. You may use sophisticated word processors to create web style pages with easily constructed links and user friendly methods for posting the pages on a web site. It is also possible to set up a web site with the aid of specialist software such as FrontPage or Adobe Pagemill. There are several programs available for PCs that simplify the creation of Help files (e.g. Help Workshop and HTML Help Workshop from Microsoft, both of which can be downloaded free from the Microsoft web site).

This type of presentation is very suitable for use on the Internet.[2]

Skills required

The skills required are distinct from those traditionally needed for writing paper-based notes for students and must be acquired. An ability to conceptualize the use of hyperlinks will grow with use, but initially it may be useful to work with someone who has experience in the field. A working knowledge is essential of the programs that

convert initially word-processed material into the file structure required by authoring, help or Internet browser programs. This has to be acquired by practice and the
help of others who already have experience, and by the use of instructional books or
the help files that come with the programs (the author has usually found books are far
more useful than the help files, possibly because they are written by people acquainted
with how students learn). This is the point at which many traditional teachers abandon the wish to create computer learning material because of the perception that the
old methods are good enough so there is no point in learning the new. For such teachers, it might be worthwhile seeking the collaboration of someone who has the skills,
accepting that their own control over the presentation of the material will never be as
complete as if they had prepared it themselves.

Level 3: creating interactive programs

Bespoke programs are needed when standard programs cannot be customized to
achieve the desired effect. They may also be appropriate when a standard program is
very expensive for the end user to buy. They are also appropriate for complex case
studies with elaborate material and wideranging interaction.

Bespoke programming requires an altogether different degree of involvement.
Although individuals can write interactive programs on their own, they tend to be relatively simple and suitable only in the context of a taught course. For success, a team
of people with different skills must be assembled. This team should consist of subject
experts (i.e. teachers), intermediaries who are familiar with teaching, interface design
and computer techniques, and software engineers.

The amount of time required to create 1 hour of instructional material is conventionally said to be at least 100 hours but, in my own experience,[1] it is probably closer
to 250 by the time the program has been thoroughly tested and evaluated. Funding is
essential for effective collaboration among team members. The major cost is in
salaries, which will depend on the country in which the work is done, but is likely to
be greater than US$ 200 000 per course in the US or western Europe. This is an enor-
mous investment of time and finance, so one must be very careful in the selection of
topics to be treated this way. For example, it is best that the subject matter is relatively
stable from year to year, such as basic epidemiologic methodology.

Level 3 requires the development of skills that are non-traditional in a higher education institution. It is extremely challenging intellectually from many points of view,
requiring ingenuity, lateral thought, problem-solving ability, an understanding of the
way students learn, and graphic design. Because of the financial and novel intellectual
demands of the subject, it is not surprising that few have attempted to write this sort
of material in the field of epidemiology. Nevertheless, this level of production is likely
to be of most benefit to students as it can involve them much more deeply in the practice of their subject than material written at levels 1 or 2.

Skills required

A team should be set up consisting of teachers, people familiar with teaching, interface design and computer techniques, and software engineers. Essential to the team is

personal enthusiasm for the project, a willingness to be involved for a lengthy period, ability to work in close collaboration (working in the same department or institution is advantageous), and certainty of financial support.

Conclusion

The creation of CAL software is as easy or difficult as you care to make it. It is almost essential for distance learning programmes. It will be absolutely essential in a few years' time when students in many countries will have computers of their own and will expect much of their communication with staff and their learning materials to be in computer-readable form. This is a time of transition: the opportunities for writing innovative epidemiologic CAL are enormous in this near virginal land.

References

[1] Available from: URL: http://www.dundee.ac.uk/cit/epical/epical.htm

[2] Available from: URL: http://www.pitt.edu/~super1/

Phillips, R. (1997) The Developer's Handbook to Interactive Multimedia. A practical guide for educational applications. Kogan Page, London.

Chapter 28

Exercises

Norman D. Noah

Introduction

Epidemiology is an ideal subject to teach by using practical exercises. Practical exercises are to epidemiology what teaching at the bedside is to clinical medicine. However, with bedside teaching, a patient with the disease that the teacher wishes to discuss generally needs to be present; with epidemiologic exercises, data obtained or a problem that occurred several years before may be used to form the basis of an epidemiologic exercise. Care must be taken, however, to ensure that the problem, and the data used to illustrate it, remain relevant. This does not preclude the use of classic historic papers for exercises, provided the message remains relevant.

A useful approach to take, or philosophy to assume, in teaching using epidemiologic exercises is to show that epidemiology is all around us. When asked to quote for securing a house to a budget, a locksmith stated that 60% of all burglaries were through the front door and 25% through the back door and that therefore these two areas should be the priorities with a limited budget. This was a clear example of applying a form of epidemiologic analysis to practical ends. In a newspaper, the numbers of murders in various areas in a given time period were superimposed on a map of the UK. An accompanying article, using information from the map, stated that London was clearly the most dangerous place in which to live, and northern Scotland (where the population is sparse) the safest. No mention was made of the base populations in any of the areas shown, and the map by itself was quite meaningless, to say nothing of the newspaper's interpretation of the statistics. This type of material can be useful as short practical teaching exercises.

This chapter will attempt to cover some of the very broad basis of teaching epidemiology to both undergraduates and postgraduates using practical exercises. By 'practical exercise' I will take to mean any teaching session which either involves a teacher giving his students a series of interlinked problems to work through, under supervision, or presenting data in any form to analyse and interpret. The emphasis will be on '*how to* teach in this way' rather than '*what* can be taught in this way'. The author's own experiences lie mainly in teaching infectious disease epidemiology, so many of the examples are taken from this speciality: the concepts and methods should be the same, and adaptable to teaching in any other epidemiologic discipline.

The principles can also be adapted for teaching statisticians, environmental health officers (sanitary inspectors), sociologists, non-medically qualified healthcare workers involved in data collection, and those with other statistical interests. In the author's experience, undergraduates just as readily understand the concepts as do postgraduates – it is only motivation towards public health that they sometimes lack! Most exercises can be adapted for these different groups: it is only in the level of detail and emphasis that changes need to be made. Thus, in an outbreak investigation exercise for undergraduates, emphasis should probably be on analysing and interpreting data in a case control or cohort study – thereby getting across the elementary principles of basic epidemiology not confined to infectious diseases. For postgraduates, the practical steps in investigating an outbreak may assume greater importance. For environmental health officers, who are expert in environmental investigation and control, but not epidemiologically trained, I would emphasize the epidemiologic principles and how to analyse exposure rates. Abramson (1992) makes a distinction between problem-solving exercises and exercises in specific techniques; most of this chapter will deal with problem-solving exercises, as those which teach specific techniques are usually best designed to be problem-solving for best results.

Teaching objectives

This chapter should enable the reader to present a practical exercise to a group of students with confidence, following the steps logically – and ensuring that the students also understand the logic of the approach to the problem. In addition, the reader should be able to make up his own practical exercises: these are often the best as they are based on one's own experiences. This also means that the teacher can build to his own strengths in teaching.

When compiling your own practical exercises, the format can be made to vary from rigid to flexible. The former has a set question and answer format in discrete parts. With the latter there is much more flexibility, especially with the answers, and it is possible to move into different areas depending on the ability and knowledge of the audience. The example below of an exercise illustrating the advantages and disadvantages of the different types of study is suitable for the flexible approach, but can be made more rigid if desired.

Teaching contents

In teaching epidemiology using practical exercises, there are two key concepts that the author has found useful – perhaps essential – in encouraging students to understand what epidemiology is all about. These are the epidemiologic quadrangle (see below), and the epidemiologic triangle of analysing by time, place, and person.

The four essentials to any epidemiologic study or investigation (the epidemiologic quadrangle) are:

- Collect
- Analyse
- Interpret
- Act.

This model assumes that the formulation of a hypothesis and the literature search have already been completed and that an epidemiologic study is about to start. Some teachers may like to add a further preliminary step for outbreak investigation: is the outbreak real or an artifact? Indeed, this is an important first step in any epidemiologic problem, as it teaches the student to consider the authenticity of any statistics before embarking on an expensive investigation.

It is helpful for the student to realize that any epidemiologic investigation can be broken down into these four steps, and opportunities can be taken in most exercises to illustrate this. These four steps follow in a logical order and can be applied to virtually any practical exercise, whether it be one on surveillance, an epidemiologic study, or an outbreak investigation. Indeed, when considering the objectives of any teaching exercise, it is useful to decide which of these steps the teacher most wants to get across to the student. Some exercises will be ideal for illustrating all four of these steps, and for showing their usefulness in dealing with a problem or investigation. Other exercises may concentrate mainly on one or two of these steps, e.g. the collection and analysis of data. The author's own preference – and strength – is for an exercise which leans heavily on the interpretation of data, because it is in this one vital step that the art of epidemiology lies – the first two steps are essentially technical and the last is practical and often political. Some examples of exercises used successfully by the author follow. They are not meant to be comprehensive.

Examples of epidemiologic exercises

Exercises on the collection of data are essentially about sources and study design: choice of type of study, sampling, design of questionnaires, avoidance of bias in collection of statistics, etc.

For choice of study, a useful approach for medical and other undergraduate students (and also for some postgraduates) is to build a 'hierarchy of studies' from weak to strong as follows:

Descriptive studies

+ Case series

+ Ecologic/correlational studies

+ Cross-sectional

Analytic studies

+ Case control

+ Cohort

+ Intervention

+ Randomized controled trial

First, present a scenario, as in the following examples: as a physician you have noticed that of your last:

+ Ten pediatric patients with leukemia, seven had been X-rayed while *in utero*.

+ Ten patients with cirrhosis of the liver, seven had a high alcohol consumption.

+ Ten patients with cancer of the lung, seven were heavy smokers.

How would you further investigate whether this association is real?

Two of the three scenarios given above are particularly relevant to developed countries, but are probably sufficiently universal to use more widely. It is important to choose an example relevant to your own country and preferably familiar to you. Ask the students to work step-by-step through the different studies possible, writing down how they would design (not do) each study, and the strengths and weaknesses of each. This could be in the form of a pre-prepared question and answer format on separate sheets of paper. In the ensuing discussion, point out that the initial observation is in itself a type of study, a case series. Its weakness may be in that it is scientifically poor, but its strength is in hypothesis generation. Indeed, many causes of disease have first been suspected in a case series. You could then discuss the different studies:

- A cross-sectional study is inappropriate in any of the examples given.
- An ecologic study could be designed for the cirrhosis/alcohol and the cancer/smoking problems. Problems of ecologic studies are many, although they are useful as supporting evidence to proceed to case control or cohort study.
- The techniques and strengths and weaknesses of case control and cohort studies for one or more of these examples can be explored.
- The practical difficulties of an intervention study could be discussed.
- Finally, the scientific perfection, and ethical imperfection, of a randomized controled trial in any of these situations, particularly the leukemia/X-ray example, can also be discussed.

In teaching undergraduates particularly, the author has found this approach and these examples invaluable in explaining the biases inherent in most ecologic studies, and the differences between a case control and a cohort study, as well as the concepts of odds ratio, relative risk, and attributable risk. There is ample scope for a flexible approach, tailoring your discussion as appropriate to the audience.

In practical exercises in which the analysis of data is the core objective, the second key concept, referred to above as the epidemiologic triangle, is used.

This means the analysis of data by:

- Time
- Place
- Person.

Person should include age, sex, occupation, and exposure if likely to be relevant. These principles of analysis are covered elsewhere in this book. Practical exercises are ideal for teaching how to analyse data. Computer programs can of course be used for analysis in teaching exercises, although the author's preference is generally for old-fashioned hand analysis, at least with beginners. For more advanced students, practical experience with inputting and analysing data using computer programs can be incorporated as part of the exercise.

Analysis is of no value without interpretation of data, which can be difficult to teach. The type of action required depends on the interpretation of data. The techniques for this will have been covered elsewhere in this book.

Some further examples of suitable types of subject matter for practical exercises follow.

Examples of material suitable as a lead-in for exercises

Sensitivity and specificity The author has found the real-life example of two pediatricians who used the reflex anal dilatation (RAD) sign to diagnose child abuse especially useful in introducing this subject, which some students find difficult. Begin by asking whether child abuse should be tolerated, and, if not (the expected answer!), what they would do about it. Invariably the students, after discussion, will present detailed criteria for suspecting such a diagnosis. Next, ask about the side effects of such a stringent policy: several innocent parents being put under suspicion and interrogated for some weeks or months, and the permanent effect this could have on their lives. Then discuss the side effects of having a policy where only when the diagnosis is clear-cut are the parents interrogated. Some children will be missed and will have serious injury or have died already. Go on to use this as a basis for an exercise on sensitivity and specificity based on your own speciality. For further reference, a useful paper on the child abuse episode discussed above was published by Harvey and Nowlan (1989).

Rates Again, choose an example from everyday life. Most car accidents occur within a mile of the driver's home. What can you do to prevent this? Answers to this tend to be interesting, but there should be an eventual realization that the statistic is meaningless as most car journeys are to within a mile of the driver's home. In a newspaper article declaiming the side effects of whooping cough vaccine the following statement was made: 'Overall, more than 30% of those with whooping cough in England and Wales have already been vaccinated against it.' This statement appears to show that whooping cough vaccine is ineffective, but a closer examination of the statement reveals that the statistic is quite meaningless. This is another useful example to start with an exercise on rates: again, choose a subject within your own expertise.

Association and causation, confounding Discuss the public health implications of the following statement: 'More attention is now being placed on emotional and psychological factors [in rearing children]. Babies who have spent time in neonatal units are disproportionately liable to child abuse.' Again, the discussion can be interesting, and the remedies even more so! However, it seems likely that social deprivation is a major confounding variable here. Another useful statement is: 'There is a strong statistically significant association between wearing nylon tights/stockings and the development of breast cancer.' In this example many of the Bradford–Hill criteria for causation are fulfilled: it is the biologic implausibility that lets it down. There are at least two confounding variables here (women and westernized women). These are other examples of lead-in for an exercise, either on confounding or on association and causation, using examples of your own.

Surveillance Choose a disease or group of diseases and ask each team to discuss a surveillance program for it/them. A short introductory review of the principles of surveillance may be required. The teams are allowed a sufficient length of time to discuss their task. This type of exercise is not usually suitable for the question and answer format, and the supervisor needs to go round the class discussing and helping. Each team will need at least 15 minutes at the end to present their plan, so this type of exercise session needs to be scheduled carefully. Useful diseases to choose are any vaccinatable disease (especially rubella), because the surveillance of vaccine uptake and side effects are good topics for discussion; hepatitis; food poisoning; influenza; several different cancers; and important rare diseases (Reye's syndrome, Creutzfeldt–Jakob disease, Guillain-Barrésyndrome, etc).

Case control *versus* cohort study Present examples of two outbreaks of hepatitis A. One follows a meal. The other is picked up by routine surveillance in a district and there is no known connection between the cases.

Supervising practical exercises

The remainder of this chapter will discuss some of the techniques for ensuring successful supervision of a practical exercise. Most of the examples are based on infectious disease epidemiology, especially outbreak exercises, which are excellent for teaching basic epidemiologic concepts, and are also relevant in most countries of the world.

Teaching method and format

Outbreak exercises, whether based on infectious disease or environmental toxins, lend themselves well to teaching students about the usefulness of a systematic approach using the epidemiologic quadrangle, and of systematic analysis by the epidemiologic triangle.

In outbreak exercises, the nature and experience of the audience should be taken into account in deciding whether it be more appropriate to take an epidemiologic approach or a management approach (Table 28.1). The epidemiologic approach column in this table illustrates the four steps of the 'quadrangle'.

The common format of serial questions and answers that the author has found particularly useful is as follows:

- ♦ Statement of problem
- ♦ First question
- ♦ Answer to first question followed by second question
- ♦ Further answers followed by questions on separate sheets of paper
- ♦ Wrap-up/denouément.

The outbreak can be made to unfold, with the student having to decide what to do next, or what data to obtain, between each part. An excellent example of this approach is included in Lowe and Kostrzewski (1973), the 'Oswego County outbreak' (originally compiled by CDC, Atlanta). It can be used as an exercise as presented, although the author has found that breaking it up into smaller parts (fact, followed by question) has been particularly helpful with his own students. It can also be adapted to any country situation: for example, in the version the author has adapted for England, the consultant in communicable disease control (CCDC), the environmental health officer, and the public health trainee have parts to play, as has the Public Health

Table 28.1 Two approaches in an outbreak exercise

Epidemiological approach	Management approach
1a. Collect the data	1. Take steps to verify the diagnosis
• Take a history	2. Immediate control if necessary
• Differential diagnosis	3. Management: setting up
• Case definition	• A control room
• Case finding	• Press office
1b. Pilot study	• Outbreak control group
• Formulate hypothesis	• Incident team
2. Analyse by time, place, and person	4. Act/control
	• Individual cases
• Descriptive study	• Local prevention
• Analytical study (to test hypothesis)	• National action
3. Interpret findings	• Change law?
4. Make conclusions	5. Write a report
5. Write a report	

Laboratory Service. This outbreak exercise is strong on teaching the epidemiologic method of outbreak investigation, as the source of the food poisoning was identified without microbiological help. The author also finds it useful in explaining the cohort approach and comparing it with a case control study. In a cohort study of food poisoning, the table is set out as shown in Table 28.2a, and the attack rates are 'food specific attack rates'. In a case control study, the table would have been set out as shown in Table 28.2b, and the rates calculated are not attack rates but 'food preference/exposure rates'. Using the table of food-specific attack rates, which the student has to compile from raw data as part of the exercise, the student can calculate the attributable and relative risks for each food item.

In practice, it is unusual to take one approach to the exclusion of the other in an outbreak practical exercise. Thus, even with medical undergraduates, steps 1, 2, and 4 of the management approach (Table 28.1) will need to be mentioned, if not in great detail. With more experienced epidemiologists the teacher may need to emphasize the management. Environmental health officers (sanitary inspectors) often need guidance on the epidemiologic investigation, being already experienced in organizing the taking of appropriate samples and in outbreak control.

For teachers who wish to revise some management issues which may surface during an exercise in outbreak investigation and control, see Mitchell (1998).

Some further examples of teaching exercises are included in Lowe and Kostrzewski (1973). The exercise on mortality statistics (pp. 125–9) teaches the student to calculate some basic rates, such as SMR, the value of age-specific death rates, and the interpretation of mortality data. This exercise uses data from Northern Ireland in 1961. It is

Table 28.2 Outbreak of food poisoning

a Cohort study: food-specific attack rates

Food item	Persons who ate specified food					Persons who did not eat specified food				Risk	
	Ill	Did not eat	Total	Attack rate (%)	Percentage ate	Ill	Not ill	Total	Attack rate (%)	Attributable	Relative

b Case control study: food preference rates

Food item	Ill				Not ill				Odds ratio
	Ate	Did not eat	Total	Percentage ate	Ate	Did not eat	Total	Percentage ate	

clearly going to be irrelevant, and possibly useless, if it is now used as published any-where in the world. However, if used as a framework for an exercise using similar data, but more recent and more relevant to the country/countries of the students, it should be a useful exercise. In the exercise the student is also asked to find and inter-pret published mortality statistics, so this searching could be built in as part of the exercise. For a shorter classroom session, some of the statistics could be provided.

For more advanced students, an unusual approach to an exercise, which can still be used today without modifying its content, is on 'A disease of obscure aetiology' (Lowe and Kostrzewski, 1973, pp. 186–202). It introduces principles of association and causation, as well as data interpretation.

The well known map of cases of cholera round the Broad Street pump as used by John Snow is a useful illustration of analysis by place.

The author has successfully conducted exercises in which the teams of students are given data to analyse overnight and to present and interpret the next day. Pemberton (1973) describes how students can be given practical work, in which they have to obtain the data themselves. Exercises can be used in which role play has a part: this can be used in interviewing exercises (Abramson, 1992). Outbreak exercises empha-sizing management can also be planned to include role play. These are useful varia-tions, suitable generally for more advanced students.

Steenland (1993) and Norell (1995) have each produced books of short exercises with descriptive text useful for self-learning. Many of the examples can be adapted for classroom teaching.

Assessing students' achievements

This can be done in various ways. Every exercise should have a list of objectives, out-lining what the exercise was planned to achieve. A brief discussion at the end can be helpful, but a more formal written assessment may be required. This is especially use-ful if there have been one or more students who have failed to participate adequately in the exercise. They may have found it too easy, or too difficult. An ideal method of assessment is a multiple choice questionnaire covering all the objectives. Not many exercises have a ready made assessment questionnaire, and in busy academic depart-ments, such forms of assessment must be rare.

In epidemiologic exercises, the interaction of the teacher with the audience is important, and should also be assessed. This is probably best done with a question-naire and a simple point scoring system which covers how good the teacher was in communicating with the audience, explaining the format and any difficult concepts, pacing the exercise, and the content of the exercise. A space for students to comment on how they would improve the exercise is valuable.

Some practical suggestions for conducting successful practical exercises

The whole point of an exercise is for the students to do some work themselves, and to work out solutions to problems. On the other hand, they will need guidance and you are the supervisor. There has to be a balance between doing too much for them, or too little. You should be able to judge fairly easily how to strike this balance, and it will vary from group to group.

Preparation

+ Be confident. To be confident, you need to do your homework and read through the exercise and the tutor's crib in advance. Look up any concepts you don't understand.

+ Prepare each exercise carefully, so that you are familiar with it. However, prepare to be flexible. Sometimes student discussions can take off at a tangent and produce some revealing insights.

+ Work out a rough timetable: this is very important. The students will feel short-changed if you have to rush through the denouément. You will need some flexibility, but keep on course for time.

+ Even though there may be an accompanying tutor's crib, think up alternative answers for each question, which may be useful for discussion. This is especially important for exercises that have been compiled elsewhere, because you can adapt it to teach to your strengths. In any case, the exercise itself will almost certainly have been prepared to someone else's strengths. It may also need to be adapted for a particular audience.

+ Even if you are using a 'ready-made' exercise, bring it to life in your discussions by illustrating from your own experiences.

+ As far as possible always use real as opposed to artificial data.

Issues of format

+ If you have decided on a particular format, go to the lecture room well in advance and set up the tables and chairs to fit your scheme. At the same time check that all the visual aids are functional and in place: projectors, pens, whiteboards, and paper. Even if ordered in advance they may not always be there. This may be a chore, but is more important than you may think!

+ The author generally finds it best to divide the students into small groups and call them teams. Even two people will make a team, three to four are ideal numbers, six or seven too large.

+ Sometimes it may be possible to introduce a sense of friendly competition between teams, which is highly recommended.

+ Exercises can also be conducted successfully dealing with the whole class as one group, or even getting students to work by themselves, although this is usually less 'fun'.

♦ Always provide a denouément, or answer page, if using a structured format for the exercise.

Conducting the exercise

♦ When the class has assembled, introduce yourself and the topic, and outline the objectives of the exercise. Except in very large classes it always helps to learn the students' names. Explain the format you are going to use, e.g. teams of four or five.

♦ If using teams, get each team to appoint a spokesperson, but ensure during the exercise that everyone gets a chance to speak. Not all teams will come to a consensus, and encourage those who have misgivings about a particular answer to voice them.

♦ An important objective for you as a leader is to make everyone feel that they have contributed.

♦ If the exercise is in the usual format of a narrative stem, leading to a question, ask one of the students to read the narrative out loud. Rotate this task. As you get to know the audience, you can choose the 'quieter' ones to read aloud.

♦ When they have read the narrative and question/s, set them a time to answer the section.

♦ In the early stages especially, they may need guidance on how to tackle the question.

♦ It is useful to plan the exercise so that the answers to the earlier questions are narrative; if you can, keep the analysis of data to the middle of the exercise.

♦ It is important that you as the supervisor go round each team as it is working, clarifying any problems impartially, and ensuring that no team is spending a lot of time doing something useless.

♦ If you find this is happening, ask them why they are doing this particular analysis, and make them think about an alternative way of doing it, or another type of analysis, if possible.

♦ This is usually more useful than pointing out that they are following the wrong path! Occasionally, however, you may find one member of a team doing his own thing, convinced he is right. If he is wrong, you may need to bring him back – firmly but gently!

♦ Sometimes you may have to break off and get the whole class to rethink what they are doing if there is a general problem.

♦ When they have finished discussing or working out one question, it is sometimes better to get each team to report to you whilst you are looking over their shoulders rather than having a general discussion. This is because some teams may modify their answers after hearing the others.

♦ Make sure every team has a chance to speak. This may be a problem sometimes if one team is obviously much weaker than the others.

Dealing with difficult students

♦ Almost invariably, there is a (usually one, but may be more) 'difficult' student.

♦ Difficult students are of different types. Few tend to be downright aggressive and constantly challenging. More often someone fails entirely to grasp the concepts, and may convey a sense of frustration to the team or the whole class. Others will decide to go their own way and analyse data differently from the method recommended.

♦ It is difficult to make rules about dealing with difficult students. Do not panic. Explain gently why they are wrong or let them do the exercise their way and compare results – their way may be better so keep an open mind. Confidence in your understanding of the exercise, and conveying this, is important here.

♦ For students who are slower than the rest and are in danger of slowing down the whole class, you may have to take them aside and try and explain, later if necessary.

♦ Always resist the temptation to make even a difficult student feel small or stupid!

Summarizing

♦ It is a good discipline to summarize at the end of each question. Many students like 'the correct answer'. This often appears in the narrative before the next question. If it is not possible to give a correct single answer, say so. Write points down using the appropriate visual aids.

♦ Try not to end with a rush. Give yourself time to summarize the exercise, and 5 minutes at the end for the students to relax after all the hard work – sometimes the most useful discussions come at this point. A short series of slides or overheads rounding off the exercise is always useful.

♦ Write down any modifications that may be useful, from discussion points that have come up during the session. Students teach you as much as you teach them.

Finally

Collect a portfolio of exercises for every occasion and audience. Examples of situations in which epidemiology can be used to gain insight abound. Some have been mentioned in this chapter. They can be particularly valuable in introducing certain concepts.

Acknowledgements

I am grateful to my colleagues and students in the London School of Hygiene & Tropical Medicine and PHLS Communicable Disease Surveillance Centre, from whom, over many years, I have learned and on whom I have practised; also, to the Centers for Disease Control in Atlanta from whom I have also learned much about the techniques described in this chapter.

References

Abramson, J. H. (1992) Teaching epidemiology in and out of the classroom. In: Olsen, J. and Trichopoulos, D. (1992) *Teaching Epidemiology*. Oxford University Press, Oxford

Harvey, I. M., Nowlan, W. A. (1989). Reflex anal dilation: a clinical epidemiological evaluation. *Pediatric and Prenatal Epidemiology* 3, 294–301.

Lowe, C. R. and Kostrzewski, J. (1973) *Epidemiology: A guide to teaching methods*. International Epidemiological Association, Churchill Livingstone, Edinburgh.

Mitchell, E. (1998) Setting up an incident room. In: Noah, N. D., O'Mahony, M. *Communicable Disease: Epidemiology and Control*. J Wiley & Sons, Chichester.

Norell, S. E. (1995) *Workbook of Epidemiology*. Oxford University Press.

Pemberton, J. (1973) Practical work in epidemiology and Community Medicine for Medical Undergraduates. *International Journal of Epidemiology* 2, 399–405.

Steenland, K. (1993) *Case Studies in Occupational Epidemiology*. Oxford University Press.

Chapter 29

Competency-based curriculum in epidemiology

Haroutune Armenian, Michael Thompson, and Jonathan Samet

Introduction

Epidemiology and biostatistics together provide the quantitative foundation for public health and clinical research. As described in earlier chapters of this book, epidemiology has been variably defined and, of course, the practice of epidemiology covers diverse activities, extending from research rooted in molecular approaches to immediate problem-solving. However, there are some essential activities that are included as part of the domain of epidemiology with every description of the discipline. These activities include gathering and using data from populations, developing study designs for investigation, and obtaining unbiased evidence for testing hypotheses.

Contemporary methods in epidemiology have their roots in public health statistics, microbiology, and social sciences. As a discipline, epidemiology is not a body of knowledge to be pursued by itself without any intent to apply it to public health problems. In fact, there are very few 'theoretical epidemiologists' who only contemplate methodology and the philosophical foundations of the field. Most methodologic developments incorporated into epidemiology have come as a response to addressing newly emerging health problems. Some examples include the introduction of the quantitative approaches in clinical assessment by P. C. A. Louis and of similar methods in public health by his students in early nineteenth century (Lilienfeld and Lilienfeld, 1979). Also, the development of the case control method received a major impetus from the investigations of the relationship of cigarette smoking and lung cancer in the mid-twentieth century.

Education in epidemiology has paralleled this course, moving with the changes in diseases and health problems of concern. In the USA, the first Department of Epidemiology was founded at the Johns Hopkins University School of Hygiene and Public Health with the appointment of Wade Hampton Frost as Professor in 1919. The development of the earliest courses in epidemiology necessitated a framework within which epidemiologic methodology could be better structured and refined. In addition to courses about the epidemiology of important diseases of the period, like tuberculosis, new courses of methodology were developed. Over time, the curriculum has expanded and has become more differentiated following the increasing specificity of epidemiologic research. Two broad goals of the curriculum remain, however: first, to prepare students for the conduct of epidemiologic research; and second, to prepare students to use epidemiologic methods and data to solve problems in public health.

The last decades of the twentieth century have seen a dramatic evolution of educational methodologies in professional education and in particular in the education of health professionals. The traditional approach to education that emphasizes the passive accumulation of knowledge has evolved to a more active learning approach that emphasizes skill development. Emphasis is increasingly placed on developing the applied skills and appropriate viewpoints for professional practice through active learning. There is increasing recognition by educators and educational institutions that knowledge alone is not enough preparation for professional practice. In education in epidemiology, evolution of this type has taken place as the discipline has evolved from a base primarily in infectious diseases to a far more expansive coverage of health problems. Thus, traditional texts of epidemiology have evolved from being compendia of the epidemiology of various infectious diseases to texts that provide general coverage of the underlying concepts and methods of epidemiology.

More recently, a competency-based approach to education in epidemiology has been promoted. These efforts mark the continuation of a process initiated by the Public Health Faculty/Agency Forum in the early 1990s (Sorensen and Bialek, 1993). In response to the Institute of Medicine report, *The Future of Public Health* (Institute of Medicine, 1988), the public health community began a concerted effort of reassessing its educational objectives and methodologies, resulting in a more practice-oriented, competency-based approach. This trend is not unique to public health: in medical education, a similar process resulted in problem-based learning curricula such as that developed several decades ago at McMaster (Donner and Bickley, 1990; Saarinen-Rahika and Binkley, 1998), while clinical medicine has recently emphasized outcome-based or evidence-based approaches (Bergman, 1995; Sheldon, 1994).

The Faculty/Agency Forum report drafted the first set of crosscutting and discipline-specific competencies for public health. As the core sciences of public health, epidemiology and biostatistics competencies were central to this effort. At schools such as Johns Hopkins, this process has been extended to produce more detailed degree and concentration-specific competencies. In fact, this process has become so central to public health education that the accrediting body for public health education, the Council for Education in Public Health (CEPH), now requires the formulation of competencies as a basis for curriculum development (CEPH, 1993). We view this requirement positively as it fits with the nature of epidemiologic practice, which is inherently action-oriented. The requirement should also promote evaluation of current teaching approaches, which have generally developed without strong linkages to formal educational methodology.

In this chapter, we present a competency-based approach to education in epidemiology. This approach matches the active and applied nature of epidemiology, whether in the research or practice setting. We suggest that this approach can facilitate overall curriculum planning and the tailoring of the curriculum to match not only the expectations of students and faculty but of the work settings where the graduates will take positions. The availability of a listing of competencies can also facilitate evaluation, providing a clear message to students as to expectations and a framework for the evaluation process regardless of the approach.

Teaching objectives and contents

What is a competency?

A competency is an active statement describing what the learner will be able to do after completion of an educational program. It is usually the result of synthesizing a learning experience (Public Health Service, 1997). Demonstration of performance of a well defined competency will require specialized knowledge as well as specific skills and well defined attitudes … can the person think like a professional, act like a professional, and behave like a professional? (Tekian *et al.*, 1999). Some of the best approaches for developing competencies are generated from experiential learning models. A competency recognizes the ability of a person to perform a well defined task. A good job description will have a listing of competencies or statements about the tasks that the person holding the job is able to perform.

A competency statement is formulated in behavioral terms, is person-referenced, and is measurable (Schalock, 1995). For example, one of the competency objectives for a course on survey research might be: 'Upon completion of this course, the student will be able to conduct a cross-sectional survey using telephone interviewing.' A poorly stated and less specific competency for the same course might read: 'At the end of this course, the student will understand how to conduct a cross-sectional survey.' In the latter example, the verb 'understand' conveys a competency that cannot readily be defined, particularly with sufficient specificity for learners. The non-specificity of the latter statement of the competency is clear in comparison to the former statement, which sets out in detail what course graduates will be able to do. Additional examples in Table 29.1 capture the active nature of properly written competencies.

Competencies can be developed at two levels. Core competencies (Appendix A) are general and address the broad-based needs of the field, while specialized competen-

Table 29.1 Examples of effectively written competency statements

Thinking like a professional

- Apply stratified and multivariate methods for data analysis to test hypotheses in a manner consistent with underlying mechanisms
- Calculate and interpret fundamental quantitative measures (OR, RR, AR, etc.)
- Develop a simple budget

Relating like a professional

- Interpret findings in a causal framework
- Synthesize data and relevant literature in a balanced fashion
- Organize and make oral presentations to professionals

Behaving like a professional

- Work in the context of a multidisciplinary research team
- Accomplish peer-review activities, including manuscript and proposal evaluation
- Respond appropriately to ethical issues in the conduct of scientific research

cies are important for various subgroups of epidemiologists or for specific contexts of the practice of epidemiology. A department of epidemiology would need to develop listings of both types of competencies.

Developing competencies

The development of an educational program that is competency-based reflects the commitment of the faculty to teach with well defined educational objectives. The purpose of a teaching program in epidemiology should not be limited to producing graduates who are just widely read intellectuals or technicians who have excellent skills, but in educating people who can effectively complete integrated tasks that are generated within a problem-solving environment. The epidemiologist needs a broad range of competencies in addition to an ability to design studies, collect data, and analyze data, which include administration, communication, and ethical conduct.

The development of competencies, properly carried out, is iterative. At the outset, input and guidance are needed from many stakeholders like current and former students, faculty, and the potential employers of graduates. With this type of input and the experience in hand, the faculty have the primary responsibility for developing the competencies. The magnitude of the task should not be underestimated. In our experience, the initial process spanned over a year before a workable set of competencies was in hand. Appendix A has a listing of the broad competencies developed at the program level by the Department of Epidemiology of the Johns Hopkins School of Hygiene and Public Health.

Before embarking on the development of a competency-based curriculum, the faculty need to be committed to the philosophy of a teaching program based on competencies. The implementation of such an approach often requires that the process of education be changed dramatically within a traditional environment. Commitment is required and the process will probably not be successful unless all the teaching faculty will participate in developing and implementing a competency-based approach. The development of a competency-based approach may have significant implications for teaching methods, requiring, for example, a shift from using a lecture-based format to one that emphasizes problem-solving in a laboratory or self-teaching environment. How should the courses be modified? What experiential components should be incorporated within the courses?

The best venue for appreciating and identifying competencies is the workplace to which students will go after receiving their degrees (Public Health Service, 1997). One can start by looking at job descriptions of epidemiologists in practice or in research. What is it that they are required to do? A preliminary list of potential competencies might be gained by having focus group discussions with epidemiologists and others who are involved or concerned with the epidemiologic practice, whether in research or public health surveillance and investigation.

An educational program, however, needs also to project to the future. Current practices do not necessarily reflect the competencies likely to be needed by an epidemiologist 5–10 years into the future or beyond. Thus, in developing competencies, the faculty need to anticipate where the cutting edge will lead. Prediction has been made ever more difficult by extremely rapid developments in some areas. Research is now possible that would not have been anticipated only a decade ago, as technologic advances in science and computing have moved the frontiers of research and application. Genetics, for example, has emerged as a theme that intersects with virtually all aspects of epidemiologic inquiry.

Past and current students represent another informative resource for developing competencies. Previous graduates of the program can offer valuable input coming from their experience following graduation. They can address strengths and weaknesses of their training in relation to expectations in their various work venues. They can be a useful sounding board for proposed competencies and curricular changes. One can present to these alumni or graduates a tentative list of competencies and ask them to assess the relative significance of these competencies to their jobs. Current students should also be consulted. Students (particularly graduate students) come to the university from a variety of backgrounds and experiences. Some of them bring to the program a rich array of competencies that have been acquired previously and the curriculum needs to acknowledge this foundation in a flexible fashion. Engaging students will help to assure that the curriculum is considered relevant to their perceived needs and expectations. As participants in the process, they are also partners in making certain that the competency-based approach succeeds. Thus, at the graduate level of education, one can encourage the faculty advisor and the student to develop together an additional list of competencies that addresses the needs of the particular student. Within the Master of Public Health Program at the School of Hygiene and Public Health of the Johns Hopkins University, over the past 5 years we have established a special requirement for all students to spend time with their advisors to define their personal educational goals. These goals are expressed in a list of personal competencies that complement the overall program goals listed as the core competencies. The process makes the student appreciate better what underlies the development of the competencies and how these competencies relate to the courses or other educational experiences.

Teaching method and format

In moving towards a competency-based curriculum, there should be a full commitment to using the competencies in an integrated educational program that encompasses all educational venues (courses, seminars, journal clubs, and even research) and evaluation. Key steps in implementation are given below.

Reassess existing courses as to consistency with competency lists

Considering that most programs are developed on an already existing set of courses within the department and that there is substantial cumulated experience and historical wisdom attached to these courses, it is important to review and reassess existing courses as to their usefulness to help the student develop specific competencies.

Revise the courses and other educational experiences by reorienting them towards teaching for competencies

Following the review above, the courses are revised by setting clear educational objectives that are consistent with the desired list of competencies already developed.

Consider alternative approaches to courses

One has also to accept that substantial learning can occur outside the framework of courses. One needs to identify alternative educational experiences that will help in achieving these competencies. Examples include experience at the workplace, project work, or the use of available audiovisual packages and teaching material.

Explain to the students the competencies and the process

Students should be engaged in the curriculum development process to assure their commitment to the final product and that their expectations for the educational program are largely met. It is also important that the student understands the rationale for the program decisions that are made and the expectations at the end of a particular educational experience.

Operating within a larger guiding framework, such as a professional practice paradigm, facilitates this process. The paradigm provides the rationale for the content, organization, structure, and sequence of the curriculum. Such frameworks may be derived from practice-based roles or theoretical models of content and should be consonant with the program's educational objectives. For example, the Master of Public Health curriculum at Johns Hopkins is geared around a problem-solving framework that prepares students as generalists and problem-solvers capable of critical response to a variety of issues. Within the practice of epidemiology, various roles such as consultant, researcher, and public health agency practitioner can be used as a framework.

Assessing students' achievements

Educational evaluation is an ongoing process for courses, students, and programs. The feedback that one gets from student and course evaluations will hopefully be reflected in revisions and improvements in the subsequent offerings of the courses. Educational evaluation is a continuous quality improvement process.

Having provided the students with an opportunity to understand and appreciate the competencies at the outset of the program, these competencies should then serve as the basis for periodic self-assessment. The self-assessment could be done either through the use of existing evaluation instruments or through a subjective review of personal confidence level in performing the various competencies that form the educational objectives.

+ How comfortable is the student about performing this particular competency?
+ Placed in a situation where the specific task needs to be implemented, does the student have the confidence that he/she will be able to perform adequately?

These are the types of questions that underlie a self-assessment process by the student.

One of the more difficult aspects of the educational process is to design examinations and other evaluation methods that test competencies rather than only assess specific knowledge or skills. However, the testing of knowledge and skills can be a component of an assessment of these competencies. Competency-based evaluation tools need to assess ability to perform. A number of approaches have been developed in health professional education that assess competencies and use approaches that are different from the traditional oral or paper and pencil examinations, such as the Observed Structured Clinical Exam (Bradley and Humphris, 1999; Tekian *et al.*, 1999).

In addition to course evaluation one needs periodically to assess the whole degree program. Some competencies are developed across courses and can be assessed only through a comprehensive evaluation or examination. A good example here is the complementary nature of biostatistics and epidemiology. For example, one may use as an educational objective a competency on data analysis but the material that teaches such a competency may be incorporated in different courses of biostatistics and epidemiology. This raises the additional issue of the need of close coordination across courses and disciplines.

The long-term evaluation of any program needs an outcome assessment. The ultimate evaluation for an educational program is the performance of the graduate on the job. In addition to measures of career success we need to develop the appropriate tools to assess retention and use of competencies by the graduates of the program over the short and long term. The maintenance of the competency-based approach should be set in an iterative process, with feedback from graduates followed by further refinement in an ongoing loop.

Conclusions

Over the past century, epidemiology has established itself as a rational scientific discipline. Competency-based education provides a framework for a more organized approach to teaching epidemiology that should enhance capabilities in relation to the expectations of current and future workplaces. The use of competencies to develop an educational program should not be seen as a fragmented activity of teaching from a list of disparate objectives. It is important to note that these competencies should be integrated within the framework of teaching the broader models of the discipline.

References

Bergman, D. A. (1995). Thriving in the 21st century: Outcome assessment, practice parameters, and accountability. *Pediatrics*, **96**, 831–5.

Bradley, P. and Humphris, G. (1999). Assessing the ability of medical students to apply evidence in practice: the potential of the OSCE. *Medical Education*, **33**, 815–17.

Council on Education for Public Health (CEPH). (1993). *Accreditation Criteria: Graduate Schools of Public Health.*

Donner, R. S. and Bickley, H. (1990). Problem-based learning: an assessment of its feasibility and cost. *Human Pathology*, **21**, 881–5.

Institute of Medicine. (1988). *The Future of Public Health*. Washington, DC: National Academy Press.

Lilienfeld, A. M. and Lilienfeld, D. E. (1979). A century of case-control studies: progress? *Journal of Chronic Disease*, **32**, 5–13.

Public Health Service (1997). *The Public Health Workforce: An Agenda for the 21st Century, A Report of the Public Health Functions Project*. USDHHS.

Saarinen-Rahika, H. and Binkley, J. M. (1998). Problem-based learning in physical therapy: a review of the literature and overview of the McMaster University experience. *Physical Therapy*, **78**, 195–207.

Schalock, R. L. (1995). *Outcome-based Evaluation*. New York: Pelmmum Press.

Sheldon, T. A. (1994). Quality: link with effectiveness. *Quality Health Care*, **3**, Suppl: 41–5.

Sorenson, A. A., Bialek, R. G. (1993). *The Public Health Faculty/Agency Forum: Linking Graduate Education and Practice, Final Report*. Gainesville: University of Florida Press.

Tekian, A., McGuire, C. H., McGaghie, W. C., and Associates. (1999). *Innovative Simulations for Assessing Professional Competence: From Paper-and-Pencil to Virtual Reality*. Chicago: University of Illinois at Chicago.

Competencies: Departmental Master's and Doctoral Degrees.

Domain I: General Knowledge

The Department is making a transition in its educational program to a competency-based approach: i.e., a consensus set of core competencies to be achieved by graduating students has been established (see following pages). These competencies will be met through coursework, the dissertation, meetings with the advisor, attendance at seminars and other meetings, and independent study. They provide an indication for you, the student, of what you should be able to do upon finishing your degree program.

This year, 1997–98, marks the second year of these competencies. As this approach evolves, the Department has been establishing venues for teaching each competency and for testing that each competency has been achieved. The competencies will serve as a framework for the comprehensive examination.

Competency	Where taught	How assessed
Describe major national and international public health problems	Advanced courses e.g. Cardiovascular, cancer, infectious disease, AIDS, tuberculosis, genetics, etc. Introductory International Health class.	Written comprehensive and oral examinations are sufficient
Describe risk factors for well established morbidity and mortality problems and the evidence in support of these factors		
Identify major historical phases of the development of epidemiological and public health thought and methods		
Review the literature and obtain an understanding of the mechanism of the problem under investigation	Epi 4, Grant Writing class. Master paper and doctoral dissertation	Class project, exams. Master and Doctoral thesis
Describe the role of epidemiology in the development of public policy		
Know the key accomplishments of epidemiology in advancing medical and public health care	Courses, seminars, and readings	Written comprehensive and oral examinations?

Domain II: Problem Identification and Planning

Competency	Where taught	How assessed
Identify public System problems for existing information	Epi 1 and Epi 2 Health Information System (?)	Class grade, comprehensive exam, thesis (proposal)
Synthesize data and relevant literature in a balanced fashion	Grant writing class, meta-analysis class Thesis preparation	Class grade, thesis (proposal)
Assess major sources of bias and variance	Epi 1 through Epi 4	Class grade, comprehensive exam, thesis
Develop an action plan with regard to further research and/or intervention	Grant writing class	Thesis (proposal), comprehensive exam and oral exam

Domain III: Information Skills

Competency	Sub-competency	Where taught	How assessed
Literature Interpretation	Able to retrieve and organize literature	Epi 4, Grant Writing class, dissertation and Master thesis	Course exams, comp exam, evaluation of grant proposal, thesis
	Able to judge, critique and interpret reports of individual epidemiological studies	Epi 1 through Epi 4, Clinical Trial class, journal clubs and other classes (?)	
	Able to review and synthesize a body of epidemiological literature and define areas of new research	Epi 4, Grant writing class, Thesis proposal	

Domain IV: Communications

Competency	Where taught	How assessed
Presentations	Able to organize and make oral presentations to professionals ranging from brief scientific presentations of research findings to longer presentations	Learning from Teaching Assistant (TA) course, being a TA, presenting at Journal clubs, taking oral exam, presenting thesis proposal (seminars), presenting papers at national meetings, defending thesis	
	Able to prepare presentation materials including outlines, slides and transparencies		
	Able to prepare poster presentations		
	Able to explain and interpret epidemiological findings for the public and the media		
Manuscripts	Able to write a manuscript	Epi 4 and thesis (sufficient)	

Domain V: Epidemiologic Consultations

Competency	Where taught	How assessed
Able to advise on epidemiological methods for other public health or clinical professionals	None. Possibly with collaboration with other epidemiological students	
Able to advise in contexts external to the public health environment	None	
Able to accomplish peer-review activities including manuscript and proposal evaluation	None	

Domain VI: Proposal Preparation (Doctoral)

Competency	Where taught	How assessed
Able to write a scientific proposal including developing specific aims and appropriate background and describing methods in needed detail	Research Management class (Joel Hill), discussion with advisors	Recommend course or workshop or Center (see below)
Able to determine personnel needs to accomplish the research project		

Domain VII: Research Conduct

Competency	Sub-competency	Where taught	How assessed
Able to develop and write a (detailed) study protocol	Familiar with elements of a study protocol	Health Survey, Grant Writing Thesis	
Recognizes ethical issues that arise in epidemiological research	Uses systematic protocol documentation	Ethic course	
	Able to recognize and develop appropriate solutions to potential ethical problems related to human subjects		
	Able to recognize and appropriately respond to ethical issues in the conduct of scientific research including fraud and plagiarism		
	Able to apply accepted conventions with regard to authorship		
Able to manage an epidemiologic study	Knows how to develop a simple budget	Grant Writing and Health Survey	
	Can monitor the status of a project	Thesis	
	Can work in the context of a multidisciplinary research team	Lab exercises and group projects	

Domain VIII: Study Design

Competency	Where taught	How assessed
Able to formulate a research question	Sequence of research methods courses, Grant Writing Course, thesis	
Able to identify an appropriate target population for testing a hypothesis		
Able to select an appropriate study design for testing hypotheses		
Able to identify potential sources of bias and variance in studies testing a particular hypothesis and to implement strategies to implement or control bias(es) and to reduce variance		
Able to specify information needs for sample size or power estimation and to calculate sample size requirements		

Domain IX: Study Conduct

Competency	Where taught	How assessed
Able to obtain participation of members of the target population	Health survey, Clinical Trial, Grant Writing, and Joel Hill's Special studies courses	Examination results, success of study
Able to prepare an application to an institutional Research Board	Thesis research involves primary data collection	
Able to develop and to assess data collection instruments (e.g. questionnaires, physical examination, lab assays, etc.)		
Able to develop and implement procedures to assure confidentiality		
Able to implement and use to project monitoring system		

Domain X: Data Management and Quality Assurance

Competency	Where taught	How assessed
Understand the principles for data management and quality assurance	Epi 2, Clinical Trials, System Survey, CME Short Course, Work-study, Dissertation (Primary data analysis)	Examination, Thesis Committee Valid study or acceptable thesis
Able to develop and implement an ongoing system for data intake and management		
Able to adapt basic principles of data management to different study designs		
Able to plan and implement quality assurance and quality control procedures for data collection in different study designs.		
Able to synthesize results of ongoing monitoring and to develop and implement corrective actions		
Understand the norms and principles of research ethics and demonstrate and ability to incorporate those principles into programs of data management and quality assurance	As above and Research ethics course (550,860) and Medical School ethics course	None (unless consider approval by CHR, IRB, or OMB)

Domain XI: Data Analysis

Competency	Where taught	How assessed
Able to conduct descriptive analyses and test hypotheses using univariate analysis	Epi sequence courses, Health Survey, Genetics Epi and Infectious Epi, Biostatistics courses, dissertation, journal clubs, and seminars	Examinations, Seminar presentation, Comprehensive and oral exams
Recognizes potential sources of bias and applies appropriate analytic techniques to assess and control these biases		
Able to identify issues needing consultation with a biostatistician		
Calculate and interpret fundamental quantitative measures (OR, RR, AR, etc.)		
Able to apply stratified and multivariate methods for data analysis to test hypothesis in a manner consistent with underlying mechanisms		
Conduct basic statistical inference and use moderately complex statistical methods such as analysis of contingency tables, logistic regression, Kaplan-Meier, Cox and other multivariate models and simple Poisson regression		
Use computer systems and analytic software packages	As above and SAS course	

Domain XII: Data Interpretation

Competency	Where taught	How assessed
Able to make inferences from results of analyses Able to interpret findings in a causal framework	Epi sequence courses, Genetics Epi, Health Survey, Infectious Epi, biostatistics courses, journal clubs, practical experience from working on research studies, dissertation	Examination thesis completion
	All epidemiology courses, background biological knowledge, literature review	Publications, dissertation

Index